2013
YEAR BOOK OF
SURGERY®

The 2013 Year Book Series

Year Book of Critical Care Medicine®: Drs Dries, Zanotti-Cavazzoni, Latenser, Martinez, Rincon, and Zwank

Year Book of Emergency Medicine®: Drs Hamilton, Bruno, Handly, Minczak, Quintana, and Ramoska

Year Book of Endocrinology®: Drs Schott, Apovian, Clarke, Eugster, Meikle, Oetgen, Ovalle, Schteingart, and Toth

Year Book of Hand and Upper Limb Surgery®: Drs Yao, Adams, Isaacs, Lee, and Rizzo

Year Book of Medicine®: Drs Barker, Garrick, Gersh, Khardori, LeRoith, Panush, Talley, and Thigpen

Year Book of Neonatal and Perinatal Medicine®: Drs Fanaroff, Benitz, Donn, Neu, Papile, and Van Marter

Year Book of Neurology and Neurosurgery®: Drs Klimo, Minagar, Gandhi, Liu, Panagariya, Rezania, Riel-Romero, Riesenburger, Robottom, Schwendimann, Shafazand, and Yang

Year Book of Obstetrics, Gynecology, and Women's Health®: Drs Dungan and Shulman

Year Book of Oncology®: Drs Arceci, Bauer, Chiorean, Gordon, Lawton, Murphy, Thigpen, and Tsao

Year Book of Ophthalmology®: Drs Rapuano, Cohen, Flanders, Hammersmith, Milman, Myers, Nagra, Nelson, Penne, Pyfer, Sergott, Shields, Talekar, and Vander

Year Book of Orthopedics®: Drs Morrey, Huddleston, Rose, Swiontkowski, and Trigg

Year Book of Otolaryngology-Head and Neck Surgery®: Drs Sindwani, Balough, Franco, Gapany, and Mitchell

Year Book of Pathology and Laboratory Medicine®: Drs Raab and Bissell

Year Book of Pediatrics®: Dr Stockman

Year Book of Plastic and Aesthetic Surgery™: Drs Miller, Boehmler, Gosman, Gutowski, Ruberg, Salisbury, and Smith

Year Book of Psychiatry and Applied Mental Health®: Drs Talbott, Ballenger, Buckley, Frances, Krupnick, and Mack

Year Book of Pulmonary Disease®: Drs Barker, Jones, Maurer, Spradley, Tanoue, and Willsie

Year Book of Sports Medicine®: Drs Shephard, Cantu, Feldman, Galea, Jankowski, Janssen, Lebrun, and Nieman

Year Book of Surgery®: Drs Behrns, Daly, Fahey, Hines, Howe, Huber, Klodell, Mozingo, and Pruett

Year Book of Urology®: Drs Andriole and Coplen

Year Book of Vascular Surgery®: Drs Gillespie, Bush, Passman, Starnes, and Watkins

2013

The Year Book of
SURGERY®

Editor-in-Chief
Kevin E. Behrns, MD
Chairman, Edward R. Woodward Professor, Department of Surgery, University of Florida, Gainesville, Florida

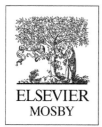

ELSEVIER
MOSBY

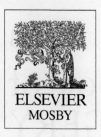

ELSEVIER
MOSBY

Senior Vice President, Content: Linda Belfus
Editor: Jessica McCool
Production Supervisor, Electronic Year Books: Donna M. Skelton
Electronic Article Manager: Michael Rainey
Illustrations and Permissions Coordinator: Dawn Vohsen

2013 EDITION

Composition by TNQ Books and Journals Pvt Ltd, India

Editorial Office:
Elsevier
1600 John F. Kennedy Blvd.
Suite 1800
Philadelphia, PA 19103-2899

International Standard Serial Number: 0090-3671
International Standard Book Number: 978-1-4557-7291-9

Printed and bound by CPI Group (UK) Ltd, Croydon, CR0 4YY

Transferred to digital print 2012

Editorial Board

Editor-in-Chief

Kevin E. Behrns, MD

Chairman, Edward R. Woodward Professor, Department of Surgery, University of Florida, Gainesville, Florida

Associate Editors

John M. Daly, MD

Harry C. Donohoo Professor of Surgery and Dean Emeritus, Temple University School of Medicine; Temple University Hospital; Fox Chase Cancer Center, Philadelphia, Pennsylvania

Thomas J. Fahey III, MD

Professor of Surgery, Weill Cornell Medical College and Chief, Endocrine Surgery, The New York Presbyterian Hospital – Weill Cornell Medical Center, New York, New York

O. Joe Hines, MD, FACS

Professor and Chief, Division of General Surgery, Robert and Kelly Day Chair in General Surgery; Director, Surgery Residency Program, Department of Surgery, David Geffen School of Medicine at the University of California, Los Angeles, Los Angeles, California

James R. Howe, M.D.

Professor of Surgery, Director, Surgical Oncology and Endocrine Surgery, Roy J. and Lucille A. Carver University of Iowa College of Medicine, Iowa City, Iowa

Thomas S. Huber, MD, PhD

Professor and Chief, Division of Vascular Surgery and Endovascular Therapy, University of Florida College of Medicine, Gainesville, Florida

Charles T. Klodell, Jr, MD

Associate Professor, Thoracic and Cardiovascular Surgery, University of Florida College of Medicine, Gainesville, Florida

David W. Mozingo, MD

Professor of Surgery and Anesthesiology, Department of Surgery, University of Florida College of Medicine; Director, Shands Burn Center, Gainesville, Florida

Timothy L. Pruett, MD

Chief of Transplantation, John S. Najarian Clinical Professor of Transplantation, Professor of Surgery and Internal Medicine, University of Minnesota, Minneapolis, Minnesota

Table of Contents

Journals Represented

Journals represented in this YEAR BOOK are listed below.

Academic Emergency Medicine
Academic Medicine
American Journal of Clinical Nutrition
American Journal of Gastroenterology
American Journal of Surgery
American Journal of Transplantation
American Surgeon
Annals of Otology Rhinology & Laryngology
Annals of Plastic Surgery
Annals of Surgery
Annals of Surgical Oncology
Annals of Thoracic Surgery
Annals of Vascular Surgery
Archives of Otolaryngology Head & Neck Surgery
Archives of Surgery
British Journal of Surgery
British Medical Journal
Burns
Cancer
Cancer Research
Chest
Circulation
Clinical Cancer Research
Clinical Infectious Diseases
Critical Care Medicine
Diabetes
Digestive Diseases and Sciences
Diseases of the Colon and Rectum
European Journal of Vascular and Endovascular Surgery
European Respiratory Journal
European Urology
Gastroenterology
Injury
Journal of Burn Care & Research
Journal of Clinical Endocrinology & Metabolism
Journal of Clinical Oncology
Journal of Gastrointestinal Surgery
Journal of Parenteral and Enteral Nutrition
Journal of Pediatrics
Journal of Pediatric Gastroenterology and Nutrition
Journal of Plastic, Reconstructive & Aesthetic Surgery
Journal of Surgical Research
Journal of the American College of Surgeons
Journal of the American Medical Association
Journal of the American Medical Association Surgery
Journal of Thoracic and Cardiovascular Surgery
Journal of Trauma and Acute Care Surgery

Journal of Vascular Surgery
Lancet
Medicine and Science in Sports and Exercise
New England Journal of Medicine
Obstetrics & Gynecology
Plastic and Reconstructive Surgery
Stroke
Surgery
Transplantation Proceedings
World Journal of Surgery
Wound Repair and Regeneration

STANDARD ABBREVIATIONS

The following terms are abbreviated in this edition: acquired immunodeficiency syndrome (AIDS), cardiopulmonary resuscitation (CPR), central nervous system (CNS), cerebrospinal fluid (CSF), computed tomography (CT), deoxyribonucleic acid (DNA), electrocardiography (ECG), health maintenance organization (HMO), human immunodeficiency virus (HIV), intensive care unit (ICU), intramuscular (IM), intravenous (IV), magnetic resonance (MR) imaging (MRI), ribonucleic acid (RNA), and ultrasound (US).

NOTE

The YEAR BOOK OF SURGERY is a literature survey service providing abstracts of articles published in the professional literature. Every effort is made to assure the accuracy of the information presented in these pages. Neither the editors nor the publisher of the YEAR BOOK OF SURGERY can be responsible for errors in the original materials. The editors' comments are their own opinions. Mention of specific products within this publication does not constitute endorsement.

To facilitate the use of the YEAR BOOK OF SURGERY as a reference tool, all illustrations and tables included in this publication are now identified as they appear in the original article. This change is meant to help the reader recognize that any illustration or table appearing in the YEAR BOOK OF SURGERY may be only one of many in the original article. For this reason, figure and table numbers appear to be out of sequence within the YEAR BOOK OF SURGERY.

Introduction

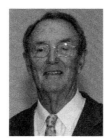

EDWARD (TED) M. COPELAND, III, MD

This introduction is dedicated to the 20 years of leadership and service that Edward (Ted) M. Copeland, III, MD provided the YEAR BOOK OF SURGERY. Dr Copeland took the reins of the YEAR BOOK editorship in 1992 and deftly led it through major transitions in surgery as only he could.

Dr Copeland is a household name in the world of surgery for his accomplishments in surgical research, oncology and mentorship of trainees and faculty because he truly commands an encyclopedic knowledge of surgery — the key to his success as a surgeon and editor. He is conversant with every aspect of surgery ranging from the physiology of nutritional repletion to the fine technical details of breast and pancreatic surgery. Few possess his knowledge and ability to clearly communicate his creative and provocative thoughts about the surgical literature.

In addition to his command of the surgical literature, Dr Copeland is a keen observer of practical knowledge. He uniquely observes and interprets operations or clinical processes, distills the content, and points out advantages and disadvantages of various approaches. This is most evident in his teachings and mentorship of residents and faculty. Dr Copeland has been wide-eyed during his tenure as a department chair and has seen what teaching tactics work and which approaches are less engaging. He has refined mentorship through these observations and regularly speaks of the lessons he learned over the years. He made a science of observing educational processes and defining mentorship through observation.

Most importantly, however, Dr Copeland communicates his thoughts clearly through the written and spoken word. His writings are a seamless blend of science and colloquial statements that emphasize teaching points. However, Dr Copeland is at his best when he is teaching in either a small or large group. As a southern gentleman and scholar, he is able to weave a lesson of surgical pathophysiology into a conversation with a hospital employee without medical training. As a trainee or faculty member, one should always be ready to receive a lesson because a nugget of knowledge is never far away when you are conversing with Dr Copeland.

Dr Copeland, thank you for sharing your wisdom with the readers of the YEAR BOOK OF SURGERY. We are clearly the recipients of wonderful words of reflection. As the editorship of the YEAR BOOK transitions, we should also thank Timothy Eberlein, MD, who made numerous insightful contributions to the YEAR BOOK. Thank you, Dr Eberlein! We feel fortunate to have two new, well-recognized surgical leaders join our editorial team — James Howe, MD, and Oscar J. (Joe) Hines, MD. Welcome Drs Howe and Hines!

Kevin E. Behrns, MD

1 General Considerations

Striving for Work-Life Balance: Effect of Marriage and Children on the Experience of 4402 US General Surgery Residents

Sullivan MC, Yeo H, Roman SA, et al (Yale School of Medicine, New Haven, CT; Memorial Sloan Kettering Cancer Ctr, NY; Duke Univ School of Medicine, Durham, NC; et al)

Ann Surg 257:571-576, 2013

Objective.—To determine how marital status and having children impact US general surgical residents' attitudes toward training and personal life.

Background.—There is a paucity of research describing how family and children affect the experience of general surgery residents.

Methods.—Cross-sectional survey involving all US categorical general surgery residents. Responses were evaluated by resident/program characteristics. Statistical analysis included the χ^2 test and hierarchical logistic regression modeling.

Results.—A total of 4402 residents were included (82.4% response rate) and categorized as married, single, or other (separated/divorced/widowed). Men were more likely to be married (57.8% vs 37.9%, $P < 0.001$) and have children (31.5% vs 12.0%, $P < 0.001$). Married residents were most likely to look forward to work ($P < 0.001$), and report happiness at work ($P < 0.001$) and a good program fit ($P < 0.001$). "Other" residents most frequently felt that work hours caused strain on family life ($P < 0.001$). Residents with children more frequently looked forward to work ($P = 0.001$), were happy at work ($P = 0.001$), and reported a good program fit ($P = 0.034$), but had strain on family life ($P < 0.001$), and worried about future finances ($P = 0.005$). On hierarchical logistic regression modeling, having children was predictive of a resident looking forward to work [odds ratio (OR): 1.22, $P = 0.035$], yet feeling that work caused family strain (OR: 1.66, $P < 0.001$); being single was associated with less strain (OR: 0.72, $P < 0.001$). The female gender was negatively associated with looking forward to work (OR: 0.81, $P = 0.007$).

Conclusions.—Residents who were married or parents reported greater satisfaction and work-life conflict. The complex effects of family on surgical

TABLE 2.—The Effect of Marital Status and Children on Surgical Residents, National Study of Expectations and Attitudes of Residents in Surgery Study (N = 4402)

Survey Item	Marital Status—% Agree				Presence of Children—% Agree		
	Married	Single	Other	P	≥1 Child	No Children	P
I look forward to coming to work everyday	69.7	64.3	59.4	<0.001	71.0	65.7	0.001
I am happy when I am at work	76.8	70.2	66.3	<0.001	77.5	72.2	0.001
I feel that I fit in well at my program	88.5	81.6	80.4	<0.001	87.1	84.4	0.034
The hours I am working are causing a strain on my family life	44.4	33.3	51.0	<0.001	52.8	34.8	<0.001
I worry about making enough money as a surgeon	37.0	37.0	42.6	0.519	40.7	35.9	0.005

residents should inform programs to target support mechanisms for their trainees (Table 2).

▶ Surgery is a stressful occupation that strains not only the surgeon but also his or her family or support system. The trainees in surgery are an especially vulnerable group because they often do not have a well-developed support system and frequently train in locations that may be remote from family. A few studies have examined factors related to stress in the resident work environment, but data examining the effect of marriage and children in residency are sparse. Sullivan et al have provided excellent survey data from more than 80% of the general surgery residents. The survey results showed that married residents with children looked forward to going to work, were happy at work, and were a good fit for their program (Table 2). However, residents with children did feel a strain on family life. Residents that were divorced, widowed, or separated noted that work hours produced a strain on family life. Female sex was negatively associated with going to work. This study is important because it identifies groups of residents that may be at risk for unhappiness at work or even depression. It is important that surgical educators provide mentoring to residents that includes modeling a work-life balance that residents see firsthand. Mentors and leaders in surgery training programs should liberally entertain residents and specifically address challenges with the work-life balance. Furthermore, identifying at-risk trainee populations and offering counseling or programs to discuss issues of personal and family strain will set an appropriate course early in trainees' careers.

K. E. Behrns, MD

Residency Training and International Medical Graduates: Coming to America No More

Traverso G, McMahon GT (Massachusetts General Hosp, Boston; Brigham and Women's Hosp, Boston, MA)
JAMA 308:2193-2194, 2012

Background.—By 2015 there will be more graduates from US medical schools than positions in residency programs. As a result, there will likely be fewer international medical graduates (IMG) who train in the United States, since most residency programs give preference to US graduates. This decrease may affect the diversity and activities of physicians who practice in the United States, with possible implications for patient care.

Postgraduate Training Effects.—About 25% of all physicians and 10% to 15% of all trainees in residency programs are IMGs currently. Existing US medical schools have expanded their enrollment and new programs have been established to meet an anticipated physician shortage. However, the number of training positions in US residency programs has not expanded correspondingly and may not because of a decline in graduate medical education funding. As a result, there are more unmatched US MD seniors, which may lead to the admission of less-qualified students, who may lower the quality of care offered by US graduates.

IMGs provide significant diversity in training and working environments. Care provided by clinicians of the same ethnicity as the patients may be of better quality and improve the patient-physician partnership, so reducing diversity could worsen existing disparities in health care. IMGs pursue training in the United States for various reasons, including the opportunity for high-quality education, better remuneration than could be expected in their native country, and a possible pathway to citizenship. If they are unable to train in the United States, IMGs may have a reduced capacity to provide high-quality care in their home countries.

Practice Activities.—Compared to US graduates, IMGs are dispro-portionately represented in areas with high infant mortality rate, lower socioeconomic status, a greater proportion of nonwhite populations, and counties classified as rural. They also work more often in the public sector and in medically underserved areas. About 10% of hospitals are considered IMG dependent. How these hospitals and the health care system itself will adapt to their decreased availability is unknown. US graduates would have to fill these more challenging roles or geographic disparities in access to care will be fostered.

If the number of training positions in the United States shrinks, fewer IMGs will fill these positions. This will affect not only the training of US candidates but also of those in other countries where IMGs return after post-graduate training. In addition, US students who attend medical school abroad may also find it difficult to reenter the United States medical system.

Conclusions.—Additional funding is needed to facilitate the growth in residency programs. Creative solutions will be needed in light of current funding source constrictions, including making primary care in rural settings and other underserved areas more attractive to US graduates, directing more recruitment and retention efforts at minority representation in US medical schools, expanding the use of nonphysician clinicians, and self-financing of postgraduate training. IMGs may also be recruited to meet primary care shortages if funding and other incentives can be obtained, perhaps including a path to citizenship for IMGs who dedicate years of primary care delivery in underserved areas.

▶ In the past several years, we have seen a significant increase in the number of new medical schools. Florida, my state of residence, is one of the leaders in establishing new medical schools, with 4 new schools created in the past 12 years. Although these new medical schools have created opportunities for medical training for undergraduate students, the number of graduate medical training positions has not increased significantly in our state. As a result, we are not training more physicians to work in Florida, and the fourth-most populous state in the United States is dependent on importing physicians. As such, we have many international medical graduates who provide necessary care to our populous—in fact, they constitute 37% of our total physician workforce.[1]

However, this physician workforce is at risk, as elegantly described by Traverso and McMahon. The increasing number of new medical schools in the US is producing enough graduates to occupy a larger proportion of our graduate medical education programs, and these US graduates crowd out international medical graduates. How does this affect surgery? In our general surgery training program, which trains 5 categorical general surgery residents per year, we annually receive about 1000 applications, approximately 600 of which are from international medical graduates. Out of this large group, we cull a few international medical graduates who may be interested in a preliminary training position. On occasion, these international trainees join us and then progress to become wonderful trainees and surgeons. Some of them have been our most stellar trainees and go on to become leaders in their professional community. Others have returned to their country where they have taken back ideas and improved the care locally. Universally, these graduates have been committed to excellence in surgery, and in this global world, this is a group of surgical trainees that should not be forgotten. They have contributed greatly to our collective success.

K. E. Behrns, MD

Reference

1. AMA Position Paper- IMG Section of Governing Council. "International medical graduates in American Medicine: contemporary challenges and opportunities." January 2010. http://www.ama-assn.org/resources/doc/img/img-workforce-paper.pdf. Accessed December 8, 2012.

Issues in General Surgery Residency Training—2012
Lewis FR, Klingensmith ME (American Board of Surgery, Philadelphia, PA; Washington Univ School of Medicine, St Louis, MO)
Ann Surg 256:553-559, 2012

Background.—Radical changes in the operations done by general surgeons have occurred over the past 20 years, but the impact on residency training has often been overlooked. The nature of these changes, their negative effects on resident training, and measures that may mitigate these effects were discussed.

Areas of Change.—Environmental and technologic changes in disease management have altered the incidence of complications, the need for surgical intervention, and treatment options in benign peptic ulcer disease, biliary tree stone disease, abdominal vascular surgery, and trauma. Current medical management and imaging advances produce fewer instances where surgery is required. In addition, laparoscopic and endoscopic surgery is often complex and not performed by general surgeons. In addition, the surgical treatment of traumatic injuries has been reduced by a markedly lower incidence of abdominal penetrating trauma and blunt trauma (often the result of automobile crashes) in the United States.

Limiting the resident's workweek to 80 hours has reduced in-hospital time by 6 months to a year in most programs. Often daytime experience is unaltered, but residents are seldom exposed to the urgent and emergent conditions seen at night and on weekends. Working at night and over weekends has often allowed residents to function more independently or autonomously, with indirect supervision, and these experiences are also being reduced.

Residents are more likely to continue their training beyond their general surgical residency than was previously the case. Interviews and observations of this trend indicate that residents feel training beyond residency is needed for them to be successful in practice and competitive in the marketplace. For practice purposes, the surgical training now lasts 6 to 7 years rather than the traditional 5 years.

Solutions.—The environmental and technologic changes have fundamentally altered the types of disease that require surgical management and how that treatment is delivered. It is unlikely that these trends will be reversed, given the positive benefits that have resulted. Things that can be changed in resident training include (1) defining and continually updating the curriculum, (2) improving the efficiency of learning, (3) using simulation and more structured teaching and assessment methods, (4) encouraging an earlier focus on specialty choices, (5) expanding laparoscopic surgery training, (6) increasing the length of the residency period, and (7) adding more skills to the surgical residency training program.

Conclusions.—Changes in general surgical practice have disrupted residency training. The assessments done by external agents who employ graduates in their practice or group, the opinions of the residents themselves, and the performance of graduates on the oral examination of the American Board of Surgery over the past 8 years testify to the significance of these issues in terms of the overall performance of recent surgical graduates. It is important that the surgical community recognize the problems and take steps to formulate effective solutions.

▶ Surgery has evolved rapidly in the last 2 decades with the introduction of minimally invasive techniques, improved critical care, and continually evolving medical therapies. These advances and the rapid dissemination of knowledge have increased the demands on surgical trainees in an era in which the duty hours have been reduced. These changes have created enormous pressure on our trainees and teachers. As Lewis and Klingensmith deftly illustrate, there are numerous challenges and opportunities to enhance surgical education, and we should instantly adopt many of these ideas to change our training paradigms. However, a substantial underlying issue, which was not discussed, permeates our culture of surgical education—we hold to the belief that all trainees learn at roughly the same pace and, therefore, the curriculum is devised in year-long blocks. Importantly, the financial underpinnings of a 12-month curriculum are substantial and not easy to address. However, if we are really in the business of training surgical residents, we should accept that not all residents learn at the same pace and that achieving competency may not come in year-long increments. It is time for us to address the funding issue of graduate medical education and to outline a curriculum that is based on competencies and not time spent on various surgical rotations. Indeed, now is the time to become efficient with both time and money, and we should develop sound proposals for funding graduate medical education that will engage the learner in an efficient, competency-based education curriculum.

K. E. Behrns, MD

Trainee satisfaction in surgery residency programs: Modern management tools ensure trainee motivation and success
von Websky MW, Oberkofler CE, Rufibach K, et al (Univ Hosp of Zurich, Switzerland; Univ of Zurich, Switzerland)
Surgery 152:794-801, 2012

Objective.—To assess trainee satisfaction in their surgery residency with a validated instrument and identify the contributing factors.

Background.—Currently, surgery is deemed unattractive by medical students and ignored by many candidates planning to enter an academic career. New insights on the rational for such lack of interest are needed. Job satisfaction is a central concept in organizational and behavioral research that is well understood by large companies such as Google, IBM, and Toyota. Similar assessment can likewise be used to improve trainee satisfaction in surgery residency.

Methods.—A survey among 2039 surgery residents was conducted in three European countries analyzing satisfaction at work using the Global Job Satisfaction Instrument (validated in Emergency Room physicians). Crucial factors covering different aspects of surgery residency where identified using the GJS instrument combined with multiple logistic regression analysis.

Results.—With an overall response rate of 23%, we identified trainee dissatisfaction in one third of residents. Factors affecting satisfaction related almost exclusively to training issues, such as assignment of surgery procedures according to skills (OR 4.2), training courses (OR 2.7), availability of a structured training curriculum (OR 2.4), bedside teaching, and availability of morbidity-mortality conferences (OR 2.3). A good working climate among residents (OR 3.7) and the option for part time work (OR 2.1) were also significant factors for trainee satisfaction. Increased working hours had a modest (OR 0.98)—though cumulative—negative effect. The sex of the trainee was not related to trainee satisfaction.

Conclusion.—Validated measurement of job satisfaction as used in the industry appears to be an efficient tool to assess trainee satisfaction in surgery residency and thereby identify the key contributing factors. Improvement of conceptual training structures and working conditions might facilitate recruitment, decrease drop-out, and attract motivated candidates with possibly better quality of care.

▶ The enthusiasm of medical students for a career in general surgery has waxed and waned over the years. Currently, in the United States, the interest in general surgery is robust, and the candidates are superb. However, on occasion, these residents become disenchanted with their training and seek positions in other specialties, or, worse yet, remain in a career path that does not suit them. Von Websky et al conducted a survey of surgical trainees in 3 European countries to determine satisfaction with training. Interestingly, one-third of the trainees were dissatisfied. Current trainees seek a structured curriculum, regular conferences and teaching rounds, case assignment based on skill or seniority level, and a good working environment. Increased work hours had a modest negative effect, and satisfaction was not related to compensation. The desires of the trainees are a bit surprising because, frankly, their wants are what every training program should provide. We must clearly foster an environment that has a foundation of education over service and seeks to continually improve the knowledge base and critical analysis skills of all our residents. The days of employing residents to provide a service are clearly over, and the balance must certainly be in favor of education. Furthermore, we must strike a compromise in duty hour limits. Many residents today do not feel they receive adequate training in terms of hours on the job, and, in fact, many simply do not accurately record duty hours. We should not place our trainees in a position that forces them to extend the duration of training either by stretching the duty hours or performing what some trainees think is an obligatory fellowship. We should continually reassess the training product and work environment and make substantive changes that will enhance the care of the patient and the education of the resident.

K. E. Behrns, MD

Professionalism in the Era of Duty Hours: Time for a Shift Change
Arora VM, Farnan JM, Humphrey HJ (Univ of Chicago, IL)
JAMA 308:2195-2196, 2012

Background.—Physicians trained before duty hour regulations were instituted may regard current physicians in training as lifestyle oriented and not as committed as they are to the medical profession. They tend to apply the tenets of "nostalgic professionalism" to the situation. This type of professionalism is defined as consistently placing the patient's or profession's interests and needs above personal needs. Medical educators face a challenge as a result, trying to reconcile this former definition of professionalism with the new model of medical training. Understanding the circumstances of modern residency training, specifically how resident actions consistent with nostalgic professionalism conflict with mandated regulations, is vital to resolving this issue.

Resident Actions.—Current residents tend to work past their shift limits even when program leaders tell them this is not appropriate. Reasons given for remaining include concern for their own patients, fear of harming patients by handing them off to the next shift, or fear about what can happen even while they may be resting. Many residents regard this behavior as professional, yet to engage in this behavior leads to the decidedly unprofessional behavior of lying about their work hours. Residents also come to work when they should not, such as when they are ill. Often they want to maintain patient care activities or do not want to inconvenience colleagues who would have to cover for them.

Residents may continue to work even after they have left the hospital. Some of the activities they pursue are remotely accessing inpatient electronic health records, following patients' progress, placing orders from off-site locations, checking laboratory results, performing dictations, and communicating about patient care on their day off. Senior residents are more likely than interns to work from home in this way. However, the Accreditation Council of Graduate Medical Education has explicitly stated that time spent working from home counts toward duty hour limits. Residents are encouraged to read and study from home to enhance medical knowledge, but delivering clinical care delivery from home complicates the definition of what is permitted and what is not.

New Professionalism Goals.—The system of residency training must fully adopt a team-based care model so that patient ownership belongs to a team rather than an individual. Residents must recognize their limitations as humans and observe the importance of maintaining their own health and alertness as part of caring for patients.

Conclusions.—Ongoing exposure to the culture of training may shape how residents view professionalism. It is important to reconcile nostalgic professionalism with modern principles of practice. Although residents are placing their obligation to the patient ahead of their own needs, behaviors that are not professional are being fostered, such as lying about work hours. A new view of professionalism needs to be emphasized that allows students to exhibit a high degree of professionalism while observing mandated shifts. Other professions have been able to manage the coexistence of high professional values and regulated shifts and may provide guidance in helping medicine to adapt as well.

▶ The era of resident duty hours has had a number of intended and unintended consequences. Arora et al address how changes in duty hours have affected professionalism. In theory, professionalism would not have been altered by duty hours. However, as the authors point out, "nostalgic professionalism"—the patient comes first—remains alive and well, but duty hour regulations have often put trainees in positions that require working beyond time limits or abandoning a patient to which they feel obligated. Subsequently, the residents cheat on their duty hour report. Has or will this create a culture of bending the truth among residents? It is not apparent that after nearly a decade of duty hour regulations that residents are untruthful, but it is also clear that we have not adequately addressed the compromised position that trainees too often face. Does it really matter if a resident spends 4—6 extra hours per week tending to an ill patient that provides a valuable educational lesson? Can we not allow mature adults enough flexibility to carefully govern their training? Although we can certainly adopt lessons learned in other professions such as nursing and the airlines, we should be more creative in our solutions and seek to instill a professionalism that indeed continues to put the patient first and realizes that sometimes rules should be bent.

K. E. Behrns, MD

Impact of Resident Participation in Surgical Operations on Postoperative Outcomes: National Surgical Quality Improvement Program
Kiran RP, Ahmed Ali U, Coffey JC, et al (Cleveland Clinic, OH; Univ of Limerick, Ireland; et al)
Ann Surg 256:469-475, 2012

Objective.—To evaluate whether resident participation in operations influences postoperative outcomes.

Background.—Identification of potential differences in outcome associated with resident participation in operations may facilitate planning from educational and health resource perspectives.

Methods.—From the National Surgical Quality Improvement Program database (2005—2007), postoperative outcomes were compared for patients with and without resident participation (RES vs no-RES). Groups were matched in a 2:1 ratio, based on age, sex, specialty, surgical procedure, morbidity probability, and important comorbidities and risk factors.

Results.—RES (40,474; 66.7%) and no-RES (20,237; 33.3%) groups were comparable for matched characteristics. Mortality was similar (0.18% vs 0.20%, $P = 0.55$). Thirty-day complications classified as "mild" (4.4% vs 3.5%, $P < 0.001$) and "surgical" (7% vs 6.2%, $P < 0.001$) were higher in RES group. Individual complications were largely similar, except superficial surgical site infection (3.0% vs 2.2%, $P < 0.001$). Operative time was longer in the RES group [mean (SD) 122 (80) vs 97 (67) minutes, $P < 0.001$]. Overall complications were lower for postgraduate year 1—2 residents than for other years. These differences persisted on multivariate analysis adjusting for confounders.

Conclusions.—Resident involvement in surgical procedures is safe. The small overall increase in mild surgical complications is mostly caused by superficial wound infections. Reasons for this are likely multifactorial but may be related to prolonged operative time.

▶ Over the last decade, multiple factors have converged and forced the examination of the impact of surgical resident participation in operations. Duty hour restrictions, the requirement for close resident supervision, payer considerations, and the quality movement have all influenced the resident participation in operations. As a result of these changes, several groups have addressed patient outcomes with resident participation in an operation. Most of these studies, which have limitations, conclude that resident participation does not significantly influence patient outcomes. Kiran et al studied the role of resident participation using the National Surgical Quality Improvement Program Database. Using this unique data collection, this study compared more than 40 000 patients with resident involvement with more than 20 000 patients who underwent operations without resident involvement. The findings suggest that resident involvement is safe. Resident involvement was associated with a slight increase in mild and surgical complications and longer operating time. The modest increase in complications was likely related to an increased superficial wound infection rate. Senior residents tended to have more complications than junior residents. This study provides convincing evidence that resident participation in surgical operations is safe. This study is important because we not only must train the next generation of surgeons, but we must train them to study the quality outcomes.

K. E. Behrns, MD

Symbiotic or Parasitic? A Review of the Literature on the Impact of Fellowships on Surgical Residents
Plerhoples TA, Greco RS, Krummel TM, et al (Inova Health System, Falls Church, VA; Stanford Univ, CA)
Ann Surg 256:904-908, 2012

Objective.—We conducted a systematic review of published literature to gain a better understanding of the impact of advanced fellowships on surgical resident training and education.

Background.—As fellowship opportunities rise, resident training may be adversely impacted.

Methods.—PubMed, MEDLINE, Scopus, BIOSIS, Web of Science, and a manual search of article bibliographies. Of the 139 citations identified through the initial electronic search and screened for possible inclusion, 23 articles were retained and accepted for this review. Data were extracted regarding surgical specialty, methodology, sample population, outcomes measured, and results.

Results.—Eight studies retrospectively compared the eras before and after the introduction of a fellowship or trended data over time. Approximately half used data from a single institution, whereas the other half used some form of national data or survey. Only 3 studies used national case data. Fourteen studies looked at general surgery, 6 at obstetrics-gynecology, 2 at urology, and 1 at otolaryngology. Only one study concluded that fellowships have a generally positive impact on resident education, whereas 9 others found a negative impact. The remaining 13 studies found mixed results (n = 6) or minimal to no impact (n = 7).

Conclusions.—The overall impact of advanced surgical fellowships on surgical resident education and training remains unclear, as most studies rely on limited data of questionable generalizability. A careful study of the national database of surgery resident case logs is essential to better understand how early surgical specialization and fellowships will impact the future of general surgery education.

▶ General surgery residency training programs are experiencing significant flux related to increasing demands for tight supervision, duty hour restrictions, the introduction of integrated training programs in surgical subspecialties, and non–Accreditation Council for Graduate Medical Education (ACGME)-approved fellowship training positions. Furthermore, an impending reduction of graduate medical education funding through the Centers for Medicare and Medicaid Services adds an additional potential threat to the current paradigm of general surgery training. Plerhoples et al performed a review of the literature to examine the effect of fellowship training positions on general surgery residency training. The review noted that a thorough study of the ACGME general surgery resident case logs to examine the number of cases performed in each index area along with an accounting of fellowship positions in each of the training programs is duly warranted. Furthermore, the authors noted that many of the past studies that examined the effect of fellowship training programs on general surgery residents noted a mixed outcome; that is, neither clear positive or negative influences were apparent. From this reviewer's point of view, fellowships should have a clear positive effect not only on the general surgery residents but the entire institution. For certain, there can be no issues related to case numbers for either the fellows or the general surgery trainees. Moreover, the experience of fellows should have a positive influence on the education of residents, and the institutional culture must demand clear educational roles for fellows in the training of general surgery residents. Fellows should be expected to raise the bar of quality clinical care, research, and education, and general surgery residents should be the recipient of these efforts.

K. E. Behrns, MD

Surgery in the Internet Era
Ancona E (Univ of Padova, Italy)
Ann Surg 256:671-674, 2012

Background.—Use of the Internet is expanding worldwide, with many countries having more than half of their citizens using this medium. Information technology is changing the way medical information is conveyed and used. Specific sectors that have been altered with respect to surgical practice include teaching, research, and patient information.

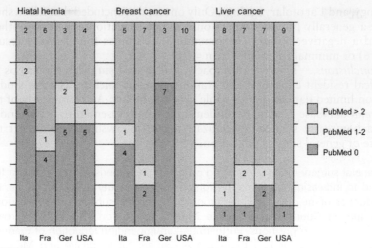

FIGURE.—Internet surfing on March 18, 2012, searching for hiatal hernia, breast cancer, and liver cancer. The number of PubMed publications in the past 10 years for each of the first 10 authors found. Fra indicates France; Ger, Germany; Ita, Italy. (Reprinted from Ancona E. Surgery in the Internet era. *Ann Surg.* 2012;256:671-674, © 2012 Southeastern Surgical Congress.)

Teaching.—Surgeon training used to be only through hands-on clinical practice. With residents working fewer hours per week, novel teaching methods based on remote learning have been developed. Studies have found no significant differences in the results of learning surgery through Internet courses compared to the conventional method, although some aspects can be conveyed only through more traditional means. Such e-learning methods are especially helpful when communicating with resident doctors in developing nations. Educators should exploit the Internet's widespread availability and adapt to the needs of today's trainee surgeons.

Research.—Via searches on the Internet, researchers can identify bibliographical material specific to their research. In addition, online research can be conducted, allowing direct involvement of different groups distributed anywhere. This opens new frontiers for the scientific community supporting surgical endeavors.

Patient Information.—Patients can access a wealth of information via the Internet, but the quality of the information varies widely. Sites are not obligated to comply with regulations about the reliability of the information, privacy issues, references to sources, tests that show the benefits of proposed treatments, or transparency concerning the commercial or noncommercial interests behind the sites. In addition, the quality of the information varies depending on what medical condition is being researched and the country of the searcher. A sample of the first 10 sites listed found that, depending on the country, information on hiatal hernia and gastroesophageal reflux was reliable in 3 and 6 listings; achalasia information was reliable in half; breast cancer information was reliable in 3 to 10; and liver and pancreas surgery information was helpful in nearly all sites, perhaps because surgeons without sufficient expertise avoid this field.

Patients may also be seeking information about the availability of surgical options in other countries for the purpose of surgical tourism. It is easy for patients to seek non-approved treatment elsewhere, "shop" for a better price on surgery, or simply find out about options that are not in the mainstream. Again, problems arise regarding the reliability of the source, since many sites offer no information on outcomes or risks.

Social media sites offer patients first-hand recounts of experiences with surgeons and procedures. These are highly useful when patients choose treatments or doctors.

Conclusions.—It is important to develop a way to monitor the content of what is posted on the Internet relevant to surgery. A code setting rules for health information on the Internet has been developed, but few Web sites have become accredited at this point. In addition, further updates to teaching programs are advisable to take advantage of the opportunities available. Medical faculties should be trained to promote professionally appropriate use of the Internet (Fig).

▶ The use of the Internet with the enormous increase in the publically available knowledge has changed how we live and has changed the world of surgery substantially as well. Many patients now arrive at their clinic appointment with printed information from the Internet. They have the information about their surgeon and are educated about their disease. Furthermore, the Internet has profoundly affected the 3 missions of academic medical centers—education, research, and clinical care. The Internet has greatly aided distribution of surgical education information and provides many educational opportunities for medical students and trainees. In addition, the Internet is a valuable resource for the conduct of surgical research, as it provides a portal for collection of data and a center for distribution of information. However, the use of the Internet for clinical purposes has had both positive and negative effects. Although patients have access to more information, the Internet has provided a substantial platform for physician and hospital marketing. Naturally, truth in advertising is in the eye of the beholder. This article by Ancona nicely shows that the results of an Internet search will not necessarily provide information from an expert in the first 10 hits (Fig 1). Should marketing on the Internet be more tightly regulated so that standards of marketing are developed? More likely, the house of surgery should provide up-to-date, factual information about diseases through our national and regional organizations and academic institutions. In addition, reputable surgeons and surgical practices should be offered as resources; currently, surgical organizations do not universally provide this information. Finally, public posting of risk-adjusted, standardized outcomes should be the goal of all surgeons.

K. E. Behrns, MD

Perioperative and anaesthetic-related mortality in developed and developing countries: A systematic review and meta-analysis
Bainbridge D, for the Evidence-based Peri-operative Clinical Outcomes Research (EPiCOR) Group (Univ of Western Ontario, London, Ontario, Canada)
Lancet 380:1075-1081, 2012

Background.—The magnitude of risk of death related to surgery and anaesthesia is not well understood. We aimed to assess whether the risk of perioperative and anaesthetic-related mortality has decreased over the past five decades and whether rates of decline have been comparable in developed and developing countries.

Methods.—We did a systematic review to identify all studies published up to February, 2011, in any language, with a sample size of over 3000 that reported perioperative mortality across a mixed surgical population who had undergone general anaesthesia. Using standard forms, two authors independently identified studies for inclusion and extracted information on rates of anaesthetic-related mortality, perioperative mortality, cardiac arrest, American Society of Anesthesiologists (ASA) physical status, geographic location, human development index (HDI), and year. The primary outcome was anaesthetic sole mortality. Secondary outcomes were anaesthetic contributory mortality, total perioperative mortality, and cardiac arrest. Meta-regression was done to ascertain weighted event rates for the outcomes.

Findings.—87 studies met the inclusion criteria, within which there were more than 21·4 million anaesthetic administrations given to patients undergoing general anaesthesia for surgery. Mortality solely attributable to anaesthesia declined over time, from 357 per million (95% CI 324—394) before the 1970s to 52 per million (42—64) in the 1970s—80s, and 34 per million

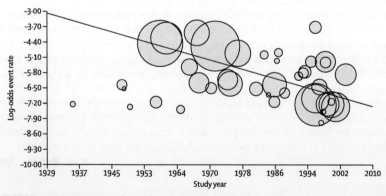

FIGURE 4.—Meta-regression for total perioperative mortality by year. Every circle represents a study; the circle size is representative of the weight of that study in the analysis. The relation between mortality and year was significant, with a significant decline over the decades (slope −0·053, 95% CI −0·054 to −0·052; *p* < 0·00001). (Reprinted from The Lancet, Bainbridge D, for the Evidence-based Peri-operative Clinical Outcomes Research (EPiCOR) Group. Perioperative and anaesthetic-related mortality in developed and developing countries: a systematic review and meta-analysis. *Lancet.* 2012;380:1075-1081. © 2012, with permission from Elsevier.)

(29–39) in the 1990s–2000s ($p < 0.00001$). Total perioperative mortality decreased over time, from 10 603 per million (95% CI 10 423–10 784) before the 1970s, to 4533 per million (4405–4664) in the 1970s–80s, and 1176 per million (1148–1205) in the 1990s–2000s ($p < 0.0001$). Meta-regression showed a significant relation between risk of perioperative and anaesthetic-related mortality and HDI (all $p < 0.00001$). Baseline risk status of patients who presented for surgery as shown by the ASA score increased over the decades ($p < 0.0001$).

Interpretation.—Despite increasing patient baseline risk, perioperative mortality has declined significantly over the past 50 years, with the greatest decline in developed countries. Global priority should be given to reducing total perioperative and anaesthetic-related mortality by evidence-based best practice in developing countries (Fig 4).

▶ As surgeons, we address questions daily about the safety of surgery and anesthesia and too frequently reply that anesthesia and surgery are incredibly safe. However, we offer this unqualified answer with few data to support our conclusion—that is, until now! Bainbridge et al carefully reviewed 87 studies that had greater than 3000 patients to assess perioperative mortality over a 50-year study period in developed and developing countries. They found that mortality attributable to anesthesia solely and total perioperative mortality decreased significantly over time (Fig 4). These findings were more pronounced in developed countries than in developing countries. Impressively, in developed countries, the mortality decreased despite increased baseline risk—related to comorbidities. This study provides excellent data that help us address patient questions related to anesthetic safety but also demonstrate the vast improvement in surgical care over time. Although these data are impressive, we will have to accomplish substantially greater gains in quality care in the next 50 years. Increasingly, we will be judged by not only our quality but the cost of delivering high-quality care. The value of care will become the yardstick by which we are measured. Obviously, the value of care may be variably defined, but nonetheless the onus will be on the surgical community to prove that we continuously improve our results and make perioperative care safer. To work toward this goal, we should scrupulously record our results and monitor progress on a regular basis. This rigorous approach must become a regular routine.

K. E. Behrns, MD

Mortality and Access to Care among Adults after State Medicaid Expansions
Sommers BD, Baicker K, Epstein AM (Harvard School of Public Health, Boston, MA)
N Engl J Med 367:1025-1034, 2012

Background.—Several states have expanded Medicaid eligibility for adults in the past decade, and the Affordable Care Act allows states to expand Medicaid dramatically in 2014. Yet the effect of such changes on adults' health remains unclear. We examined whether Medicaid expansions were associated with changes in mortality and other health-related measures.

Methods.—We compared three states that substantially expanded adult Medicaid eligibility since 2000 (New York, Maine, and Arizona) with neighboring states without expansions. The sample consisted of adults between the ages of 20 and 64 years who were observed 5 years before and after the expansions, from 1997 through 2007. The primary outcome was all-cause county-level mortality among 68,012 year- and county-specific observations in the Compressed Mortality File of the Centers for Disease Control and Prevention. Secondary outcomes were rates of insurance coverage, delayed care because of costs, and self-reported health among 169,124 persons in the Current Population Survey and 192,148 persons in the Behavioral Risk Factor Surveillance System.

Results.—Medicaid expansions were associated with a significant reduction in adjusted all-cause mortality (by 19.6 deaths per 100,000 adults, for a relative reduction of 6.1%; $P = 0.001$). Mortality reductions were greatest among older adults, nonwhites, and residents of poorer counties. Expansions increased Medicaid coverage (by 2.2 percentage points, for a relative increase of 24.7%; $P = 0.01$), decreased rates of uninsurance (by 3.2 percentage points, for a relative reduction of 14.7%; $P < 0.001$), decreased rates of delayed care because of costs (by 2.9 percentage points, for a relative reduction of 21.3%; $P = 0.002$), and increased rates of self-reported health status of "excellent:" or "very good" (by 2.2 percentage points, for a relative increase of 3.4%; $P = 0.04$).

Conclusions.—State Medicaid expansions to cover low-income adults were significantly associated with reduced mortality as well as improved coverage, access to care, and self-reported health.

▶ The passage of the Affordable Care Act caused consternation in the medical community, largely because by the year 2014 millions of additional patients will be enrolled in the already voluminous Medicaid program. One of the most commonly raised questions is, "How can we take care of these additional patients?" Although this is an important question, the real question is, "Will this provide better health to our nation's citizens who historically have had less care?" Sommers et al have taken a major step forward in addressing this question by conducting a well-designed study that examined the health of patients before and after the expansion of Medicaid in 3 states. Neighboring states that did not expand Medicaid services served as controls. The results showed that Medicaid expansion resulted in reduced mortality for these patients (Fig 1 in the original article). Mortality reduction was most evident in older and non-white patients and individuals from poorer counties. Why is this important for surgeons? First and foremost, surgeons have always placed quality of care as the top priority, and there can be no quality of care without access to care. In addition, perhaps preventive care will ultimately change the surgical population and we will see fewer patients present with complex disease and untreated comorbidities. Obviously, this would be a welcome change in practice, and perhaps we could care for an increased number of patients if some of the patients were less ill. Only time will tell how this major change in health care delivery will play out.

K. E. Behrns, MD

Importance of Perioperative Glycemic Control in General Surgery: A Report From the Surgical Care and Outcomes Assessment Program
Kwon S, Thompson R, Dellinger P, et al (Univ of Washington, Seattle; Harborview Med Ctr, Seattle, WA; et al)
Ann Surg 257:8-14, 2013

Objective.—To determine the relationship of perioperative hyperglycemia and insulin administration on outcomes in elective colon/rectal and bariatric operations.

Background.—There is limited evidence to characterize the impact of perioperative hyperglycemia and insulin on adverse outcomes in patients, with and without diabetes, undergoing general surgical procedures.

Methods.—The Surgical Care and Outcomes Assessment Program is a Washington State quality improvement benchmarking-based initiative. We evaluated the relationship of perioperative hyperglycemia (>180 mg/dL) and insulin administration on mortality, reoperative interventions, and infections for patients undergoing elective colorectal and bariatric surgery at 47 participating hospitals between fourth quarter of 2005 and fourth quarter of 2010.

Results.—Of the 11,633 patients (55.4 ± 15.3 years; 65.7% women) with a serum glucose determination on the day of surgery, postoperative day 1, or postoperative day 2, 29.1% of patients were hyperglycemic.

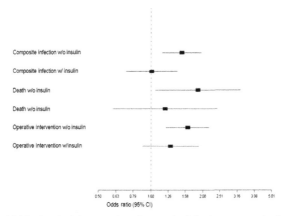

FIGURE 2.—Multivariate logistic regression of composite infections, reoperative interventions, and inpatient mortality rates for hyperglycemia (>180 mg/dL) on the day of surgery with and without adjustment for administration of insulin. (Reprinted from Kwon S, Thompson R, Dellinger P, et al. Importance of perioperative glycemic control in general surgery: a report from the surgical care and outcomes assessment program. *Ann Surg.* 2013;257:8-14, © 2012, Southeastern Surgical Congress.)

After controlling for clinical factors, those with hyperglycemia had a significantly increased risk of infection [odds ratio (OR) 2.0; 95% confidence interval (CI), 1.63—2.44], reoperative interventions (OR, 1.8; 95% CI, 1.41—2.3), and death (OR, 2.71; 95% CI, 1.72—4.28). Increased risk of poor outcomes was observed both for patients with and without diabetes. Those with hyperglycemia on the day of surgery who received insulin had no significant increase in infections (OR, 1.01; 95% CI, 0.72—1.42), reoperative interventions (OR, 1.29; 95% CI, 0.89—1.89), or deaths (OR, 1.21; 95% CI, 0.61—2.42). A dose-effect relationship was found between the effectiveness of insulin-related glucose control (worst 180—250 mg/dL, best <130 mg/dL) and adverse outcomes.

Conclusions.—Perioperative hyperglycemia was associated with adverse outcomes in general surgery patients with and without diabetes. However, patients with hyperglycemia who received insulin were at no greater risk than those with normal blood glucoses. Perioperative glucose evaluation and insulin administration in patients with hyperglycemia are important quality targets (Fig 2).

▶ Perioperative glucose control has been studied intensely in the last several years because regulated glucose control is highly associated with patient complications. This association was first identified in cardiac surgery patients and in patients in the intensive care unit. The effects of postoperative hyperglycemia in general surgery patients have not been studied thoroughly. However, Kwon et al examined more than 11 633 medical records in the state of Washington through the Surgical Care and Outcomes Assessment Program and noted that the effect of postoperative hyperglycemia in patients undergoing bariatric surgery and colon and rectal surgery were profound. Patients with hyperglycemia on the day of surgery or postoperative days 1 or 2 had a significantly increased risk of death, postoperative infection, and the need for reoperation. Interestingly, those patients with day-of-surgery hyperglycemia that was treated with insulin did not have an increased risk of death, infection, or reoperation (Fig 2). Even though this is a retrospective study, the message of this work speaks volumes; glucose control is well within our boundaries for improving patient outcomes. Furthermore, this work begs the question of preoperative control of hyperglycemia. Perhaps we should not perform major abdominal surgery until we have adequately controlled blood glucose. This work not only advances our knowledge but should make us cognizant of the untoward effects of poorly treated hyperglycemia in the postoperative patient.

K. E. Behrns, MD

"First Do No Harm": Balancing Competing Priorities in Surgical Practice
Leung A, Luu S, Regehr G, et al (Univ Health Network and Univ of Toronto, Ontario, Canada; Univ of British Columbia, Vancouver, Canada; et al)
Acad Med 87:1368-1374, 2012

Purpose.—To explore surgeons' perceptions of the factors that influence their intraoperative decision making, and implications for professional self-regulation and patient safety.

Method.—Semistructured interviews were conducted with 39 academic surgeons from various specialties at four hospitals associated with the University of Toronto Faculty of Medicine. Purposive and theoretical sampling was performed until saturation was achieved. Thematic analysis of the transcripts was conducted using a constructivist grounded-theory approach and was iteratively elaborated and refined as data collection progressed. A preexisting theoretical professionalism framework was particularly useful in describing the emergent themes; thus, the analysis was both inductive and deductive.

Results.—Several factors that surgeons described as influencing their decision making are widely accepted ("avowed," or in patients' best interests). Some are considered reasonable for managing multiple priorities external to the patient but are not discussed openly ("unavowed," e.g., teaching pressures). Others are actively denied and consider the surgeon's best interests rather than the patient's ("disavowed," e.g., reputation). Surgeons acknowledged tension in balancing avowed factors with unavowed and disavowed factors; when directly asked, they found it difficult to acknowledge that unavowed and disavowed factors could lead to patient harm.

Conclusions.—Some factors that are not directly related to the patient enter into surgeons' intraoperative decision making. Although these are probably reasonable to consider within "real-world" practice, they are not sanctioned in current patient care constructs or taught to trainees. Acknowledging unavowed and disavowed factors as sources of pressure in practice may foster critical self-reflection and transparency when discussing surgical errors.

▶ In 1999, the Institute of Medicine issued the report "To Err is Human" with a follow-up publication entitled "Crossing the Quality Chasm" in 2001. These publications placed emphasis on avoidable or potentially avoidable injuries to patients and highlighted the need to address patient safety. The quality movement has altered considerably the practice of medicine, with many programs focused on avoiding harm. Surgical care has been no exception to the quality movement even though surgical practices have long scrutinized results through mechanisms such as morbidity and mortality conference. Central to high-quality care is surgical decision-making. Leung et al provide an interesting analysis of emotional components of surgical decision-making. Although the focus of high-quality surgical care has been placed largely on the surgeon's results, little attention has been paid to the environment in which the surgeon makes decisions. Surgical decision-making in the operating room occurs in a complex environment with multiple pressures to wisely use resources, yet provide excellent care and perhaps teach trainees or staff. Many hospital programs have been created to address quality issues either specifically or in a broader context. However, few, if any, programs address the emotional environment that may influence decision-making that affects patient outcome. This article highlights issues in decision-making that too frequently are unaddressed. The pressure to produce not only quality care but to meet volume targets has increased markedly with decreased reimbursement. Clearly, this situation often inherently puts the surgeon, a major revenue producer, in conflict. It is imperative that health care systems render high-quality patient care by fostering excellent decision-making through enhancement of the work environment.

K. E. Behrns, MD

An Observational Study of the Frequency, Severity, and Etiology of Failures in Postoperative Care After Major Elective General Surgery

Symons NRA, Almoudaris AM, Nagpal K, et al (Imperial College London, UK)
Ann Surg 257:1-5, 2013

Objective.—To investigate the nature of process failures in postoperative care, to assess their frequency and preventability, and to explore their relationship to adverse events.

Background.—Adverse events are common and are frequently caused by failures in the process of care. These processes are often evaluated independently using clinical audit. There is little understanding of process failures in terms of their overall frequency, relative risk, and cumulative effect on the surgical patient.

Methods.—Patients were observed daily from the first postoperative day until discharge by an independent surgeon. Field notes on the circumstances surrounding any nonroutine or atypical event were recorded. Field notes were assessed by 2 surgeons to identify failures in the process of care. Preventability, the degree of harm caused to the patient, and the underlying etiology of process failures were evaluated by 2 independent surgeons.

Results.—Fifty patients undergoing major elective general surgery were observed for a total of 659 days of postoperative care. A total of 256 process failures were identified, of which 85% were preventable and 51% directly led to patient harm. Process failures occurred in all aspects of care, the most frequent being medication prescribing and administration, management of lines, tubes, and drains, and pain control interventions. Process failures accounted for 57% of all preventable adverse events. Communication failures and delays were the main etiologies, leading to 54% of process failures.

Conclusions.—Process failures are common in postoperative care, are highly preventable, and frequently cause harm to patients. Interventions to prevent process failures will improve the reliability of surgical postoperative care and have the potential to reduce hospital stay.

▶ Surgeons have long reported harm to patients through morbidity and mortality conferences (M&M), and, more recently, through quality programs such as the Surgical Care Improvement Project (SCIP) and the National Surgical Quality Improvement Project (NSQIP). However, as practicing surgeons, we know that although M&M, SCIP, and NSQIP capture a large number of untoward events in the perioperative period, the number of what we deem "small deviations in care" is tremendous. How many times have we ordered a peripheral intravenous line (IV) on morning rounds only to find out that on afternoon rounds the IV could not be placed for myriad reasons? In addition, during this period the patient missed ordered doses of narcotics, antibiotics, or other medications. Generally, we do not count these deviations in care processes or acknowledge them in a public forum. However, Symons et al report these types of deviations of care processes in 50 patients that underwent gastrointestinal surgery. They found 256 processes of care failures, of which 85% were preventable and 51% were associated with harm. Not surprisingly, most of these failures were associated with the administration of medications and the management of drains, tubes, and IV lines. Furthermore, communication errors and delays in care were at the root of many of these process deviations. Although this is an observational study, which nonetheless is laborious, the message is of paramount importance because it highlights the rudimentary foundation of our patient care delivery system that permits 4.5 process errors per patient in the postoperative period. This study speaks to the need for a completely revamped care delivery system that is less dependent on human analysis and interpretation and more frequently guided by technological aids that constantly remind us of a standard of care delivery.

K. E. Behrns, MD

Simulation-Based Trial of Surgical-Crisis Checklists
Arriaga AF, Bader AM, Wong JM, et al (Harvard School of Public Health, Boston, MA; et al)
N Engl J Med 368:246-253, 2013

Background.—Operating-room crises (e.g., cardiac arrest and massive hemorrhage) are common events in large hospitals but can be rare for individual clinicians. Successful management is difficult and complex. We sought to evaluate a tool to improve adherence to evidence-based best practices during such events.

Methods.—Operating-room teams from three institutions (one academic medical center and two community hospitals) participated in a series of surgical-crisis scenarios in a simulated operating room. Each team was randomly assigned to manage half the scenarios with a set of crisis checklists and the remaining scenarios from memory alone. The primary outcome measure was failure to adhere to critical processes of care. Participants were also surveyed regarding their perceptions of the usefulness and clinical relevance of the checklists.

Results.—A total of 17 operating-room teams participated in 106 simulated surgical-crisis scenarios. Failure to adhere to lifesaving processes of care was less common during simulations when checklists were available (6% of steps missed when checklists were available vs. 23% when they were unavailable, $P < 0.001$). The results were similar in a multivariate model that accounted for clustering within teams, with adjustment for institution, scenario, and learning and fatigue effects (adjusted relative risk, 0.28; 95% confidence interval, 0.18 to 0.42; $P < 0.001$). Every team performed better when the crisis checklists were available than when they were not. A total of 97% of the participants reported that if one of these crises occurred while they were undergoing an operation, they would want the checklist used.

Conclusions.—In a high-fidelity simulation study, checklist use was associated with significant improvement in the management of operating-room crises. These findings suggest that checklists for use during operating-room crises have the potential to improve surgical care. (Funded by the Agency for Healthcare Research and Quality.)

▶ Patient safety in the operating room and other complex care environments is of obvious paramount importance, but as care providers, we have only scratched the surface of systematically assessing safety in this complex, high-risk care venue. Think for a minute about the complex nature of the operating room environment in the context of patient safety. First, the patient, nearly by definition, is quite ill because only surgery (not a medication) is the treatment. Furthermore, the physical environment in the operating room is complex, with sophisticated equipment that must function properly for safe patient care. Moreover, the team of care providers in the operating room is diverse with unique skill sets, training, and expectations. The care of a patient in the operating room becomes even more complicated when a crisis occurs. In many operating rooms (hopefully all), checklists are used as a reminder of the processes of care that should be employed before starting and concluding an operation. However, we often do not use checklists in crisis management in the operating room. These authors demonstrate clearly in a simulated setting that the use of checklists in clinical scenarios that are often chaotic is warranted. These data demonstrate that the use of checklists results in a more systematic approach to crisis intervention. Importantly, although not studied directly, the use of team training and rehearsing the management of a critically ill patient are valuable. Unfortunately, the engagement of surgeons in this study was disappointingly low. As leaders in the operating room, we should embrace the use of checklists and team training and participate in the studies necessary to enhance the care of the patient.

K. E. Behrns, MD

Ensuring Physicians' Competence—Is Maintenance of Certification the Answer?

Iglehart JK, Baron RB (Univ of California, San Francisco)
N Engl J Med 367:2543-2549, 2012

Background.—Physicians are faced with serious challenges in initiatives that are designed to correlate the goals of learning with the delivery of better care and measures of accountability. The maintenance of certification (MOC) program sponsored by the American Board of Medical Specialties (ABMS) is the most contentious of these. MOC programs require most certified specialists to be recertified periodically, usually every 10 years, through the successful completion of a four-part assessment testing their medical knowledge, clinical competence, and communication skills with patients. Problems in the MOC design and implementation were outlined along with possible improvements.

MOC System.—The MOC process is based on six domains jointly developed and approved by the ABMS and the Accreditation Council for Graduate Medical Education (ACGME): medical knowledge, patient care and procedural skills, interpersonal and communication skills, professionalism, practice-based learning and improvement, and systems-based practice. These competencies apply to residents and fellows alike. They are used by medical and other health professional schools to structure curricula, enhance assessment, and define interprofessional collaboration and by the Joint Commission in its requirements for hospitals to assess the competence of physicians on their staffs. These six competencies also underlie the four MOC components that form the preferred model to maintain certification. The four parts are (1) licensure and professional standing, (2) lifelong learning and self-assessment, (3) cognitive expertise, and (4) assessment of practice performance.

Changes.—The fourth area exhibits that greatest differences in implementation between specialties. A new approach to part four allows physicians who participate in quality-improvement programs sponsored by their institutions to receive MOC credits. The Mayo Clinic and 10 other organizations are MOC portfolio participants, drawing physicians to join in and hopefully strengthening the MOC program. Individual boards are also revising their MOC programs, with the most significant approaches being a greater effort to be continuous and requiring the more regular participation of diplomates. The ABMS has also recognized the value of minimizing redundant data-collection tasks for physicians and raising the profile of MOC. MOC is increasingly being aligned with other efforts to improve quality of care and clinical competence, including offering physicians a modest bonus for more frequent participation in MOC and reporting quality measures to Medicare's Physician Quality Reporting System (PQRS). Participation in both MOC and PQRS earns additional bonus money, whereas nonparticipation entails lowered Medicare fees. MOC is also aligned with the Federation of State Medical Boards (FSMB).

Conclusions.—The medical profession cannot eliminate MOC and return to honor-system self-regulation. What will make the MOC process less burdensome is having MOC count for all the entities that will be judging physician performance. The ABMS and its boards must actively and openly respond to concerns regarding the MOC system and step up efforts to collaborate with organizations to form a system that meets the needs for professionalism, government regulation, and market issues.

▶ Since the publication of the Institute of Medicine reports, To Err is Human: Building a Safer Health System in 1999 and Crossing the Quality Chasm: A New Health System for the 21st Century in 2001, the medical community has sharpened the focus on delivery of quality health care. The public, as a prime stakeholder in health care outcomes, is also intensely interested in the quality of care and, in particular, the competence of their physicians. A national approach to ensure physician competence is Maintenance of Certification (MOC), which was developed by the American Board of Medical Specialists and its 24-member boards. MOC is based on the 6 competencies that underlie the training of all physicians: medical knowledge, patient care and procedural skills, interpersonal and communication skills, professionalism, practice-based learning and improvement, and systems-based practice. The American Board of Surgery requires a 3-year cycle based on 4 parts of MOC. MOC part 1 mandates a current state license and good professional standing in the provider's health care community, part 2 is driven by continuing medical education that is directed at lifelong learning and self-assessment, part 3 tests cognitive experience through a recertification examination every 10 years, and part 4 is focused on assessment of practice performance. Although MOC has met with some resistance, our focus as a surgical community should be directed at developing the regulations that are pertinent to our practice rather than having policy dictated to us. Nowhere is this more evident than in MOC part 4, which is directed at the quality of care we deliver. Simple participation in quality programs will not suffice for driving quality of care in our practices. We should be intimately involved in developing quality programs that are directed at quality issues that affect our patients. This should be the goal of MOC part 4, which is likely to undergo substantial revision over the next several years.

K. E. Behrns, MD

Budget Sequestration and the U.S. Health Sector
McDonough JE (Harvard School of Public Health, Boston, MA)
N Engl J Med 2013 [Epub ahead of print]

Background.—On March 1 across-the-board cuts in most federal agencies and programs began because the Congress and President Obama were unable to agree on a plan to reduce the budget deficit. These cuts (termed sequestration) were put in place to reduce the deficit by $1.2 trillion between 2013 and 2021. Equal cuts of $42.67 billion are being made from defense-related and nondefense parts of the 2013 budget over the last

7 months of the 2013 fiscal year. These are being implemented by the Office of Management and Budget (OMB) and represent about 13% from nonexempt defense programs and about 9% from nonexempt nondefense programs. The effect of these cuts on the US health sector was explored.

Overview of Sequestration Effects.—The cuts will not fall equally on all health-related government programs. Certain programs such as Medicare and community health centers will have 2% reductions, whereas nonexempt and nondefense discretionary funding will be reduced between 7.6% and 8.2%. Medicaid and the Veterans Health Administration are exempt. Thirty-five percent of the sequester cuts will involve nondefense discretionary purposes.

Specific Programs Affected.—Medicare funding will be cut by 2% by reducing payments to hospitals, physicians, and other health care providers and insurers who participate in Medicare Advantage (Part C). These cuts take place just as Medicare is beginning the full implementation of savings and cuts required by the Affordable Care Act (ACA).

The National Institutes of Health (NIH) will have an 8.2% across-the-board reduction that will delay or stop scientific projects. To avoid having to reduce the number of grants and renewals the NIH makes, reductions will be made in nearly all extramural and intramural programs.

The Centers for Disease Control and Prevention (CDC) will have reductions of 8% to 10%. The CDC estimates it will fund 424,000 fewer HIV tests and 50,000 fewer immunizations for adults and children, eliminate tuberculosis programs in 11 states, shutter the National Healthcare Safety Network, eliminate the Cities Readiness Initiative, and find 150 fewer outbreaks of food-borne disease.

The Food and Drug Administration expects it will conduct 2100 fewer inspections at domestic and foreign food manufacturers. The Substance Abuse and Mental Health Services Administration will cut the Mental Health Block Grant program, which will eliminate services for 373,000 adults and children and cut inpatient admissions for addiction by 109,000. The Indian Health Service will cover 3000 fewer inpatient admissions and 804,000 fewer outpatient visits. The Health Resources and Services Administration will deliver AIDS drug-assistance services to 7400 fewer patients.

Conclusions.—The sequestration and uncertainty about federal policy threaten further improvement in the US economy. If the cuts remain in place, some experts predict that real growth in the gross domestic product will be reduced by 0.5 to 0.7 percentage points in 2013. This reduction in services is harming vital health care functions at all levels.

▶ This article presents a poignant review of the effects of the budget sequestration on US health care. How is sequestration pertinent to surgeons? Two effects will be most evident. First, reimbursement for medicare patients will be reduced 2% to hospitals and physicians. Although 2% may seem trivial, for a busy group practice this will undoubtedly mean loss of personnel. For example, our academic group practice will likely need to reduce our support staff by 2 positions because of the decrement in Medicare funding. Thus, patient quality of care related to access could be affected. Obviously, this is an undesirable situation. Second, funding to the National Institutes of Health (NIH) will be reduced 8.2% or $1.55 billion in 2013. For the extramural grant program, this either means that the number of awards will be reduced or the dollars per award will be dropped. Locally, we have seen recently 2 NIH notifications of awards reduced by 20% to 25%. What does this mean? Practically, either experiments are cut or laboratory personnel are decreased in number. Neither situation is palatable. Notably, the cuts to Medicare and the NIH come in the face of decreased state funding for indigent patients and, almost universally, decreased state support for academic initiatives. Furthermore, the Affordable Care Act is largely exempt from sequestration. Undoubtedly, this will mean that a smaller workforce will be required to see an increasing number of patients for less reimbursement. Politics aside, clearly it is time for us to advocate for our patients, our discipline, and to continue scientific investigation to not only maintain but also improve the health of those in our nation.

K. E. Behrns, MD

2 Trauma

Battlefield trauma care then and now: A decade of Tactical Combat Casualty Care
Butler FK Jr, Blackbourne LH (US Army Inst of Surgical Res, Fort Sam Houston, TX)
J Trauma Acute Care Surg 73:S395-S402, 2012

Maughon reported in 1970 that 193 of a cohort of 2,600 casualties that were killed in action in Vietnam died of isolated extremity hemorrhage. The percentage of fatalities that resulted from exsanguination from extremity wounds was 7.9%; this was the leading cause of preventable death among US military casualties in the Vietnam War. Maughon commented at the time that little progress had been made in battlefield trauma care in the last 100 years. A sobering postscript to Maughon's observations in 1970 is found in the preventable death analyses done by Holcomb et al. and Kelly et al. in the current conflicts. Holcomb et al. found a 15% incidence of potentially preventable fatalities in his article that reviewed all Special Operations deaths in Iraq and Afghanistan from the initiation of hostilities until November 2004. He found that 25% (3 of 12) fatalities with potentially survivable injuries might have been saved by the simple application of a tourniquet. The larger causes of death analysis by Kelly et al. studied 982 fatalities from the first 5 years of the conflicts in Afghanistan and Iraq. He documented that 77 of 232 potentially preventable deaths from the Armed Forces Medical Examiner records resulted from failure to use a tourniquet; exsanguination from isolated extremity wounds thus caused 7.8% of the combat-related deaths reported in the article of Kelly et al. The failure to make progress in addressing the leading cause of preventable deaths on the battlefield in the 30 years between the Vietnam and Afghanistan wars, despite the ready availability of the requisite technology, dramatically underscores Maughon's point about the lack of progress in battlefield trauma care.

▶ In this article, the authors provide an excellent review of the progress of battlefield care for the critically injured soldier and provide insights as to why so much progress has been made in the past decade. The most obvious answer is the continuing presence of America's longest armed conflict, which has allowed the benefits of lifesaving innovations in combat trauma care to be seen in near real time and thus accelerate the transition process. The other factor, however, has been the tri-service Committee on Tactical Combat Casualty Care (CoTCCC), which was begun in 2001 as a US Special Operations Command biomedical research effort to ensure that emerging technology and information are incorporated into the TCCC guidelines on an ongoing basis. This group has provided an intense and sustained tri-service effort to update battlefield trauma care best practice guidelines. The presence of both military and civilian trauma experts, medical researchers, medical educators, and combat medical personnel on the CoTCCC positions the group uniquely well to accomplish this task. With the advancements in hospital care and evacuation techniques, the US military and its coalition partners now have the best definitive care and evacuation capabilities for the management of combat trauma in history. This is truly exceptional progress.

D. W. Mozingo, MD

Influence of Resident Involvement on Trauma Care Outcomes
Bukur M, Singer MB, Chung R, et al (Cedars-Sinai Med Ctr, Los Angeles, CA)
Arch Surg 147:856-862, 2012

Hypothesis.—Discrepancies exist in complications and outcomes at teaching trauma centers (TTCs) vs nonteaching TCs (NTCs).

Design.—Retrospective review of the National Trauma Data Bank research data sets (January 1, 2007, through December 31, 2008).

Setting.—Level II TCs.

Patients.—Patients at TTCs were compared with patients at NTCs using demographic, clinical, and outcome data. Regression modeling was used to adjust for confounding factors to determine the effect of house staff presence on failure to rescue, defined as mortality after an in-house complication.

Main Outcome Measures.—The primary outcome measures were major complications, in-hospital mortality, and failure to rescue.

Results.—In total, 162 687 patients were available for analysis, 36 713 of whom (22.6%) were admitted to NTCs. Compared with patients admitted to TTCs, patients admitted to NTCs were older (52.8 vs 50.7 years), had more severe head injuries (8.3% vs 7.8%), and were more likely to undergo immediate operation (15.0% vs 13.2%) or ICU admission (28.1% vs 22.8%) ($P < .01$ for all). The mean Injury Severity Scores were similar between the groups (10.1 for patients admitted to NTCs vs 10.4 for patients admitted to TTCs, $P < .01$). Compared with patients admitted to TTCs, patients admitted to NTCs experienced fewer complications (adjusted odds ratio [aOR], 0.63; $P < .01$), had a lower adjusted mortality rate (aOR, 0.87; $P = .01$), and were less likely to experience failure to rescue (aOR, 0.81; $P = .01$).

Conclusions.—Admission to level II TTCs is associated with an increased risk for major complications and a higher rate of failure to rescue compared with admission to level II NTCs. Further investigation of the differences in care provided by level II TTCs vs NTCs may identify areas for improvement in residency training and processes of care.

▶ In this retrospective review of the National Trauma Data Bank, the authors compared outcomes of patients cared for in level 2 trauma centers with and without residency training programs. They found that those trauma centers with training programs were associated with worse outcomes measured by in-hospital complications, failure to rescue, and higher in-hospital mortality rates.

It is important to acknowledge several limitations of this study. As with any retrospective study, you cannot establish a direct cause-and-effect relationship but report only associations between the variables examined. Multiple limitations are inherent in using the National Trauma Data Bank as a source. The National Trauma Data Bank is a sample of information voluntarily reported by trauma centers, with basic issues about the quality of data reported, level of detail provided, and number of variables available. Some improvements have been noted with the more recent datasets. Significant numbers of hospitals that contribute data to the National Trauma Data Bank do not code any complications, and because the National Trauma Data Bank does not audit hospital data, it is not possible to determine whether data regarding complications are distributed evenly or accurately between teaching trauma centers and nonteaching trauma centers. In general, this study does speak for more diligent exploration of the influence of trainees in our current setting on patient outcomes.

D. W. Mozingo, MD

Repeat imaging in trauma transfers: A retrospective analysis of computed tomography scans repeated upon arrival to a Level I trauma center
Emick DM, Carey TS, Charles AG, et al (Univ of North Carolina at Chapel Hill; et al)
J Trauma Acute Care Surg 72:1255-1262, 2012

Background.—The repetition of computed tomography (CT) imaging in caring for injured patients transferred between institutions is common, but it is not well studied. Our objective is to quantify and describe the characteristics associated with repeating chest and abdominal CT images for patients transferred to trauma centers and to determine whether repeat imaging leads to delays in definitive care or disparate outcomes.

Methods.—This is a retrospective review of adult, blunt trauma patients transferred to two Level I trauma centers between January 2004 and May 2008 who underwent CT imaging of the chest, abdomen, or both.

Results.—60% of patients had at least one study repeated upon arrival to the trauma center. Variables associated with repeat imaging include Injury Severity Scores between 24 and 33 versus <15 (odds radio [OR], 1.6; 95% confidence interval [CI], 1.05—2.4), transfer to University of North Carolina (OR, 1.5; 95% CI, 1.01—2.2), transport by helicopter (OR, 1.6; 95% CI, 1.2—2.2), transfer in any year before 2008 (OR, 2.4; 95% CI, 1.6—3.6 for 2007; OR, 3.4; 95% CI, 2.2—5.3 for 2006; OR, 3.0; 95% CI, 1.8—5.0 for 2005; OR, 2.8; 95% CI, 1.7—4.7 for 2004), and triage alert level higher than the least severe level III (OR, 1.6; 95% CI, 1.01—2.7 for level II; OR, 2.2; 95% CI, 1.2—4.1 for level I). In adjusted models, there was no evidence that repeat imaging neither shortened the total time to definitive care nor altered patient outcomes.

Conclusions.—Injured patients often undergo imaging that gets repeated, adding cost and radiation exposure while not significantly altering outcomes. The current policy push to digitize medical records must include provisions for the interoperability and use of imaging software.

Level of Evidence.—III, therapeutic study.

▶ With increasing reliance on images obtained by computed tomography (CT) for diagnosis and the widespread availability of technology, CT imaging before transfer and repetition of studies upon arrival to a trauma center are common. A number of factors may account for the repetition of studies. Patients may be transferred with only a written interpretation of CT images but no actual images, images sent on digital media may be incompatible with the receiving hospital's informatics system, and the images themselves may be suboptimal or become damaged during transfer. There are also perceived administrative hurdles to obtain an official radiology interpretation of images taken elsewhere, surgeon preference, and a change in the patient's clinical condition.

In this article, the authors studied repetition of chest and abdominal CT scans upon arrival to a level I trauma center and found that there were identifiable patient and system factors associated with a higher risk of repeat imaging. Repeat imaging substantially increases a patient's individual exposure to potentially harmful radiation and increases resource utilization for the institution with costs that are often not reimbursed. Although there is often a firm clinical indication for repeating a head CT scan, chest and abdominal imaging in blunt trauma patients rarely substantially changes over the course of a few hours without an associated change in clinical condition. The authors could not identify any difference in outcomes for patients who underwent repeat imaging compared with those who had imaging at only 1 institution.

D. W. Mozingo, MD

Administer tranexamic acid early to injured patients at risk of substantial bleeding

Gruen RL, Reade MC (The Alfred and Monash Univ, Melbourne, Victoria, Australia; Univ of Queensland, Brisbane, Australia)
BMJ 345:e7133, 2012

Haemorrhage is the principal cause of 30-40% of all trauma deaths, and half of these occur before admission to hospital. Many bleeding patients develop coagulopathy, making control of haemorrhage more difficult. In some patients this coagulopathy develops early and seems to be associated with excessive fibrinolysis and breakdown of clots. Current protocols for massive transfusions of blood products (variably defined as >10 red cell units or >50% blood volume in 24 hours, or >5 units in four hours) to patients with haemorrhagic shock prescribe plasma and cryoprecipitate to replace lost, consumed, diluted, or dysfunctional clotting factors, but these do not specifically treat fibrinolysis. There is now compelling evidence that tranexamic acid (1 g loading dose plus 1 g over eight hours), a relatively safe and inexpensive antifibrinolytic, should be administered within three hours of injury in patients at risk of severe bleeding.

▶ Tranexamic acid seems to work by inhibiting lysine-binding sites on plasminogen, preventing its conversion to plasmin. Plasmin has potential fibrinolytic, inflammatory, and neurotoxic effects. The observed reduction in bleeding probably results from reduced fibrinolysis and, therefore, reduced clot breakdown. Like surgery, severe trauma and hemorrhage can accelerate fibrinolysis, which contributes to acute traumatic coagulopathy. In a systematic review of antifibrinolytic drugs in trauma, the only trial to assess hemorrhage was the randomized, placebo-controlled CRASH-2 trial, which evaluated the effects of tranexamic acid in 20 211 adult trauma patients with or at risk of bleeding in 274 hospitals in 40 countries.[1] Tranexamic acid given within 8 hours of injury reduced all-cause mortality from 16.0% to 14.5%, and the risk of death resulting from bleeding from 5.7% to 4.9%. The authors of this article recommend administering tranexamic acid 1 g intravenously in 100 mL normal saline over 10 minutes then 1 g over 8 hours, starting as early as possible and no later than 3 hours after injury, to trauma patients who have or are at risk of major hemorrhage. Prehospital services with capacity for drug administration should consider incorporating its administration into protocols for trauma care in severe cases with strict medical oversight.

D. W. Mozingo, MD

Reference

1. Shakur H, Roberts I, Bautista R, et al. Effects of tranexamic acid on death, vascular occlusive events, and blood transfusion in trauma patients with significant haemorrhage (CRASH-2): a randomised, placebo-controlled trial. *Lancet*. 2010; 376:23-32.

Damage control resuscitation: Early decision strategies in abdominal gunshot wounds using an easy "ABCD" mnemonic
Ordoñez CA, Badiel M, Pino LF, et al (Fundación Valle del Lili, Cali, Colombia; et al)
J Trauma Acute Care Surg 73:1074-1078, 2012

Background.—Early damage-control resuscitation (DCR) indicators have not been clearly discerned in patients with penetrating abdominal trauma. Our objective was to identify these clinical indicators that could standardize a DCR initiation policy in this subset of patients.

Methods.—Prospective data collection from January 2003 to October 2010 at a Level I trauma center in Cali, Colombia. All adult (>15 years) patients with abdominal gunshot wounds (GSWs) were included. They were divided into two groups: those who underwent DCR and those who did not. Both groups were compared by demographics, clinical variables, severity scores, and overall mortality. Other scores were compared with our newly devised model using the area under the receiver operating characteristic curve (AUROC).

Results.—There was a total of 331 abdominal GSWs. Of these, a total of 162 (49%) underwent DCR. The overall mortality was 11.2%. Multivariate analysis identified (A) acidosis (base deficit $\geq$ 8); (B) blood loss (hemoperitoneum > 1,500 mL); (C) cold (temperature < 35°C); (D) damage (New Injury Severity Score > 35) as significant clinical indicators that aided in the decision process of early implementation of DCR. The Trauma-Associated Severe Hemorrhage (AUROC, 0.8333), McLaughlin (AUROC, 0.8148), ABC (AUROC, 0.7372) scores and our ABCD mnemonic (AUROC, 0.8745) were all good predictors of DCR, and the difference between them was statistically significant ($p < 0.001$).

Conclusion.—We have identified (A) acidosis (base deficit $\geq$ 8); (B) blood loss (hemoperitoneum > 1,500 mL); (C) cold (temperature < 35°C); (D) damage (New Injury Severity Score > 35) as significant clinical indicators that aided in the decision process of early implementation of DCR for patients with abdominal GSWs.

Level of Evidence.—Prognostic/epidemiologic study, level III.

▶ This is an interesting prospective study of a case series of patients with abdominal gunshot wounds from a single institution with the purpose of creating a simple mnemonic based on a compendium of observations and currently available scoring systems for predicting when to institute damage-control resuscitation. A useful model for damage-control resuscitation in trauma must be based on information that is rapidly available, concrete, and simply applicable. We evaluated several physiologic and laboratory variables that were readily available and identified that temperature less than 35°C, initial hemoperitoneum of greater than 1500 mL, New Injury Severity Score of greater than 35, and a base deficit of 8 or greater are significant clinical indicators that could aid in the decision process of early implementation of damage-control resuscitation for patients with abdominal gunshot wounds in a civilian population. All of these indicators have been included in a simple, injury-specific "ABCD" mnemonic that can accurately identify the need for damage-control resuscitation in these patients compared with those previously published scores.

D. W. Mozingo, MD

Defining geriatric trauma: When does age make a difference?
Goodmanson NW, Rosengart MR, Barnato AE, et al (Univ of Pittsburgh Med Ctr, PA)
Surgery 152:668-675, 2012

Background.—Injured elderly patients experience high rates of undertriage to trauma centers (TCs) whereas debate continues regarding the age defining a geriatric trauma patient. We sought to identify when mortality risk increases in injured patients as the result of age alone to determine whether TC care was associated with improved outcomes for these patients and to estimate the added admissions burden to TCs using an age threshold for triage.

Methods.—We performed a retrospective cohort study of injured patients treated at TCs and non-TCs in Pennsylvania from April 1, 2001, to March 31, 2005. Patients were included if they were between 19 and 100 years of age and had sustained minimal injury (Injury Severity Score < 9). The primary outcome was in-hospital mortality. We analyzed age as a predictor of mortality by using the fractional polynomial method.

Results.—A total of 104,015 patients were included. Mortality risk significantly increased at 57 years (odds ratio 5.58; 95% confidence interval 1.07−29.0; P =.04) relative to 19-year-old patients. TC care was associated with a decreased mortality risk compared with non-TC care (odds ratio 0.83; 95% confidence interval 0.69−0.99; P =.04). Using an age of 70 as a threshold for mandatory triage, we estimated TCs could expect an annual increase of approximately one additional admission per day.

Conclusion.—Age is a significant risk factor for mortality in trauma patients, and TC care improves outcomes even in older, minimally injured patients. An age threshold should be considered as a criterion for TC triage. Use of the clinically relevant age of 70 as this threshold would not impose a substantial increase on annual TC admissions.

▶ Elderly trauma patients differ significantly from their younger counterparts, having a greater number of pre-existing comorbidities, a greater risk of complications, and an increased probability of mortality. The findings in this selection suggest that older age is an excellent candidate for a triage criterion, yet debate persists regarding the exact age beyond which a trauma patient is considered elderly. The objectives of this study were to identify when age becomes an independent risk factor for mortality in trauma patients and to determine whether care in a trauma center is superior to that in a nontrauma center for elderly trauma patients with minimal injury severity. The authors hypothesized that age is an independent risk factor for mortality in trauma patients and that care in a trauma center, compared with that in a nontrauma center, is associated with reduced mortality for elderly patients, independent of injury severity. They secondarily determined the increased burden of admission for trauma centers by using an increasing threshold age as a mandatory criterion for transport to a trauma center. Using an age threshold of 70 years, the authors estimated that 244 patients would need to be transferred to a trauma center to save one additional life; this amounts to approximately one added patient per trauma center per day in Pennsylvania. This may be a statistically correct result, however, the full impact, both financial and logistical, needs to be considered when proposing increasing the transfers of this complex population to trauma centers.

D. W. Mozingo, MD

Negative Laparotomy in Trauma: Are We Getting Better?

Schnüriger B, Lam L, Inaba K, et al (Univ of Southern California, Los Angeles)
Am Surg 78:1219-1223, 2012

One of the trauma surgeons' daily challenges is the balancing act between negative laparotomy and missed abdominal injury. We opted to characterize the indications that prompted a negative trauma exploratory laparotomy and the rate of missed abdominal injuries in an effort to optimize patient selection for laparotomy. At the Los Angeles County + University of Southern California Medical Center, negative laparotomies and missed injuries are consecutively captured and reviewed at the weekly mortality + morbidity (MM) conferences. All written reports of the MM meetings from January 2003 to December 2008 were reviewed to identify all patients who underwent a negative laparotomy or a laparotomy as a result of an initially missed abdominal injury. Over the 6-year study period, a total of 1871 laparotomies were performed, of which 73 (3.9%) were negative. The rate of missed injuries requiring subsequent laparotomy was 1.3 per cent (25 of 1871). The negative laparotomy rate and the rate of missed injuries did not vary significantly during the study period (2.8 to 4.7%, $P = 0.875$, and 0.7 to 2.9%, $P = 0.689$). Penetrating mechanisms accounted for the majority of negative laparotomies (58.9%). The primary indication for negative laparotomy was peritonitis (54.8%) followed by hypotension (28.8%) and suspicious computed tomographic scan findings (27.4%). The complication rate after negative laparotomy was 14.5 per cent, and of these, 10.1 per cent were directly related to the procedure. A low but steady rate of negative laparotomies and missed abdominal injuries after

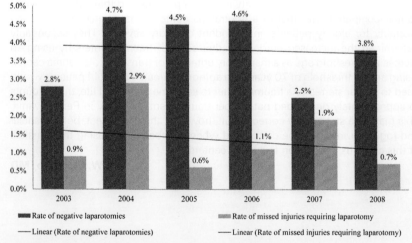

FIGURE.—Rates of negative laparotomies and laparotomies resulting from missed injuries over the study period. (Reprinted from Schnüriger B, Lam L, Inaba K, et al. Negative laparotomy in trauma: are we getting better? *Am Surg.* 2012;78:1219-1223, with permission from Southeastern Surgical Congress.)

trauma remains. Negative laparotomies and missed abdominal injuries when they occur are still associated with significant complication rates and a prolonged length of stay (Fig).

▶ The optimal timing and indications for exploratory laparotomy in penetrating or blunt trauma continue to be elusive, and the decision to go to the operating room remains a challenging diagnostic dilemma for surgeons. Commonly accepted indications for exploratory laparotomy include peritonitis on examination, hypotension in penetrating abdominal trauma, and hypotension combined with free fluid visualized with ultrasonography for blunt trauma. These criteria, however, still result in false-positive and false-negative laparotomies. With more patients being managed nonoperatively, there is always a danger of delay in diagnosis and missed injury. This study finds that an aggressive strategy of nonoperative management for appropriate patients results in a low (1.3%) rate of missed injuries, and that these patients experience no greater risk of complications compared with patients undergoing negative laparotomies. The figure depicts the change in negative laparotomy over time.

D. W. Mozingo, MD

Age should be considered in the decision making of prophylactic splenic angioembolization in nonoperative management of blunt splenic trauma: A study of 208 consecutive civilian trauma patients
Brault-Noble G, Charbit J, Chardon P, et al (Lapeyronie Univ Hosp, Montpellier, France; et al)
J Trauma Acute Care Surg 73:1213-1220, 2012

Background.—A strategy of prophylactic splenic angioembolization using observation failure risk (OFR) computed tomographic (CT) scan criteria has been proposed recently. The main aim of the present study was to evaluate the relevance of the criteria in terms of delayed splenic rupture in patients with blunt splenic injury.

Methods.—All patients with blunt splenic injuries admitted consecutively between January 2005 and January 2010 to our institution were included. Clinical, CT scan, and angiographic data, initial management, and outcome were noted. Patients managed expectantly were classified according to OFR CT scan criteria (high OFR was defined by at least one of the following CT scan signs: blush, pseudoaneurysm, Organ Injury Scale [OIS] grade III with a large hemoperitoneum, and OIS grade IV or 5). Initial management success was especially studied.

Results.—Among the 208 patients included, 161 (77%) were treated by observation (35 OIS grade I, 64 OIS grade II, 33 OIS grade III, 18 OIS grade IV, and 11 OIS grade V) and 129 (80%) were men, with a mean (SD) age of 36.1 (18.7) years and a mean (SD) Injury Severity Score of 20.8 (15.4). Forty-nine patients (30%) had high OFR CT scan criteria. Thirteen patients (8%) experienced observation failure. High OFR CT scan criteria (odds ratio, 11; 95% confidence interval, 2.5–47.5) and patients

50 years and older (odds ratio, 33.9; 95% confidence interval, 6.2–185.5) were independent factors related to observation failure. The positive predictive value of OFR CT scan criteria for observation failure was 18%, and the negative predictive value was 96%. The corresponding values were 67% and 90%, respectively, in patients 50 years and older and 3% and 99%, respectively, in patients younger than 50 years.

Conclusion.—OFR CT scan criteria lack specificity to predict observation failure, mainly in patients younger than 50 years. Age should be considered when identifying patients requiring prophylactic splenic angioembolization.

Level of Evidence.—Diagnostic study, level III (Fig 1, Table 5).

▶ Nonoperative management is the standard initial treatment of blunt splenic trauma in all patients without hemodynamic instability. In patients who present

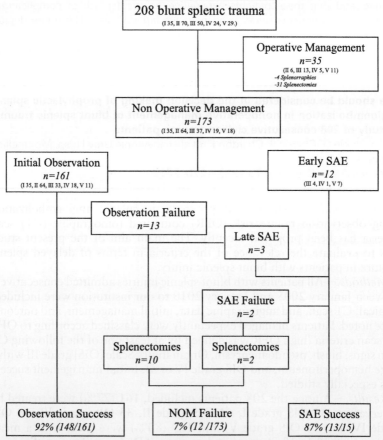

FIGURE 1.—Flowchart showing initial management of all the 208 patients with BST and their outcome. (Reprinted from Brault-Noble G, Charbit J, Chardon P, et al. Age should be considered in the decision making of prophylactic splenic angioembolization in nonoperative management of blunt splenic trauma: a study of 208 consecutive civilian trauma patients. *J Trauma Acute Care Surg.* 2012;73:1213-1220, with permission from Lippincott Williams & Wilkins.)

TABLE 5.—Logistic Regression Analysis of Risk Factors Affecting Observation Failure

	OR (95% CI)	*p*
Age ≥50 y	33.9 (6.2–185.5)	<0.0001
High OFR CT scan criteria*	11 (2.5–47.5)	0.001

Model logit including all categorical variables at admission with *p* = 0.2; age ≥ 50 years (yes/no), OFR CT scan criteria (high/low risk), and AAST grade (I–V). AAST-grade variable was deleted from the model because it was significantly related with OFR CT scan criteria variable.
AAST, American Association for the Surgery of Trauma.[10]
Editor's Note: Please refer to original journal article for full references.
*CT scan criteria from Sabe et al[6]: patients at high risk of NOM failure being defined as having at least one of the following criteria: (1) AAST grade IV or V, (2) ICE, (3) pseudoaneurysm, and (4) AAST grade III with large hemoperitoneum.

with clinical signs of splenic bleeding, an initial hemostatic treatment by splenic artery embolization increases the success of nonoperative management and splenic salvage rates. Age is an independent predictor of successful treatment and should be considered to increase the predictive value of delayed splenic rupture. In patients older than 50 years of age, the observation failure risk (OFR) computed tomographic (CT) scan criteria should be used in the screening of patients at risk of splenic rupture who might benefit for prophylactic splenic artery embolization. Patients younger than 50 years of age without any initial sign of exsanguination seem to have a low risk of delayed splenic bleeding; consequently, even in the presence of high OFR CT scan criteria, initial prophylactic splenic artery embolization does not seem justified. Fig 1 and Table 5 present the overall outcome of the study patients and the risk of nonoperative management failure in older patients, respectively.

D. W. Mozingo, MD

A model for predicting primary blast lung injury
Macfadden LN, Chan PC, Ho KH-H, et al (L-3 Communications/JAYCOR, San Diego, CA)
J Trauma Acute Care Surg 73:1121-1129, 2012

Background.—This article presents a model-based method for predicting primary blast injury. On the basis of the normalized work injury mechanism from previous work, this method presents a new model that accounts for the effects of blast orientation and species difference.
Methods.—The analysis used test data from a series of extensive experimental studies sponsored by the US Army Medical Research and Materiel Command. In these studies, more than 1200 sheep were exposed to air blast in free-field and confined enclosures, and lung injuries were quantified as the percentage of surface area contused. Blast overpressure data were collected using blast test devices placed at matching locations to represent loadings to the thorax. Adopting the modified Lobdell model with further modifications specifically for blast and scaling, the thorax deformation

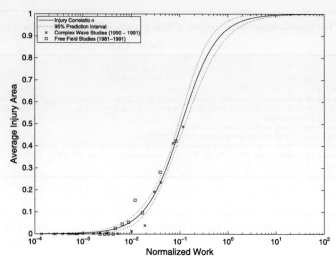

FIGURE 3.—Correlation of lung area injured with normalized work. The area was determined by averaging the injured areas of individual animals (binned into groups of 40). (Reprinted from MacFadden LN, Chan PC, Ho KH-H, et al. A model for predicting primary blast lung injury. *J Trauma Acute Care Surg.* 2012;73:1121-1129, with permission from Lippincott Williams & Wilkins.)

histories for the left, chest, and right sides of the thorax were calculated for all sheep subjects. Using the calculated thorax velocities, effective normalized work was computed for each test subject representing the irreversible work performed on the lung tissues normalized by lung volume and ambient pressure.

Results.—Dose-response curves for four categories of injuries (trace, slight, moderate, and severe) were developed by performing log-logistic correlations of the computed normalized work with the injury outcomes, including the effect of multiple shots. A blast lethality correlation was also established.

Conclusion.—Validated by sheep data, the present work revalidates the previous understanding and findings of the blast lung injury mechanism and provides an anthropomorphic model for primary blast injury prediction that can be used for occupational and survivability analysis.

Level of Evidence.—Economic and decision analysis, level III (Fig 3).

▶ Primary blast injuries comprise a small percentage of combat injuries and casualties. When the blast overpressure results in a primary blast injury to the lung, the physiologic damage can be significant and even lethal. The number and severity of blast lung injuries has increased in the recent military operations in Iraq and Afghanistan. Pulmonary contusions are typically observed after exposure to a blast overpressure incident.

The focus of this article is to present a mechanistic model of gross lung injury resulting from blast overpressure. Pulmonary injuries from blast overpressures or underpressures are the most common critical injuries to people near a blast. The data used in this study showed that free field blasts resulted in lower levels of injury compared with the complex wave tests. In addition, soldiers in combat are often wearing body armor that can provide protection against primary blast lung injury. It is also important to note that pulmonary blast injuries rarely occur independently. Fragment injuries, burn injuries, and blunt trauma are also often observed because of a blast. The animal model presented here focused solely on the mechanism behind primary blast injury to the lung. Fig 3 is included to demonstrate the correlation between blast intensity and the severity of injury. This model can be used in conjunction with other models that predict primary blast injury to other body systems. A well-developed model of blast injury as described in this article will help make the study of this rare but serious injury more feasible.

D. W. Mozingo, MD

ACGME case logs: Surgery resident experience in operative trauma for two decades

Drake FT, Van Eaton EG, Huntington CR, et al (Univ of Washington Med Ctr, Seattle; Harborview Med Ctr, Seattle, WA; et al)
J Trauma Acute Care Surg 73:1500-1506, 2012

Background.—Surgery resident education is based on experiential training, which is influenced by changes in clinical management strategies, technical and technologic advances, and administrative regulations. Trauma care has been exposed to each of these factors, prompting concerns about resident experience in operative trauma. The current study analyzed the reported volume of operative trauma for the last two decades; to our knowledge, this is the first evaluation of nationwide trends during such an extended time line.

Methods.—The Accreditation Council for Graduate Medical Education (ACGME) database of operative logs was queried from academic year (AY) 1989–1990 to 2009–2010 to identify shifts in trauma operative experience. Annual case log data for each cohort of graduating surgery residents were combined into approximately 5-year blocks, designated Period I (AY1989–1990 to AY1993–1994), Period II (AY1994–1995 to AY1998–1999), Period III (AY1999–2000 to AY2002–2003), and Period IV (AY2003–2004 to AY2009–2010). The latter two periods were delineated by the year in which duty hour restrictions were implemented.

Results.—Overall general surgery caseload increased from Period I to Period II ($p < 0.001$), remained stable from Period II to Period III, and decreased from Period III to Period IV ($p < 0.001$). However, for ACGME-designated trauma cases, there were significant declines from Period I to Period II (75.5 vs. 54.5 cases, $p < 0.001$) and Period II to Period III (54.5 vs. 39.3 cases, $p < 0.001$) but no difference between Period III and Period IV (39.3 vs. 39.4 cases). Graduating residents in Period I performed, on average, 31 intra-abdominal trauma operations, including approximately five spleen and four liver operations. Residents in Period IV

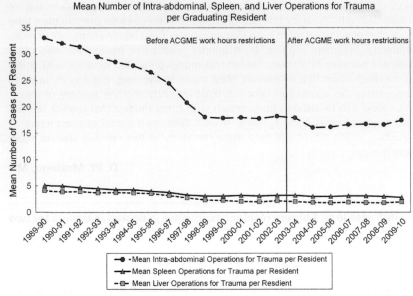

FIGURE 3.—Mean number of intra-abdominal, spleen, and liver operations for trauma per graduating resident. The "Intra-abdominal Trauma" category was generated from subtotals of operations for esophageal, gastric, duodenal, small bowel, colon, splenic, hepatic, kidney, and pancreatic trauma, as well as repair of the abdominal aorta or vena cava and cases coded as trauma laparotomy or laparoscopy. (Reprinted from Drake FT, Van Eaton EG, Huntington CR, et al. ACGME case logs: surgery resident experience in operative trauma for two decades. *J Trauma Acute Care Surg.* 2012;73:1500-1506, with permission from Lippincott Williams & Wilkins.)

performed 17 intra-abdominal trauma operations, including three spleen and approximately two liver operations.

Conclusion.—Recent general surgery trainees perform fewer trauma operations than previous trainees. The majority of this decline occurred before implementation of work-hour restrictions. Although these changes reflect concurrent changes in management of trauma, surgical educators must meet the challenge of training residents in procedures less frequently performed.

Level of Evidence.—Epidemiologic study, level III; therapeutic study, level IV (Fig 3).

▶ General surgery residents learn to manage trauma through a broad exposure, including operative experience and nonoperative management. There is concern that changes in surgical education, changes in the epidemiology of trauma, and the evolution toward a nonoperative approach to blunt solid organ trauma may reduce the residents' educational experience. In this selection, the authors sought to quantify these changes through a review of the Accreditation Council for Graduate Medical Education's database of graduating residents' operative case logs. This represents the aggregated nationwide experience of all graduating surgery residents. Previous reviews of resident experience in operative trauma have been based on single-institution data or have focused on the era before implementation of work-hour restrictions. This case log data shows that as blunt trauma and solid organ injury has become an increasingly nonoperative condition, resident experience in operative trauma has also diminished. Fig 3 is included to show the time-based nature of this finding. Work-hour restrictions did not contribute substantially to the changes seen over the last 2 decades. They may, however, complicate efforts to increase resident experience in operative trauma. Such a reduction in experience may represent a limitation in preparedness for general surgeons who care for trauma patients, which may be especially pertinent to those who will practice in areas remote from high-level trauma centers. Alternatively, with the evolution of acute care surgical training, more operative trauma experience may be gained by those surgeons choosing this specialty.

D. W. Mozingo, MD

Delayed Diagnosis of Hand Injuries in Polytrauma Patients
Adkinson JM, Shafqat MS, Eid SM, et al (Lehigh Valley Health Network, Allentown, PA)
Ann Plast Surg 69:442-445, 2012

Trauma patients are at high risk for delayed diagnosis of injuries, including those to the hand, with reports in the literature as high as 50%. As a result, patients may have prolonged disability and longer hospital stays with associated increased costs. Our objective was to elucidate risk factors for the delayed diagnosis of hand injuries.

A review was performed from 2000 through 2009, assessing for age, sex, blood alcohol level, Glasgow Coma Score (GCS), Injury Severity Score (ISS), mechanism, injury type, length of stay, and timing of hand injury diagnosis.

In this study, 36,568 patients were identified; 738 meeting criteria; 21.7% of patients had delayed diagnoses with 91.3% of patients diagnosed by the day after admission. Delayed diagnoses were more than 2 times higher for severely injured patients. Patients with delayed diagnoses had a lower GCS and a higher ISS and length of hospitalization.

With a decreased GCS and elevated ISS, patients are at risk for delayed diagnoses of hand injuries. A focused tertiary survey is mandatory, particularly in patients with an altered mental status or with multiple injuries (Table 5).

▶ Injury or intoxication causing impaired mental status is often noted to delay the diagnosis of traumatic injuries because of the associated unreliable clinical examination. In this selection, the authors identified patients with a decreased Glasgow Coma Score (GCS), elevated Injury Severity Score (ISS), and elevated blood alcohol levels who were noted to have delayed diagnosis of hand injury. However, only GCS and ISS levels were found to be statistically significant. With a decreased GCS, a patient would be less able to communicate an occult injury which is consistent with other missed injuries. The ISS levels (described here as mild, moderate, and severe) correlate with the relative severity of injury to multiple body systems. As such, an elevated ISS indicates that the clinicians

TABLE 5.—Delayed Diagnosis by ISS Category Crosstabulation ($P < 0.001$)

| Injury Severity Score Category | Delayed Diagnosis [n (%)] | | Total [n (%)] |
	Yes	No	
Mild	50 (14.4)	298 (85.6)	348 (47.2)
Moderate	33 (24.1)	104 (75.9)	137 (18.6)
Severe	77 (30.4)	176 (69.6)	253 (34.3)

associated with emergency care of the patient would be focused on more severe, life-threatening injuries. Subtle clinical findings associated with an underlying hand injury may then be easily missed. Table 5 is included in this selection, showing the stratification of missed hand injuries by ISS. Because the delayed diagnosis of hand injuries has significant physical and economic implications for patients, every effort should be made to expedite diagnosis in the injured patient. A standardized evaluation of the trauma patient with a focused tertiary survey is essential, particularly in patients with an altered mental status or multiple injuries.

D. W. Mozingo, MD

A prehospital shock index for trauma correlates with measures of hospital resource use and mortality
McNab A, Burns B, Bhullar I, et al (Univ of Florida College of Medicine–Jacksonville)
Surgery 152:473-476, 2012

Background.—The assessment and treatment of trauma patients begins in the prehospital environment. Studies have validated the shock index as a correlate for mortality and the identification of shock in trauma patients. We investigated the use of the first shock index obtained in the prehospital environment and the first shock index obtained upon arrival in the trauma center as correlates for other outcomes to evaluate its usefulness as a triage tool.

Methods.—This is a retrospective review of data from a level I trauma center. Prehospital and trauma center shock indices for 16,269 patients were evaluated as correlates for duration of hospital stay, duration of stay in the intensive care unit, the number of ventilator days, blood product use, and destination of transfer from the trauma center.

Results.—Pearson correlation coefficients revealed that the relationship of prehospital and trauma center shock indices were correlates for duration of hospital stay, duration of stay in the intensive care unit, the number of ventilator days, and blood product use. A chi-square analysis found that shock indices ≥ 0.9 indicate a higher likelihood of disposition to the intensive care unit, operating room, or death.

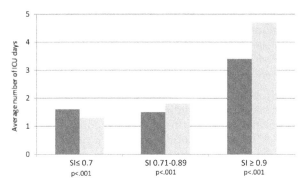

FIGURE 2.—Average number of surgical intensive care unit days associated with shock indices (*dark gray*, prehospital; *light gray*, trauma center). *SI*, Shock index. (Reprinted from Surgery. McNab A, Burns B, Bhullar I, et al. A prehospital shock index for trauma correlates with measures of hospital resource use and mortality. *Surgery.* 2012;152:473-476, Copyright 2012, with permission from Elsevier.)

Conclusion.—A prehospital shock index for trauma correlates with measures of hospital resource use and mortality. A prospective study is needed to determine the use of this measure as a triage tool (Fig 2).

▶ Trauma is the leading cause of death for patients younger than 45 years of age and the fourth-leading cause of death for all ages. Assessment and treatment of trauma patients begins in the prehospital environment upon arrival of emergency medical personnel and is essential in the presence of life-threatening injuries. Despite current triage criteria, trauma continues to be a leading cause of morbidity and mortality, showing the need for an improved prehospital screening system. The data and analyses in this selection indicate that higher prehospital and trauma center shock index (SI) are associated with a longer duration of hospital stay, a longer duration of stay in the intensive care unit (ICU), more ventilator days, more blood product use, and mortality. The SI is the ratio of heart rate to systolic blood pressure. Fig 2 is included as an example of the increasing ICU days associated with increasing SI. An elevated SI is also associated with more frequent disposition to the ICU or operating room directly from the emergency department. These data indicate that prehospital SI is as useful as trauma center SI for anticipation of all measured outcome variables. Considering these positive correlations, prehospital SI should be investigated with a prospective observational study to evaluate its use as a predictor of outcomes and resource utilization.

D. W. Mozingo, MD

An Objective Study of the Impact of the Electronic Medical Record on Outcomes in Trauma Patients

Schenarts PJ, Goettler CE, White MA, et al (East Carolina Univ, Greenville, NC)
Am Surg 78:1249-1254, 2012

It is commonly believed that the electronic medical record (EMR) will improve patient outcomes. However, there is scant published literature to support this claim and no studies in any surgical population. Our hypothesis was that the EMR would not improve objective outcome measures in patients with traumatic injury. Prospectively collected data from our university-based Level I trauma center was retrospectively reviewed. Demographic, injury severity as well as outcomes and complications data were compared for all patients admitted over a 20-month period before introduction of the EMR and a 20-month period after full, hospital-wide use of the EMR. Implementation of the EMR was associated with a decreased hospital length of stay, $P = 0.02$; intensive care unit length of stay, $P = 0.001$; ventilator days, $P = 0.002$; acute respiratory distress syndrome, $P = 0.006$, pneumonia, $P = 0.008$; myocardial infarction, $P = 0.001$; line infection,

TABLE.—Comparison of Demographic, Outcomes, and Complications Data*

	Pre-EMR (n = 3,161)	Post-EMR (n = 2,835)	P Value
Age (years)	38.8	40.9	<0.001
Male gender	69.9%	69.7%	NS
Blunt mechanism	85.4%	83.1%	0.03
Highest activation level	29.7%	29.5%	NS
Injury Severity Score	13.7	12.8	<0.001
Hospital LOS (days)	7.9	7.1	0.02
ICU LOS (days)	7.4	6.0	0.001
Ventilator days	8.2	6.2	0.002
Airway complication	22 (0.7%)	20 (0.7%)	NS
ARDS	64 (2.0%)	20 (1.1%)	0.006
Pneumonia	238 (7.5%)	165 (5.8%)	0.008
Pulmonary embolus	14 (0.4%)	11 (0.4%)	NS
DVT	13 (0.4%)	18 (0.6%)	NS
Myocardial infarction	23 (0.7%)	4 (0.1%)	0.001
Cardiac arrest	55 (1.7%)	41 (1.5%)	NS
Line infection	18 (0.6%)	6 (0.1%)	0.03
Septicemia	64 (2.0%)	19 (0.7%)	0.000
Late urinary tract infection	145 (4.6%)	157 (5.5%)	NS
Wound infection	50 (1.6%)	39 (1.4%)	NS
Other infection	33 (1.1%)	36 (1.3%)	NS
Renal failure—dialysis	27 (0.9%)	5 (0.2%)	0.000
Hepatobiliary	3 (0.1%)	8 (0.3%)	NS
Upper GI bleeding	11 (0.4%)	5 (0.2%)	NS
Drug complication	20 (0.6%)	5 (0.2%)	0.001
Delay in diagnosis	95 (3.0%)	61 (2.2%)	0.04
Decubitus ulcer	62 (2.0%)	94 (3.3%)	0.001
Mortality	6.0%	5.8%	NS

EMR, electronic medical record; LOS, length of stay; ICU, intensive care unit; ARDS, acute respiratory distress syndrome; DVT, deep vein thrombosis; GI, gastrointestinal; NS, nonsignificant.

*Demographic and outcomes data presented as mean or percent. Complications data presented as number of occurrences (percent).

$P = 0.03$; septicemia, $P = 0.000$; renal failure, $P = 0.000$; drug complication, $P = 0.001$; and delay in diagnosis, $P = 0.04$. There was no difference in mortality, unexpected cardiac arrest, missed injury, pulmonary embolism/deep vein thrombosis, or late urinary tract infection. This is the first study to investigate the impact of the EMR in surgical patients. Although there was an improvement in some complications, the overall impact was inconsistent (Table).

▶ The electronic medical record has been touted to improve quality and patient safety, increase adherence to evidence-based guidelines, improve legibility, provide real-time accessibility to a patient's entire medical record, and decrease cost. As a result of these patient-focused benefits, many stakeholders have called for widespread implementation of the electronic medical record. A demonstration of the support for this initiative can be found in the American Recovery and Reinvestment Act of 2009, which included $17 billion in incentives for providers to switch to the electronic medical record and another $2 billion to develop electronic medical record standards and best practice guidelines. Following the implementation of the electronic medical record system, studies investigating the effectiveness of the electronic medical record have yielded varying results. Because no previous studies existed on a purely surgical population, the authors of this article sought to investigate the impact of the electronic medical record on traumatically injured patients using preintervention and postintervention study designs. The Table demonstrates the inconsistent impact of implementation of an electronic medical record on the outcome of trauma patients. The authors provide an in-depth analysis of how some of these outcomes may improve with an electronic medical record and others may not. One complicating factor could be that they only measured the first 2 years following implementation. The learning curve may be a bit longer than that.

D. W. Mozingo, MD

Evaluation and management of geriatric trauma: An Eastern Association for the Surgery of Trauma practice management guideline
Calland JF, Ingraham AM, Martin N, et al (Univ of Virginia, Charlottesville; Univ of Cincinnati, OH; Jefferson Univ School of Medicine, Philadelphia, PA; et al)
J Trauma Acute Care Surg 73:S345-S350, 2012

Background.—Aging patients constitute an increasing proportion of patients treated at trauma centers. Previous and existing guidelines addressing care of the injured elder have not adequately addressed emerging data regarding optimal means for undertaking triage decisions, correcting coagulopathy, and the limitations of supraphysiologic resuscitation.

Methods.—More than 400 MEDLINE citations published between the years 2000 and 2008 were identified and screened. A total of 90 references were selected for the evidentiary table followed by consensus-based discussions regarding the level of evidence and the strength of recommendations that could be derived from the related findings of the individual studies.

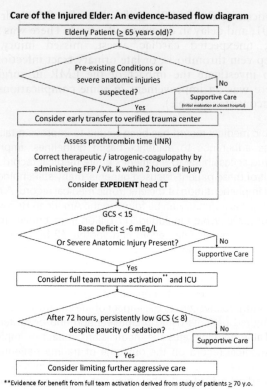

Care of the Injured Elder: An evidence-based flow diagram

Elderly Patient (≥ 65 years old)?

Pre-existing Conditions or severe anatomic injuries suspected? — No → **Supportive Care** (Initial evaluation at closest hospital)

Yes

Consider early transfer to verified trauma center

Assess prothrombin time (INR)

Correct therapeutic / iatrogenic-coagulopathy by administering FFP / Vit. K within 2 hours of injury

Consider **EXPEDIENT** head CT

GCS < 15
Base Deficit ≤ -6 mEq/L
Or Severe Anatomic Injury Present? — No → Supportive Care

Yes

Consider full team trauma activation** and ICU

After 72 hours, persistently low GCS (≤ 8) despite paucity of sedation? — No → Supportive Care

Yes

Consider limiting further aggressive care

**Evidence for benefit from full team activation derived from study of patients ≥ 70 y.o.

FIGURE.—Care of the injured elder: An evidence-based flow program. (Reprinted from Calland JF, Ingraham AM, Martin N, et al. Evaluation and management of geriatric trauma: an eastern association for the surgery of trauma practice management guideline. *J Trauma Acute Care Surg.* 2012;73:S345-S350, Lippincott Williams & Wilkins.)

Results.—In general, a lower threshold for trauma activation should be used for injured patients aged 65 years or older who are evaluated at trauma centers. Furthermore, elderly patients with at least one body system with an AIS score of 3 or higher or a base deficit of −6 or less should be treated at trauma centers, preferably in intensive care units staffed by surgeon-intensivists. In addition, all elderly patients who receive daily therapeutic anticoagulation should have appropriate assessment of their coagulation profile and cross-sectional imaging of the brain as soon as possible after admission where appropriate. In patients aged 65 years or older with a Glasgow Coma Scale (GCS) score less than 8, if substantial improvement in GCS is not realized within 72 hours of injury, consideration should be given to limiting further aggressive therapeutic interventions.

Conclusion.—Effective evidence-based care of aging patients necessitates aggressive triage, correction of coagulopathy, and limitation of care when clinical evidence points toward an overwhelming likelihood of poor long-term prognosis (Fig).

▶ One of the main topics addressed by this patient management guideline is the manner in which elderly patients are triaged to trauma centers and, if triaged to a trauma center, whether they should routinely receive a trauma activation level of initial care. Ample evidence demonstrates that injured elderly patients are less likely to receive care at trauma centers despite being at increased risk for adverse outcomes following injury because of limited cardiovascular reserve, comorbidities, and general frailty. Although independent risk for postinjury mortality may begin at a much younger age, the authors of this analysis have chosen to limit their recommendations to those patients aged 65 years or older. This threshold is consistent with the assumptions and designations of existing trauma centers regarding advancing age. The figure is included here to provide an evidence-based care flow diagram. Elderly patients should receive care at centers that have devoted specific resources to attaining excellence in the care of the injured using similar criteria to those used in younger patients. Pre-existing conditions and severe anatomic injuries dramatically increase the risk of poor outcome in elderly patients.

D. W. Mozingo, MD

Changes in massive transfusion over time: An early shift in the right direction?
Kautza BC, The Inflammation and the Host Response to Injury Investigators (Univ of Pittsburgh Med Ctr, PA; et al)
J Trauma Acute Care Surg 72:106-111, 2012

Background.—Increasing evidence suggests that high fresh frozen plasma:packed red blood cell (FFP:PRBC) and platelet:PRBC (PLT:PRBC) transfusion ratios may prevent or reduce the morbidity associated with early coagulopathy which complicates massive transfusion (MT). We sought to characterize changes in resuscitation which have occurred over time in a cohort severely injured patients requiring MT.

Methods.—Data were obtained from a multicenter prospective cohort study evaluating outcomes in blunt injured adults with hemorrhagic shock. MT was defined as requiring ≥ 10 units PRBCs within 24 hours postinjury. Mean PRBC, FFP, and PLT requirements (per unit; 6 hours, 12 hours, and 24 hours) were determined over time (2004−2009). Sub-MT, those patients just below the threshold for MT, were defined as requiring ≥ 7 and <10 units PRBCs in the initial 24 hours. The percent of resuscitation given at 6 hours relative to 24 hours total (6 of 24%) was determined and compared across "early" (admission until December 2007) and "recent" (after December 2007) periods for each component.

Results.—Over the study time period (2004−2009) for the MT group (n = 526), initial base deficit and presenting international normalized ratio were unchanged, while Injury Severity Score was significantly higher. The

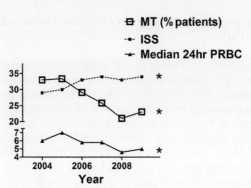

FIGURE 1.—Incidence of MT, median 24-hour PRBC requirement, and ISS for the entire enrolled cohort over time (2004–2009); *p < 0.05. MT, massive transfusion; ISS, Injury Severity Score; PRBC, packed red blood cells. (Reprinted from Kautza BC, The Inflammation and the Host Response to Injury Investigators. Changes in massive transfusion over time: an early shift in the right direction? *J Trauma Acute Care Surg.* 2012;72:106-111, with permission from Lippincott Williams & Wilkins.)

percent of patients who required MT overall significantly decreased over time. No significant differences were found over time for six-hour, 12-hour, or 24-hour FFP:PRBC and PLT:PRBC transfusion ratios in MT patients. Sub-MT patients (n = 344) had significantly higher six-hour FFP:PRBC ratios and significantly higher six-hour,12-hour, and 24-hour PLT:PRBC ratios in the recent time period. The six h/24 h% total for FFP and PLT transfusion was significantly greater in the recent time period. (FFP: 54% vs. 70%; $p = 0.004$ and PLT 46% vs. 61%; $p = 0.048$).

Conclusion.—In a severely injured cohort requiring MT, FFP:PRBC and PLT:PRBC ratios have not changed over time, whereas the rate of MT overall has significantly decreased. During the recent time period (after December 2007), significantly higher transfusion ratios and a greater percent of 6-hour/24-hour FFP and PLT were found in the sub-MT group, those patients just below the PRBC transfusion threshold definition of MT. These data suggest early, more aggressive attainment of high transfusions ratios may reduce the requirement for MT and may shift overall blood requirements below those which currently define MT. Further prospective evidence is required to verify these findings (Fig 1).

▶ The effects of coagulopathy, hypothermia, and acidosis have long been known as important markers for mortality after traumatic hemorrhage. The main objective of this study was to demonstrate how this recent evidence has impacted massive transfusion practice and to determine whether changes have occurred over time regarding the achievement of high component transfusion ratios and the timing of such transfusions in a cohort of severely injured patients requiring massive transfusion. The authors of this article hypothesized that significant changes in massive transfusion resuscitation practice have occurred over time and that earlier, more aggressive attainment of high fresh frozen plasma:packed red blood cell and platelet:packed red blood cell transfusion ratios have occurred in more recent time periods corresponding to the expanding literature on massive transfusion resuscitation. Data were derived from the ongoing multicenter prospective cohort study known as the Inflammation and the Host Response to Injury Large Scale Collaborative Program. The data presented suggest earlier, more aggressive attainment of high transfusion ratios, and component transfusion may reduce the requirement for massive transfusion and may shift overall blood requirements below those that currently define massive transfusion. Fig 1 demonstrates these changes over time. Future studies documenting changes in massive transfusion practice are needed to verify these findings and to continue monitoring and progress with the ultimate goal of improving outcome for these severely injured patients.

D. W. Mozingo, MD

3 Burns

Obesity and Burns
Goutos I, Sadideen H, Pandya AA, et al (John Radcliffe Hosp, Headington, Oxford, UK; King's College London Med School, Strand, UK; et al)
J Burn Care Res 33:471-482, 2012

The population of overweight patients presenting to burn facilities is expected to increase significantly over the next decades due to the global epidemic of obesity. Excess adiposity mediates alterations to key physiological responses and poses challenges to the optimal management of burns. The purpose of this study is to document the general epidemiological aspects of thermal injuries in the obese population, outline relevant physiological aspects associated with obesity, and draw attention to topics relating to the management, rehabilitation, and prognosis of burns in this emerging subpopulation of patients.

▶ Obesity is a worldwide epidemic, and health care professionals are increasingly faced with challenges relating to the management of overweight burn patients. Excess adipose tissue is now considered an active immune organ responsible for the release of proinflammatory mediators, which enhances the systemic inflammatory response to burn trauma. Obesity is accompanied by a host of alterations in key physiologic processes, whose ramifications influence both the acute management and rehabilitation of patients with thermal injuries. Appreciation of the individual characteristics of this subpopulation of burn victims will allow better treatment planning and provision of care with a view to improving survival and long-term functional outcomes. It is apparent that obesity has a large impact on all aspects of acute burn care and rehabilitation. Determination of a more accurate method to calculate the total body surface area of burn by using modern imaging techniques will undoubtedly be a great contribution in tailoring fluid therapy. Also, advances in the quest for optimal resuscitation endpoints are likely to benefit obese patients who are particularly prone to derangements in fluid balance. Obesity, now recognized as a chronic inflammatory state, represents an interesting pharmacologic arena in an attempt to counteract the superimposed morbidity on the burn-related hypermetabolic response.

D. W. Mozingo, MD

Objective estimates of the probability of death in acute burn injury: A proposed Taiwan burn score

Chen C-C, Chen L-C, Wen B-S, et al (Taipei Veterans General Hosp and Natl Yang-Ming Univ, Taipei City, Taiwan; Tamkang Univ, New Taipei City, Taiwan)
J Trauma Acute Care Surg 73:1583-1589, 2012

Background.—This study aimed to develop an objective model for predicting mortality after burn injury in Taiwan.

Methods.—From 1997 to 2010, 23,147 patients with acute burn injury in 44 hospitals were retrospectively reviewed. Variables examined were age, sex, depth and extent of burn, inhalation injury, flushing time, hospital admission and referral status, intensive care unit admission, and mortality. Logistic regression analyses were used to evaluate risk factors. Model performance and calibration was evaluated by measures of discrimination and goodness-of-fit statistic, respectively. A nomogram of four major risk factors was used to calculate the probability of mortality.

Results.—Only 22,665 patients (mean [SD] age, 31.05 [22.67] years; mean second-degree and third-degree burn sizes, 8.67% [10.64%] and 3.25% [10.91%], respectively) survived until discharge, for a mortality rate of 2.08%.

Conclusion.—Burn depth is an important predictive factor for mortality. An objective model can help estimate the probability of death in acute burn injury.

Level of Evidence.—Prognostic study, level II.

▶ The survival rates of burn injury have increased steadily over the decades. This can be attributed to numerous factors, including vigorous fluid resuscitation, early eschar excision and grafting, introduction of effective topical and systemic antibiotics, and advances in critical care and nutrition. In 1961, the Baux score (age + total body surface area [TBSA]) was developed as a model for predicting burn mortality. However, this classic scoring system, which contains only 2 factors, age and percentage of body surface area burned, is too simple for contemporary use. Additionally, inhalation injury has been recognized as an important contributor to mortality in many other reports. The authors of this article developed a simple formula encompassing 4 factors—age, burn injury, inhalation injury, and burn size of greater than 20% TBSA—with good performance and calibration. One should be very cautious and only use such predictors as an adjunct to clinical assessment in the evaluation of the severity of illness and the risk of mortality in critical patients. Prediction of outcome from burn injury is useful for prognostic determinations, triage of patients, and allocation of resources. It is also helpful for the clinician to understand the relative contribution of specific prognostic factors and to reduce the reliance on clinical intuition.

D. W. Mozingo, MD

Adapting to Life After Burn Injury—Reflections on Care

Dahl O, Wickman M, Wengström Y (Karolinska Institutet, Stockholm, Sweden)
J Burn Care Res 33:595-605, 2012

A burn injury is an unforeseen event that means physical and psychological trauma for the person afflicted. The trauma experienced by different individuals varies greatly, as do perceived problems during care, rehabilitation, and throughout the remainder of life. The purpose of this study was to explore burn patients' experiences of adapting to life after burn injury to acquire a deeper understanding of the most important issues for patients when providing care during and after a burn injury. A qualitative approach was applied, and interviews were conducted with 12 adult burn patients (8 men and 4 women) 6 to 12 months postburn. The interviews were analyzed using Kvales' method for structuring analysis and comprised a close reading and interpretation of the texts. Analysis focused on the personal experiences of burn patients living after burn injury and treatment. Struggling with the consequences of burn injury and how patients perceived life today after treatment are important issues for adapting to life after burn injury. New experiences of a fragile body, coping with daily life, and reflections of burn care were also prominent themes. Patients with burn injuries need adequate repeated information about the plan for their care, about the physiological changes, and more support to handle the trauma event. The patients would also like to be more involved in their care. A program of support and preparatory work to help the patient to cope with the new bodily sensations and new body image is necessary and should begin during hospital care. A multidisciplinary team approach for pain treatment needs to be prioritized. In addition, multidisciplinary follow-up after burns need to include patients with minor burns.

▶ The findings in this selection indicate that patients with burn injuries need more information about the plan for their care and that they would also like to be more involved in their care. Patients need adequate repeated information of what has happened physiologically, what feelings can occur in relation to this injury, and the expected care trajectory related to their injury. A burn injury is an unforeseen event that constitutes physical as well as psychological trauma for the person afflicted. The trauma experienced by different individuals varies greatly, as do perceived problems during care and rehabilitation throughout the remainder of life. Even after hospital discharge, the burn injury causes major limitations that extend well beyond the physical area to include emotional, social, and relational aspects. Improvements in burn care have resulted in decreased mortality, and more people with massive burns are surviving. Even with expert multidisciplinary and high-quality acute care and follow-up, burn survivors frequently have cosmetic and functional impairments that can never be completely corrected. A program of support and preparatory work to help the patients cope with the new bodily sensations and new body image is necessary and should begin during hospital care. To reach this goal is a challenge in today's pace of patient care, but it is of great importance to the overall recovery of our patients.

D. W. Mozingo, MD

A Review of the Use of Human Albumin in Burn Patients

Cartotto R, Callum J (Univ of Toronto, Canada)

J Burn Care Res 33:702-717, 2012

This review article examines the use of human albumin (HA) in burn treatment. Generally, there are two scenarios where HA may be administered: acutely as a volume expander during burn shock resuscitation and chronically following resuscitation to correct hypoalbuminemia. Although colloids were the cornerstone of the earliest burn resuscitation formulas, HA was in fact rarely used. More recently however, with the recognition of fluid creep, HA usage during resuscitation has increased. Animal studies demonstrate that during acute fluid resuscitation, administration of colloids, including albumin (ALB), have no ability to arrest the formation of burn wound edema, but they do reduce edema formation in the nonburn soft tissues and help preserve intravascular volume and reduce resuscitation fluid requirements with no apparent increase in extravascular water accumulation in the lung. Human studies suggest that immediate use of ALB during acute resuscitation achieves adequate resuscitation using a lower total overall volume requirement, transiently provides better maintenance of intravascular volume and cardiac output, produces less overall edema gain than crystalloid resuscitation alone but may be associated with increased extravascular lung water accumulation during the first postburn week. However, many questions remain unanswered, and modern, large-scale prospective studies are desperately needed. Maintenance of normal serum ALB levels through continuous supplementation of HA following burn resuscitation is even less well understood. Although this approach makes physiologic sense, the limited amount of available data from human burn studies reveal that chronic ALB supplementation is expensive and may not result in any major clinical benefits. Again, modernized prospective studies are greatly needed in this area.

▶ Controversy continues to surround the use of human albumin in the treatment of patients with major burn injuries. Originally, colloids were the cornerstone of most of the fluid resuscitation formulas for the acutely burned patient although plasma, rather than albumin, was the predominant colloid used. Colloid-based resuscitation strategies were eventually replaced by formulas that relied predominantly on crystalloids, but recent intensive interest in volume-sparing strategies to correct fluid creep during resuscitation have resulted in renewed enthusiasm for the use of colloids. Concerns surrounding the cost and safety of plasma have led many to consider albumin as the colloid of choice. Unfortunately, there appears to be no uniform consensus on how and when, or even whether, to initiate albumin during acute fluid resuscitation. Most of the major studies on albumin during burn resuscitation were conducted more than 2 decades ago, and modern, large, randomized, controlled trials in this area are nonexistent. One might consider implementing albumin treatment in patients when a trigger volume of crystalloid solution is reached rather than a time-based protocol. This may result in a reduction in total volume fluid required for resuscitation in those patients who are most fluid avid and avoid colloid administration in those whose capillary leak is less pronounced. This selection is an excellent review of the history and summation of current knowledge of burn fluid resuscitation.

D. W. Mozingo, MD

Evaluation of biofilm production and characterization of genes encoding type III secretion system among *Pseudomonas aeruginosa* isolated from burn patients
Jabalameli F, Mirsalehian A, Khoramian B, et al (Tehran Univ of Med Sciences, Iran; et al)
Burns 38:1192-1197, 2012

Pseudomonas aeruginosa is one of the common pathogenic causes of serious infections in burn patients throughout the world. Type III secretion toxins are thought to promote the dissemination of *P. aeruginosa* from the site of infection, the bacterial evasion of the host immune response and inhibition of DNA synthesis leading to host cell death. A total of 96 isolates of *P. aeruginosa* were collected from wound infections of burn patients, from April to July 2010. Antimicrobial susceptibility of the isolates were determined by disk agar diffusion method. Polymerase chain reaction (PCR)-based method was used for targeting the genes encoding the type III secretion toxins.

The quantitative determination of biofilm-forming capacity was determined by a colorimetric microtiter plate assay. All the isolates were resistant to cefixime and ceftriaxone. More than 90% of the isolates were resistant to amikacin, carbenicillin, cefepime, cefotaxime, cefpodoxime, gatifloxacin, gentamicin, piperacillin/tazobactam, ticarcillin and tobramycin. All the isolates carried the *exoT* gene, 95% carried *exoY*, 64.5% carried *exoU* and 29% carried the *exoS* gene. Most of the isolates (58%) carried both *exoY* and *exoU* genes while 24% showed the concomitant presence of *exoS* and *exoY* and 1% carried both *exoS* and *exoU*. Coexistence of *exoS*, *exoY* and *exoU* was seen in 4% of the isolates. Biofilm formation was seen in more than 96% of the isolates among which 47% were strong biofilm producers, 26% were moderate and 22.9% were weak biofilm formers. In conclusion, the findings of this study show that the genes, particularly the *exoU* gene, encoding the type III secretion toxins, are commonly disseminated among the *P. aeruginosa* strains isolated from burn patients.

▶ *Pseudomonas aeruginosa* is an opportunistic pathogen that is able to cause pulmonary, bloodstream, urinary tract, surgical site, and soft tissue infections. It is one of the common pathogenic causes of serious infections in burn patients throughout the world. Biofilm is a complex aggregation of microorganisms in an exopolysaccharide matrix. *P. aeruginosa* is thought to exist as a biofilm during infections in acute burn wounds. The formation of biofilm facilitates microbial survival in hostile environments, protects the bacteria from the host immune response, and enhances their resistance to antibiotics. In this study, more than 96% of the isolates produced biofilm, among which, 47.9% showed strong biofilm formation, 26% formed moderate biofilms, and 22.9% showed weak biofilm formation. There was no correlation between the patterns of biofilm production and cytotoxin encoding genes. The authors found that the type III secretion toxin-encoding genes, in particular the exoUgene, are commonly disseminated among the *P. aeruginosa* strains isolated from burn patients. Finally, a high prevalence of biofilm producer isolates, implicated in burn patients, is a serious problem that makes the treatment of wound infections difficult and complicated.

D. W. Mozingo, MD

Early coagulopathy of major burns
Mitra B, Wasiak J, Cameron PA, et al (Monash Univ, Melbourne, Victoria, Australia; et al)
Injury 44:40-43, 2013

Introduction and Aims.—The pathophysiology and time-course of coagulopathy post major burns are inadequately understood. The aims of this study were to review the incidence of acute coagulopathy post major burns, potential contributing factors associated with this coagulopathy and outcome of patients who developed early coagulopathy.

Methods.—A retrospective review of all patients with major burns (≥20% total body surface area (TBSA)) presenting to a tertiary burns referral centre was conducted. Data on demographic, injury characteristics and fluid resuscitation practices were recorded and tested for association with coagulopathy (INR > 1.5 or aPTT > 60 s) at hospital presentation and within 24 h of burns injury. Mortality, intensive care unit (ICU) admission, mechanical ventilation and blood product usage were primary endpoints.

Results.—There were 99 patients who met the inclusion criteria with 36 (16) %TBSA burns. Coagulopathy was present in only three patients on presentation, but 37 (37%) patients developed early onset (within 24 h of injury) coagulopathy. Early onset coagulopathy was independently associated with %TBSA burnt ($p < 0.001$) and volume of fluid administered ($p = 0.005$). Early onset coagulopathy was associated with higher volumes of blood and blood product administration, ICU admission and prolonged mechanical ventilation.

Conclusions.—Post major burns, a very low proportion of patients presented with coagulopathy, but a substantial proportion of patients developed coagulopathy within 24 h. This and the association of coagulopathy with the volume of fluid resuscitation suggest dilution as a major cause of the early coagulopathy of major burns.

▶ Coagulopathy presents as a potentially preventable, measurable, and treatable complication of burn injury. An initial moderate decrease in coagulation factors occurs after burn injury and correlates to a rise in partial thromboplastin time and prothrombin times. Dilution by intravenous resuscitation fluid administration had been postulated as a potential mechanism. The authors of this selection have shown a significant association between early-onset coagulopathy and larger volumes of fluid administration, thereby generating the hypothesis of being able to prevent coagulopathy through judicious fluid administration regimes. Although there is probably a component of dilutional coagulopathy related to large volume fluid administration, there are likely other mechanisms involved. D-dimers are elevated in patients with extensive burn, suggesting a consumptive coagulopathy. Additionally, the significant inflammatory response increases the synthesis of acute-phase proteins while reducing the synthesis of others such as albumin and clotting factors. The authors have derived much information from a retrospective review, but a prospective approach would provide more useful information.

D. W. Mozingo, MD

A Rationale for Significant Cost Savings in Patients Suffering Home Oxygen Burns: Despite Many Comorbid Conditions, Only Modest Care Is Necessary

Vercruysse GA, Ingram WL (Univ of Arizona School of Medicine, Tucson; Emory Univ, Atlanta, GA)
J Burn Care Res 33:e268-e274, 2012

Increasingly, patients are being evaluated for burns related to home oxygen use. Although the majority of burns are minor, referral to a burn unit regardless of depth or size is still common. The care of this population was reviewed to determine the feasibility and potential saving if such patients could be managed by nonburn-trained surgeons. Prospectively collected data on 5103 consecutive patients admitted to an urban tertiary burn center between April 1997 and September 2010 was reviewed. Data collected included age, TBSA burned, comorbidities, mode of admission, distance transported, mode of transport, number requiring surgery, length of stay, and outcome. Of 5103 admissions, 64 were for home oxygen burns. Patients had a mean age of 62.5 years and five comorbidities. They suffered a mean 4% TBSA burn, and all were mostly superficial, of partial thickness, and healed without surgery. Patients had a mean length of stay of 2 days and required one follow-up visit. Twenty-seven percent were transferred from another facility after initial care, and 28% arrived intubated. Twenty-two percent were transported by helicopter, and 61% arrived intubated. Eighty percent of ventilated patients were extubated within 8 hours of admission, and all within 24 hours. Average distance by helicopter transport was 57 miles, and cost $12,500.00. Large savings could be realized if patients cared for by local physicians were educated in basic burn care. This would be more palatable with good communication between the community hospital and burn center, with consultation on an as-needed basis.

▶ The authors of this selection noted a trend toward increasing numbers of patients suffering from home oxygen burns. Of the 64 patients with home oxygen burns in this 14-year database, more than half (36) were admitted during the final 3 years of the study. This trend seems logical, given the number of adults reaching ages at which the use of home oxygen becomes more prevalent. At the University of Florida, we have noted a similar trend, as we currently admit 1 to 2 patients per month. In treating these patients, it must be remembered that nasal cannulae are made of plastic and often burn when part of a home oxygen fire. Small fragments of the plastic cannula may be found in the nose and can be removed with forceps. Carbon deposits from the burned cannula are often found in the nose and the mouth. This is sometimes mistaken for carbonaceous sputum. These patients always have singed nasal hairs, but this is a direct injury and is not an indication of significant smoke inhalation. Patients can almost always breathe through their mouth easily if their nasal passages become occluded by edema or secretions. In these patients, the most common cause of shortness of breath is exacerbation of an underlying medical condition. The combination of pain, surprise, and fear can cause bronchospasm. Treatment with bronchodilating aerosols and small doses of intravenous opioids for pain often improves symptoms significantly.

D. W. Mozingo, MD

Clinical effectiveness of dermal substitution in burns by topical negative pressure: A multicenter randomized controlled trial

Bloemen MCT, van der Wal MBA, Verhaegen PDHM, et al (Association of Dutch Burn Ctrs, Beverwijk, The Netherlands)
Wound Repair Regen 20:797-805, 2012

Previous research has shown clinical effectiveness of dermal substitution; however, in burn wounds, only limited effect has been shown. A problem in burn wounds is the reduced take of the autograft, when the substitute and graft are applied in one procedure. Recently, application of topical negative pressure (TNP) was shown to improve graft take. The aim of this study was to investigate if application of a dermal substitute in combination with TNP improves scar quality after burns. In a four-armed multicenter randomized controlled trial, a split-skin graft with or without a dermal substitute and with or without TNP was compared in patients with deep dermal or full-thickness burns requiring skin transplantation. Graft take and rate of wound epithelialization were evaluated. Three and 12 months postoperatively, scar parameters were measured. The results of 86 patients showed that graft take and epithelialization did not reveal significant differences.

Significantly fewer wounds in the TNP group showed postoperative contamination, compared to other groups. Highest elasticity was measured in scars treated with the substitute and TNP, which was significantly better compared to scars treated with the substitute alone. Concluding, this randomized controlled trial shows the effectiveness of dermal substitution combined with TNP in burns, based on extensive wound and scar measurements.

▶ In this selection, a multicenter, randomized, controlled trial investigated long-term effects of dermal substitution combined with topical negative pressure in acute burn wounds. Most important, it was shown that scars treated with dermal substitution and topical negative pressure were significantly more elastic compared with scars treated with the substitute alone. In addition, successful application of a dermal substitute in a 1-stage grafting procedure was shown: both graft take and wound epithelialization were comparable in the 4 groups. Furthermore, significantly lower postoperative wound contamination was shown in wounds treated with topical negative pressure alone compared with other groups. Finally, scar pigmentation was significantly more similar to normal skin in scars treated with topical negative pressure alone compared with the other groups at 12 months postoperatively. The benefits to the wounds were shown with an extensive array of reliable and valid wound and scar measurements. The beneficial effect of the dermal substitute in combination with topical negative pressure was shown on long-term scar elasticity. There are some limitations to this study. Because of the multicenter setting, site-specific adjustment for measurement tools used in each burn center was proven necessary in the analysis. Also, clinicians and patients could not be blinded.

D. W. Mozingo, MD

Burn Disaster Response Planning in New York City: Updated Recommendations for Best Practices
Leahy NE, Yurt RW, Lazar EJ, et al (New York Presbyterian Hosp; Weill Cornell Med College, NY; et al)
J Burn Care Res 33:587-594, 2012

Since its inception in 2006, the New York City (NYC) Task Force for Patients with Burns has continued to develop a city-wide and regional response plan that addressed the triage, treatment, transportation of 50/ million (400) adult and pediatric victims for 3 to 5 days after a large-scale burn disaster within NYC until such time that a burn center bed and transportation could be secured. The following presents updated recommendations on these planning efforts. Previously published literature, project deliverables, and meeting documents for the period of 2009—2010 were reviewed. A numerical simulation was designed to evaluate the triage algorithm developed for this plan. A new, secondary triage scoring algorithm, based on co-morbidities and predicted outcomes, was created to prioritize

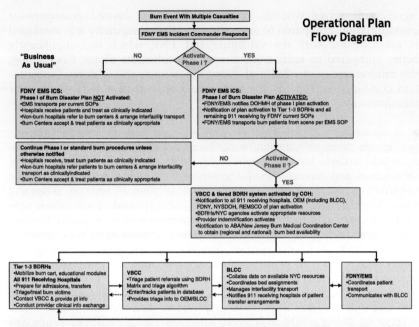

FIGURE 2.—Operational plan overview. (Reprinted from Leahy NE, Yurt RW, Lazar EJ, et al. Burn disaster response planning in New York City: updated recommendations for best practices. *J Burn Care Res*. 2012;33:587-594, with permission from the American Burn Association.)

multiple patients within a given acuity and predicted survivability cohort. Recommendations for a centralized patient and resource tracking database, plan operations, activation thresholds, mass triage, communications, data flow, staffing, resource utilization, provider indemnification, and stakeholder roles and responsibilities were specified. Educational modules for prehospital providers and nonburn center nurses and physicians who would provide interim care to burn injured disaster victims were created and pilot tested. These updated best practice recommendations provide a strong foundation for further planning efforts, and as of February 2011, serve as the frame work for the NYC Burn Surge Response Plan that has been incorporated into the New York State Burn Plan (Fig 2).

▶ In this selection, the authors provide updated recommendations for best practices and offer a detailed outline for plan operations, stakeholder roles and responsibilities, provider education, communications pathways, data management, legal protection, and public health policy in the event of a large-scale burn disaster. Although this plan is limited in scope to burn-injured patients, it provides both specific steps and general operating principles for a city-wide and regional response plan that capitalizes on the multiagency cooperation required to coordinate resources and maximize patient outcomes that may be adapted to other disaster response planning efforts. Many states and regional plans have been developed to address burn disasters, but many are still in their infancy. Although this plan is the first of its kind for the New York City (NYC) region and is limited in scope to a burn disaster response only, it offers guidance on operationalizing general principles that may pertain to other emergency preparedness planning groups both within NYC and outside jurisdictions. Such groups may consider modifying these principles to meet the unique population, resource, or geographic needs for a specific preparedness response or region. This plan, in part, resembles the Gulf States' plan for hurricane readiness on which the Southern burn region bases its preparedness activities. Fig 2 shows the operational plan overview.

D. W. Mozingo, MD

A Survey of Invasive Catheter Practices in U.S. Burn Centers
Sheridan RL, Neely AN, Castillo MA, et al (Shriners Hosps for Children®— Boston, MA; Shriners Hosps for Children®—Cincinnati, OH; Army Inst of Surgical Res, Fort Sam Houston, TX; et al)
J Burn Care Res 33:741-746, 2012

Burn-specific guidelines for optimal catheter rotation, catheter type, insertion methods, and catheter site care do not exist, and practices vary widely from one burn unit to another. The purpose of this study was to define current practices and identify areas of practice variation for future clinical investigation. An online survey was sent to the directors of 123 U.S. burn centers. The survey consisted of 23 questions related to specific practices in placement and maintenance of central venous catheters (CVCs), arterial catheters, and peripherally inserted central catheters (PICCs). The overall response rate was 36%; response rate from verified centers was 52%. Geographic representation was wide. CVC and arterial catheter replacement varied from every 3 days (24% of sites) to only for overt infection (24% of sites); 23% of sites did not use the femoral position for CVC placement. Nearly 60% of units used some kind of antiseptic catheter. Physicians inserted the majority of catheters, and 22% of sites used nonphysicians for at least some insertions. Ultrasound was routinely used by less than 50% of units. A wide variety of post-insertion dressing protocols were followed. PICCs were used in some critically injured patients in 37% of units; the majority of these users did not rotate PICCs. Thus, it can be surmised that wide practice variation exists among burn centers with regard to insertion and maintenance of invasive catheters. Areas with particular variability that would be appropriate targets of clinical investigation are line rotation protocols, catheter site care protocols, and use of PICCs in acute burns (Fig 3).

▶ Existing practice guidelines designed to minimize invasive catheter infections and insertion-related complications are widely followed in general adult and pediatric intensive care units; however, burn care providers view the needs of patients in burn intensive care units as unique. There is a wide range of practices related to the use of central venous catheters in burn patients. These beliefs are based on the frequent need to place catheters through burn-injured skin and

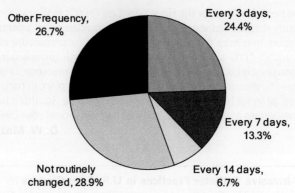

FIGURE 3.—Routine catheter change frequency. (Reprinted from Sheridan RL, Neely AN, Castillo MA, et al. A survey of invasive catheter practices in U.S. burn centers. *J Burn Care Res.* 2012;33:741-746, with permission from the American Burn Association.)

the frequent occurrence of bacteremia related to burn wound manipulation. Widely accepted burn-specific guidelines for optimal catheter rotation, catheter type, insertion methods, and catheter site care do not exist. Fig 3 is an example of this variation. Despite recent emphasis on standardization and protocols in critical care, wide practice variation remains among burn centers with regard to insertion and maintenance of invasive catheters. Future multicenter studies to determine optimal central venous catheter use and care might include the role of peripherally inserted central catheters, line rotation protocols, impact of antiseptic catheters, and catheter site care protocols.

D. W. Mozingo, MD

Long-Term Propranolol Use in Severely Burned Pediatric Patients: A Randomized Controlled Study

Herndon DN, Rodriguez NA, Diaz EC, et al (Shriners Hosps for Children—Galveston, TX; et al)
Ann Surg 256:402-411, 2012

Objective.—To determine the safety and efficacy of propranolol given for 1 year on cardiac function, resting energy expenditure, and body composition in a prospective, randomized, single-center, controlled study in pediatric patients with large burns.

Background.—Severe burns trigger a hypermetabolic response that persists for up to 2 years postburn. Propranolol given for 1 month postburn blunts this response. Whether propranolol administration for 1 year after injury provides a continued benefit is currently unclear.

Methods.—One-hundred seventy-nine pediatric patients with more than 30% total body surface area burns were randomized to control (n = 89) or 4 mg/kg/d propranolol (n = 90) for 12 months postburn. Changes in resting energy expenditure, cardiac function, and body composition were measured

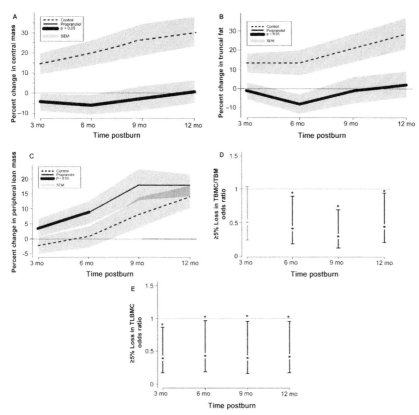

FIGURE 3.—Effect of propranolol on body composition. Percentage of change in central mass (A), truncal fat (B), and peripheral lean mass (C). In all panels, data are expressed as the percentage of change from patient baseline and are shown as the Loess smoothed trend, with shading indicating standard error of the mean. (D, E) Comparison of the likelihood of losing 5% or more of (D) total bone mineral content/total body mass and (E) total lumbar bone mineral content in control and propranolol-treated patients. Data are expressed as the odds ratios. *Significant difference at $P < 0.05$. (Reprinted from Herndon DN, Rodriguez NA, Diaz EC, et al. Long-term propranolol use in severely burned pediatric patients: a randomized controlled study. *Ann Surg*. 2012;256:402-411, © 2012, Southeastern Surgical Congress.)

acutely at 3, 6, 9, and 12 months postburn. Statistical analyses included techniques that adjusted for non-normality, repeated-measures, and regression analyses. $P < 0.05$ was considered significant.

Results.—Long-term propranolol treatment significantly reduced the percentage of the predicted heart rate and percentage of the predicted resting energy expenditure, decreased accumulation of central mass and central fat, prevented bone loss, and improved lean body mass accretion. There were very few adverse effects from the dose of propranolol used.

Conclusions.—Propranolol treatment for 12 months after thermal injury, ameliorates the hyperdynamic, hypermetabolic, hypercatabolic, and osteopenic responses in pediatric patients. This study is registered at clinicaltrials.gov: NCT00675714 (Fig 3).

▶ Propranolol, a nonselective β-adrenergic receptor antagonist, mitigates the actions of plasma catecholamines and significantly reduces the hyperdynamic and hypermetabolic states in patients with acute burn injury. One of the secondary endpoints of the study was peripheral lean body mass, which showed a 10% improvement in the propranolol group compared with the control group. This finding is in keeping with previous studies showing a decrease in protein degradation. The effect on lean body mass is demonstrated in Fig 3. Also in this study, the beneficial effects of propranolol could be extended to bone, with less pronounced bone loss over the study period. This is an excellent study in children and needs to be repeated in the adult population. Application of this treatment may extend to other conditions with chronic catabolic states other than burns.

D. W. Mozingo, MD

An Experience in the Management of the Open Abdomen in Severely Injured Burn Patients
Hardin MO, Mace JE, Ritchie JD, et al (United States Army Inst of Surgical Res, Fort Sam Houston, TX)
J Burn Care Res 33:491-496, 2012

Few descriptions of temporary abdominal closure for planned relaparotomy have been reported in burned patients. The purpose of this study is to describe our experience and outcomes in the management of burned patients with an open abdomen. The authors performed a retrospective review of all admissions to our burn center from March 2003 to June 2008, identifying patients treated by laparotomy with temporary abdominal closure. The authors collected data on patient demographics, indication for laparotomy, methods of temporary and definitive abdominal closure, and outcomes. Of 2,104 patients admitted, 38 underwent a laparotomy with temporary abdominal closure. Their median TBSA was 55%, and the incidence of inhalation injury was 58%. Abdominal compartment syndrome was the most common indication for laparotomy (82%) followed by abdominal trauma (16%). The in-hospital mortality associated with an open abdomen was 68%. Temporary abdominal closure was performed most commonly using negative pressure wound therapy (90%). Fascial closure was performed in 21 patients but was associated with a 38% rate of failure requiring reexploration. Of 12 survivors, fascial closure was achieved in seven patients and five were managed with a planned ventral hernia. Burned patients who necessitate an open abdomen management strategy have a high morbidity and mortality. Fascial closure was associated with a high rate of failure but was successful in a select group of patients. Definitive abdominal closure with a planned ventral hernia was associated with no

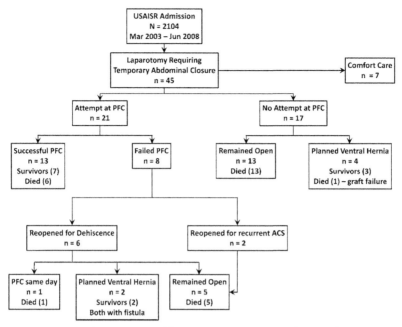

FIGURE.—Consort diagram. (Reprinted from Hardin MO, Mace JE, Ritchie JD, et al. An experience in the management of the open abdomen in severely injured burn patients. *J Burn Care Res.* 2012;33:491-496, with permission from American Burn Association.)

increased mortality and remains an option when "tension-free" fascial closure cannot be achieved (Fig).

▶ In the current era of damage control surgery, the practice of planned relaparotomy to address intra-abdominal issues that remain after stabilization of a critically ill patient has become commonplace. The open abdomen is a complex problem in severely burned patients and has been associated with high morbidity and mortality. The authors of this article found that the development of an enterocutaneous fistula was associated with an increased duration of an open abdomen. No patient with the complication of fistula had definitive abdominal coverage before 35 days following laparotomy. Multiple logistic regression analysis demonstrated that the risk of a fistula formation doubled for every 5 days the abdomen remained open. The risk of injury to the underlying, fragile granulating bowel and subsequent fistula formation remains a significant factor in the desire to provide definitive closure of the abdomen as soon as possible. The figure is included here to describe the ultimate outcome of patients with the complication of open abdomen.

D. W. Mozingo, MD

A new algorithm to allow early prediction of mortality in elderly burn patients

Davis JS, Prescott AT, Varas RP, et al (Univ of Miami Burn Ctr, FL)
Burns 38:1114-1118, 2012

Introduction.—The elderly are the fastest growing population segment, and particularly susceptible to burns. Predicting outcomes for these patients remains difficult. Our objective was to identify early predictors of mortality in elderly burn patients.

Methods.—Our Burn Center's prospective database was reviewed for burn patients 60+ treated in the past 10 years. Predictor variables were identified by correlative analysis and subsequently entered into a multivariate logistic regression analysis examining survival to discharge.

Results.—203 patients of 1343 (15%) were eligible for analysis. The average age was 72 ± 10 (range 60−102) and the average total body surface area (TBSA) burned was $23 \pm 18\%$ (range 1−95). Age, TBSA, base deficit, pO_2, respiratory rate, Glasgow Coma Score (GCS), and Revised Trauma Score (RTS, based on systolic blood pressure, respiratory rate, and GCS) all correlated with mortality ($p \leq 0.05$). Using multiple logistic regression analysis, a model with age, TBSA and RTS was calculated, demonstrating:

increased risk of mortality $= \beta_0 + 1.12(\text{age}) + 1.094(\text{TBSA}) + 0.718(\text{RTS})$

In this model, β_0 is a constant that equals -8.32.

Conclusions.—Predicting outcomes in elderly burn patients is difficult. A model using age, TBSA, and RTS can, immediately upon patient arrival, help identify patients with decreased chances of survival, further guiding end-of-life decisions (Table 1).

▶ The Miami Model, by virtue of incorporating Revised Trauma Score into its calculations, allows the clinician to incorporate patient physiologic derangements into a predictive model, along with the standard age and total body surface area burn. Moreover, this model demonstrated noninferiority when tested against the

TABLE 1.—Correlative Analysis of Early Survival Predictors

Predictor	Included Values, n (%)	Mean $\pm$ SD	Alive, n (%)	Deceased, n (%)	R^{2a}	p Value[§]
Age	203 (100%)	70 ± 10	120 (59%)	83 (41%)	0.25	<0.001
TBSA	185 (91%)	23 ± 18	104 (56%)	81 (44%)	0.49	<0.001
Base deficit	178 (88%)	-3 ± 5	99 (56%)	79 (44%)	−0.29	<0.001
pO_2	178 (88%)	95 ± 8.5	99 (56%)	79 (44%)	0.27	<0.001
Respiratory rate	202 (99.5%)	19 ± 6	120 (59%)	82 (41%)	−0.19	0.008
GCS	201 (99%)	13 ± 3.1	120 (60%)	81 (40%)	−0.39	<0.001
RTS	199 (98%)	7.4 ± 1.2	120 (60%)	81 (40%)	−0.36	<0.001

TBSA, total body surface area; pO_2, arterial blood oxygenation; GCS, Glasgow Coma Scale; RTS, Revised Trauma Score.
[a]R^2 is Pearson's coefficient, a standard measure in linear regressions that refers to proportion of variability in the data that is accounted for by the statistical model. A value between 0 and 1 indicates a positive, linear relationship between outcomes and their predicted values.
[§]p-Values refer to the significance of the association between predictor variable and mortality in the univariate analysis.

Baux Score. As such, the Miami Model is a valuable addition to the clinician's armamentarium when assessing patient mortality risk. This retrospective cohort study is subject to certain limitations. The data collected and analyzed come from one institution and cannot, therefore, be controlled for institution-specific practices and management. The small sample size, often at issue in studies analyzing relatively small cohorts of patients, may limit the applicability of this study. Further studies will be necessary to validate the regression model against other patient populations. Each patient presents a unique case, and decisions regarding end-of-life care must be based on individual factors that are often beyond the scope of any predictive tools. Nevertheless, when providing information to patients and their families, presenting a range of population outcomes may assist the clinician in educating them.

D. W. Mozingo, MD

A Comparison of Dexmedetomidine and Midazolam for Sedation in Severe Pediatric Burn Injury

Fagin A, Palmieri T, Greenhalgh D, et al (Univ of California Davis, Sacramento; Shriners Hosp for Children, Sacramento, CA)
J Burn Care Res 33:759-763, 2012

Dexmedetomidine (DEX) is an α-adrenergic agonist that has been used for sedation during invasive procedures and endotracheal intubation. In pediatric burn injury, DEX has been shown to be safe as a long-term sedative in the intensive care unit (ICU). However, comparison of DEX with traditional sedatives, such as midazolam, for sedation in pediatric burn injury has not been performed. The purpose of this study was to compare DEX with midazolam in terms of sedation, efficacy, and side effects in children with burn injury. A retrospective review of all children with a TBSA burn injury $\geq 20\%$ admitted from December 2008 to September 2010 was performed. Children who received a continuous DEX infusion were compared with children receiving a continuous midazolam infusion. Data collected included: age, TBSA burn, ventilator days, ICU days, hypotensive episodes, bradycardic episodes, and Richmond Agitation Score (RAS). A total of 21 patients who received DEX infusions were compared with 21 age-matched and burn size—matched patients who received midazolam infusions. Of the 21 DEX patients, nine also received midazolam infusions, eight prior to DEX and one after. These patients did not receive DEX and midazolam simultaneously. There was no difference in age (6.9 vs 6.4 years), TBSA (45.5 vs 49.2%), ICU days (45.3 vs 55.4), and ventilator days (38.5 vs 45.5) between the DEX and midazolam patients, respectively. The mean duration of infusion was 22.5 ± 24.9 days for DEX and 20.1 ± 24.8 days for midazolam. DEX patients had a mean RAS of −0.91 ± 0.8. Midazolam patients were more sedated with a mean RAS of −1.33 ± 0.7. Only one episode of bradycardia was noted in the DEX group. The DEX group had fewer hypotensive episodes (mean arterial pressure < 60 mm Hg) while on infusion compared with the midazolam group

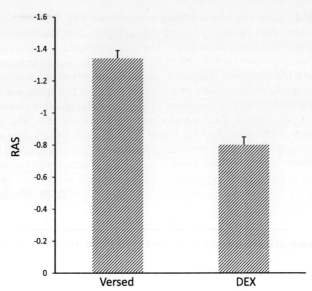

FIGURE.—Mean daily Richmond Agitation Score (RAS). (Reprinted from Fagin A, Palmieri T, Greenhalgh D, et al. A comparison of dexmedetomidine and midazolam for sedation in severe pediatric burn injury. *J Burn Care Res*. 2012;33:759-763, with permission from the American Burn Association.)

(15.8 vs 29.7 episodes). Thus, it can be surmised that DEX is a safe and effective sedative for pediatric burn patients. Compared to midazolam, DEX may provide more effective sedation and less sedation-related hypotension (Fig).

▶ Adequate analgesia and sedation are important during the care of critically injured burn patients. Sedation in children can be even more difficult to achieve because of parental separation, stranger fear, incomprehension, and degree of perceived situational control. Severely injured pediatric burn patients experience both pain and anxiety for weeks. Also, burns can alter the pharmacokinetics and pharmacodynamics of many drugs. Dexmedetomidine (DEX) is primarily used as a short-term adjunct to anesthesia. Intranasal DEX has been shown to be more effective than oral midazolam at inducing sleep and is comparable for conditions at induction, emergence from anesthesia, or postoperative pain. Also, DEX is used for short-term sedation for both noninvasive and invasive procedures. In this study, the investigators compared DEX with midazolam for sedation in pediatric burn injury. Their practice is to administer DEX to patients as first-line sedation, so most of the controls were historical. There was only about a 1-year difference in their dates of admission, and their practice has not substantially changed in that time. Their findings suggest that DEX is safe and effective and may be able to minimize hypotensive episodes with minimal risk of bradycardia. A prospective, randomized trial is warranted to prove the efficacy and safety of DEX for long-term use in severely burned pediatric patients.

D. W. Mozingo, MD

A randomized, controlled, double-blind prospective trial with a Lipido-Colloid Technology-Nano-OligoSaccharide Factor wound dressing in the local management of venous leg ulcers

Meaume S, on behalf of the CHALLENGE Study Group (Rothschild Univ Hosp, Paris, France; et al)

Wound Repair Regen 20:500-511, 2012

Venous leg ulcers (VLUs) are the most prevalent chronic wounds in western countries with a heavy socioeconomic impact. Compression therapy is the etiologic treatment of VLU but until now no wound dressing has been shown to be more effective than another. The aim of this study was to assess the efficacy of a new dressing in the management of VLU. Adult patients presenting a noninfected VLU and receiving effective compression therapy were enrolled in this randomized, controlled, double-blind trial. The VLUs were assessed every 2 weeks for 8 weeks. The primary study outcome was the relative Wound Area Reduction (WAR, in %), and the secondary objectives were absolute WAR, healing rate, and percentage of wounds with >40% surface area reduction. One hundred eighty-seven patients were randomly allocated to treatment groups. Median WAR was 58.3% in the Lipido-Colloid Technology-Nano-OligoSaccharide Factor (TLC-NOSF) dressing group (test group) and 31.6% in the TLC dressing group (control group) (difference: -26.7%; 95% confidence interval: -38.3 to -15.1%; $p = 0.002$). All other efficacy outcomes were also significant in favor of the TLC-NOSF dressing group. Clinical outcomes for patients treated with the new dressing are superior to those patients treated with the TLC dressing (without NOSF compound), suggesting a strong promotion of the VLU healing process.

▶ Venous leg ulcers are very common in the United States population with its high prevalence of obesity. The development of venous leg ulcers leads to major morbidity, loss of productivity, and financial losses to individuals and the health care system. As the authors point out, compression therapy has been the mainstay of outpatient therapy, but its success is quite variable. Thus, newer treatments are indicated to accelerate the healing process, reduce morbidity, and improve patient outcomes. Matrix metalloproteinases (MMP 2 and MMP 9) have been implicated in the ongoing creation of venous leg ulcers and their resistance to healing. Thus, substances (Nano-Oligosaccharide Factor—impregnated dressing) to inhibit these proteases have been studied to augment the healing process in these ulcers. This prospective, randomized, blinded trial accrued adequate patients into 2 comparable groups and evaluated healing every 2 weeks for 8 weeks. Wound area reduction was significantly greater in the experimental group than in the control, and other factors, such as patient acceptability and painless dressing changes, favored the experimental group. It is important to note that wound compression remained the mainstay of therapy in both groups of patients. This is a well-carried out study, and its results should make major differences in how we care for patients with venous leg ulcers.

J. M. Daly, MD

A randomised prospective study of split skin graft donor site dressings: AWBAT-D™ vs. Duoderm®

Solanki NS, MacKie IP, Greenwood JE (Royal Adelaide Hosp, South Australia, Australia; Frenchay Hosp, Bristol, UK)
Burns 38:889-898, 2012

Objective.—To assess patient comfort and wound-healing efficacy of a new, purpose-designed biosynthetic material (AWBAT-D™) in the healing of split-skin graft donor sites in comparison with our standard dressing, Duoderm®.

Materials and Methods.—We conducted a prospective randomised controlled trial of donor site dressings, comparing AWBAT-D™ with our standard dressing, Duoderm®. Patients were randomly allocated to have their donor site dressed with one of these materials. Outcome measures included pain scores at rest and during dressing changes, time to re-epithelialisation, time to discharge, scarring and infection. Results were assessed for significance using the Mann–Whitney U-test (non-parametric data) and the Chi-Square test (parametric data).

Results.—Fourteen patients were recruited with 8 donor sites in each group. The mean pain scores at rest and during dressing changes were not found to be significantly different between the two groups ($P = 0.99$ and $P = 0.90$ respectively). The median time to re-epithelialisation was shorter in the Duoderm® group at 11 days compared to 17 days in the AWBAT-D™ group ($P = 0.007$). The median time to discharge was not significantly different ($P = 0.38$). No infection or scarring has been observed.

Conclusions.—Based on these early results, AWBAT-D™ appears to have slower donor site healing and does not provide significant improvements in postoperative pain or discharge time compared to Duoderm®. There is no evidence at this stage that our standard donor site dressing should be changed.

▶ Over the years, many attempts have been made to find inert or biologic materials that would accelerate the healing of burn wound donor sites while providing comfort for the patient during the healing process. The healing process can be ascertained somewhat in animal studies, but randomized, controlled trials need to be conducted in humans. In the burn setting, it could be possible to use each patient as his or her own control, but logistics, anatomy, and extent of burn often preclude this type of trial. In the described study, 20 patients were initially planned, but only 14 were entered, and only one patient served as his own control. Although this limits the conclusions somewhat, the authors hypothesized that the experimental wound dressing (AWBAT-D) would improve comfort and healing. Instead, they found that Duoderm (the control dressing) caused less pain and had equivalent healing to that of the AWBAT-D group. Thus, although the study was underpowered to determine if experimental treatment was better than control, it was powered adequately to show control better than experimental. These results again show how important it is to perform randomized, controlled studies where possible. While blinding of the treatments would be preferred, it is impossible in this clinical situation.

J. M. Daly, MD

Angiogenin expression in burn blister fluid: Implications for its role in burn wound neovascularization
Pan S-C, Wu L-W, Chen C-L, et al (Natl Cheng Kung Univ, Tainan, Taiwan; Natl Cheng Kung Univ Med College and Hosp, Tainan, Taiwan)
Wound Repair Regen 20:731-739, 2012

Deep partial thickness burn (DPTB) wound fluids have a greater propensity for establishing neovascularization than did superficial partial thickness burn (SPTB) wound fluids in our previous study. To investigate the factors responsible for this activity, cytokine array and enzyme-linked immunosorbent assay were used to perform an expression analysis of angiogenic factors in burn fluid. Although present in approximately equal amounts in both SPTB and DPTB blister fluids from burn patients, angiogenin does appear to be involved in the ability of DPTB blister fluid to promote neovascularization in vitro and in vivo. Angiogenin alone was sufficient to induce endothelial differentiation of circulating angiogenic cells (CAC) without vascular endothelial growth factor A involvement. In addition, angiogenin was positively associated with CAC differentiation in the burn blister fluid. Blocking the effect of angiogenin in burn blister fluids resulted in a significant reduction of endothelial cell proliferation, CAC differentiation, and new blood vessel formation in vivo. Moreover, immunohistochemistry revealed that high angiogenin expression colocalizes with high vascularity in human burn wounds at day 7, further supporting our hypothesis that angiogenin is involved in burn wound neovascularization.

▶ The ability to control the healing process in burn patients is critically important. Skin coverage reduces the chances of infection and lessens the catabolic activity in the patient. However, controlling the healing process means a great deal to the final cosmetic result for the patient. Thus, this report lends insight into the factors that may control burn wound healing, at least to some extent.

As noted, the burn blister fluid from deep partial-thickness burns appeared to stimulate new capillary formation more than blister fluid from superficially burned areas. Angiogenin seemed to be the factor involved because it induced endothelial differentiation of circulating angiogenic cells, and blocking angiogenin inhibits such differentiation. It is interesting that interferon blocks angiogenin, and this may be a mechanism whereby the healing process could be controlled so that excessive scar formation does not occur.

J. M. Daly, MD

Accelerated Wound Healing with Topical Application of Complement C5

Sinno H, Malhotra M, Lutfy J, et al (McGill Univ, Montreal, Quebec, Canada)
Plast Reconstr Surg 130:523-529, 2012

Background.—Delayed-healing traumatic, surgical, and chronic wounds can be detrimental to patients and the health care system. The authors set out to investigate the effects of complement C5, a naturally occurring chemotactic cytokine, on wounds.

Methods.—The authors examined the effects of complement C5 on the rat paired skin incision model. Each rat served as its own control where topical collagen was applied to one incision and 100 nM of C5 in collagen vehicle was applied to the other incision. Rats were killed on days 3 ($n = 6$), 7 ($n = 6$), and 28 ($n = 5$) after wounding.

Results.—There was a statistically significant, 65 percent increase in maximum wound breaking strength with the topical application of C5 at day 3 ($p < 0.01$). The increase persisted to 14 percent at 7 days after wounding ($p < 0.05$). When compared with the sham group, the C5-treated wound strength increased by 83 percent at day 3 and 64 percent at day 7. There was no change in breaking strength at 28 days. Western blot analysis demonstrated a significant increase in collagen and fibronectin content in the C5-treated wounds.

Conclusions.—Topical application of C5 to skin wounds significantly increases wound healing maximum breaking strength as early as 3 days and up to 7 days after wounding. C5 accelerated wound healing by at least 4 days in the first week of wounding. This was correlated with an increase in vascular permeability, increased inflammatory cell recruitment, subsequent fibroblast migration, and increased collagen deposition.

▶ The authors studied the effects of C5 applied to skin wounds in rats using another skin wound treated with collagen in the same rat as a control. The C5-treated wounds showed statistically improved tensile strength at days 3 and 5 compared with collagen-treated wounds, but the results may not be clinically relevant when examining differences shown in Fig 1 of the original article, and there were no differences at day 28. One wonders if there might have been differences noted at days 14 or 21. There were also biochemical increased levels of collagen and fibronectin in the C5-treated wounds compared with controls. The mechanisms of action for this application of C5 to the wounds are unclear. Do C5 levels locally increase significantly, and for what period of time? For how long after wounding does the C5 need to be applied and when should it start? Clearly, further work needs to be done to define the role of C5 in wound management.

J. M. Daly, MD

Antibacterial Efficacy of Silver-Impregnated Polyelectrolyte Multilayers Immobilized on a Biological Dressing in a Murine Wound Infection Model

Guthrie KM, Agarwal A, Tackes DS, et al (Univ of Wisconsin, Madison; et al)
Ann Surg 256:371-377, 2012

Objective.—To investigate the antibacterial effect of augmenting a biological dressing with polymer films containing silver nanoparticles.

Background.—Biological dressings, such as Biobrane, are commonly used for treating partial-thickness wounds and burn injuries. Biological dressings have several advantages over traditional wound dressings. However, as many as 19% of wounds treated with Biobrane become infected, and, once infected, the Biobrane must be removed and a traditional dressing approach should be employed. Silver is a commonly used antimicrobial in wound care products, but current technology uses cytotoxic concentrations of silver in these dressings. We have developed a novel and facile technology that allows immobilization of bioactive molecules on the surfaces of soft materials, demonstrated here by augmentation of Biobrane with nanoparticulate silver. Surfaces modified with nanometer-thick polyelectrolyte multilayers (PEMs) impregnated with silver nanoparticles have been shown previously to result in in vitro antibacterial activity against *Staphylococcus epidermidis* at loadings of silver that are noncytotoxic.

Methods.—We demonstrated that silver-impregnated PEMs can be nondestructively immobilized onto the surface of Biobrane (Biobrane-Ag) and determined the in vitro antibacterial activity of Biobrane-Ag with *Staphylococcus aureus*. In this study, we used an in vivo wound infection model in mice induced by topical inoculation of S aureus onto full-thickness 6-mm diameter wounds. After 72 hours, bacterial quantification was performed.

Results.—Wounds treated with Biobrane-Ag had significantly ($P < 0.001$) fewer colony-forming units than wounds treated with unmodified Biobrane (more than 4 $\log_{10}$ difference).

Conclusions.—The results of our study indicate that immobilizing silver-impregnated PEMs on the wound-contact surface of Biobrane significantly reduces bacterial bioburden in full-thickness murine skin wounds. Further research will investigate whether this construct can be considered for human use.

▶ Infection of a burn wound leads to major morbidity, such as turning a superficial partial thickness burn into a much deeper thickness wound and dramatically increasing the time to complete healing. Thus, the use of antibacterial substances on dressings has become the mainstay of burn wound treatment to obviate infection. The use of biologic dressings shortens healing times and improves patient comfort, but there is still an appreciable wound infection rate. These authors sought to combine the efficacious properties of biologic dressings with a new approach to antibacterial treatment of open wounds by using silver bioactive particles impregnated in Biobrane. Previous in vitro studies found positive benefits in reducing bacterial counts using this material. This in vivo animal study found significantly reduced bacterial counts after use of the modified Biobrane compared with the control. Further studies are needed to determine safety and then test efficacy in humans.

J. M. Daly, MD

A Novel Autologous Cell-Based Therapy to Promote Diabetic Wound Healing

Castilla DM, Liu Z-J, Tian R, et al (Univ of Miami, FL)
Ann Surg 256:560-572, 2012

Objectives.—We have previously shown that stromal cell—derived factor-1α (SDF-1α) is downregulated within diabetic cutaneous wounds, and that direct application of recombinant SDF-1α increases wound closure rates, neovascularization, and endothelial progenitor cell (EPC) recruitment. However, increased wound levels of exogenous SDF-1α results in elevated systemic levels of this proangiogenic chemokine that raises concerns for tumorigenesis and inflammation. We now seek to test the efficacy of a novel, safer cell-based therapy (CBT) employing *ex vivo* primed bone marrow-derived stem cells (BMDSC) with SDF-1α. We also elucidate the mechanism of action of this new approach for accelerating diabetic wound healing.

Methods.—Unfractionated BMDSC from diabetic Lepr$^{db/db}$ mice were incubated for 20 hours with SDF-1α (100 ng/mL) or bovine serum albumin (control). Pretreated BMDSC (1 × 10) were injected subcutaneously into full-thickness skin wounds in Lepr$^{db/db}$ mice (n = 8 per group). Wound closure rates, capillary density, and the recruitment of EPC were assessed with serial photography, DiI perfusion, confocal microscopy, and immunohistochemistry. The expression of molecular targets, which may mediate prohealing/proangiogenic effects of SDF-1α—primed BMDSC was evaluated by polymerase chain reaction array and immunoblotting assay. The biological function of a potential mediator was tested in a mouse wound-healing model. Serum SDF-1α levels were measured with enzyme-linked immunosorbent assay (ELISA).

Results.—SDF-1α—primed BMDSC significantly promote wound healing (P < 0.0001), neovascularization (P = 0.0028), and EPC recruitment (P = 0.0059). Gene/protein expression studies demonstrate upregulation of Ephrin Receptor B4 and plasminogen as downstream targets potentially mediating the prohealing and proangiogenic responses. *Ex vivo* BMDSC activation and the subsequent inoculation of cells into wounds does not increase systemic SDF-1α levels.

Conclusions.—We report a novel CBT that is highly effective in promoting healing and neovascularization in a murine model of type 2 diabetes. Furthermore, we identify new molecular targets that may be important for advancing the field of wound healing.

▶ It is well known that wound healing is significantly impaired in diabetic patients. Investigators continue to seek the Holy Grail in finding the factor or factors that can be given locally or systemically to accelerate healing in diabetic subjects. Biochemical and mineral substances as well as growth factors have been applied in animal models, and many have been successful but with some drawbacks. The authors noted that stromal cell—derived growth factor-1α (SDF-1α) is diminished in diabetic skin wounds, and local application of SDF-1α increased local and systemic levels that might increase tumor cell growth or increase inflammation. Their cell-based approach is novel in that they were able to up-regulate bone marrow—derived stem cells (BMDSC) 4-fold after 20 hours' incubation with SDF-1α. When these cells were applied to cutaneous wounds in genetically diabetic mice, their wounds healed significantly faster than controls by measurement and by evaluating capillary ingrowth. In addition, they noted no increase in SDF-1α systemic levels. Thus, they found significant improvement in wound closure rates, epithelialization, numbers of endothelial progenitor cells, and capillary ingrowth in the SDF-1α—stimulated BMDSCs than with the nonprimed cells. This novel approach leads the way for other cell-based therapies to improve wound healing in diabetic subjects.

J. M. Daly, MD

4 Critical Care

Systematic review and meta-analysis of outcomes following emergency surgery for *Clostridium difficile* colitis
Bhangu A, on behalf of the West Midlands Research Collaborative (Queen Elizabeth Hosp, Edgbaston, Birmingham, UK)
Br J Surg 99:1501-1513, 2012

Background.—Only a small proportion of patients with severe *Clostridium difficile* infection (CDI) undergo emergency surgery, the timing and nature of which is unclear. The aim of this study was to describe the operations performed and to identify factors predictive of death following emergency surgery for CDI.

Methods.—A systematic review of published literature was performed for studies comparing survivors and non-survivors of emergency surgery for CDI. Meta-analysis was carried out for 30-day and in-hospital mortality.

Results.—Overall 31 studies were included, which presented data on a total of 1433 patients undergoing emergency surgery for CDI. Some $1 \cdot 1$ per cent of all patients with CDI and $29 \cdot 9$ per cent with severe CDI underwent emergency surgery, although rates varied between studies ($0 \cdot 2 - 7 \cdot 6$ and $2 \cdot 2 - 86$ per cent respectively). The most commonly performed operation was total colectomy with end ileostomy ($89 \cdot 0$ per cent, 1247 of 1401 detailed surgical procedures). When total colectomy with end ileostomy was not performed, reoperation to resect further bowel was needed in $15 \cdot 9$ per cent (20 of 126). Where described, the 30-day mortality rate was $41 \cdot 3$ per cent (160 of 387). Meta-analysis of high-quality studies revealed that the strongest predictors of postoperative death were those relating to preoperative physiological status: preoperative intubation, acute renal failure, multiple organ failure and shock requiring vasopressors.

Conclusion.—This systematic review supports total colectomy with end ileostomy as the primary surgical treatment for patients with severe CDI; other surgical procedures are associated with high rates of reoperation and mortality. Less extensive surgery may have a role in selected patients with earlier-stage disease.

▶ Establishing the standards of surgical care for patients who fail medical treatment for *Clostridium difficile* infection represents a significant challenge, because prospective, randomized trials are unlikely to be completed. Systematic review of small observational studies may provide the only clinical data to guide management.

This systematic review confirmed that postoperative mortality rates are high after surgery for *C. difficile* infection. It was also found that reoperation, defined as further bowel resection, may be expected in 15.9% of patients not undergoing total colectomy with end ileostomy at the first operative procedure. Certain preoperative physiological indicators, including shock requiring vasopressors, preoperative intubation, acute renal failure, and multiple organ failure, were identified as the most important identifiable predictors of postoperative death. Importantly, white blood cell count was not shown to be a significant predictor of death in patients undergoing emergency surgery. This systematic review supports total colectomy with end ileostomy as the primary surgical treatment in patients with severe disease, including multiple organ failure, because there is a high rate of reoperation coupled with a high risk of death following other surgical procedures. Less extensive surgery, such as loop ileostomy and colonic washout, may have a role in selected patients with earlier stage disease or impending organ failure. Comorbid illness and advanced age (over 75 years) have a significant influence on survival. A raised white blood cell count does not reliably predict survival in patients already selected for surgery.

D. W. Mozingo, MD

Arginine vasopressin: The future of pressure-support resuscitation in hemorrhagic shock
Anand T, Skinner R (Kern Med Ctr, Bakersfield, CA)
J Surg Res 178:321-329, 2012

Background.—Arginine vasopressin (AVP) is a key player in maintaining the intravascular volume and pressure during hemorrhagic shock. During the past 2 decades, animal studies, case reports, and reviews have documented the minimized blood loss and improved perfusion pressures in those receiving pressure support with AVP.

Materials and Methods.—A PubMed search of studies was conducted with the terms: "AVP," "arginine vasopressin," "antidiuretic hormone," "hemorrhagic shock," "hemorrhage," "circulatory shock," "fluid resuscitation," "trauma," "massive transfusion protocol," "physiology," "cerebral," "renal," "cardiac," "perfusion," "dose," and "hypotension." The studies were located by a search of a combination of these terms. Also, within-PubMed, citations relating to the studies gathered from the initial search were explored. Reports discussing vasopressin in hemorrhagic states were considered. No predetermined limit was used to choose or exclude articles.

Results.—AVP is an important hormone in osmoregulation and blood pressure. During stress, such as hemorrhage, the levels have been shown to rapidly decrease. Furthermore numerous animal studies and limited human studies have shown that circulatory support with AVP is linked to improved outcomes. No large human prospective studies are available to guide its use at present, but some of its effectiveness seems to lie in its ability to increase calcium sensitivity in acidotic environs, thereby allowing for more effective maintenance of vascular tone than catecholamines. It also redirects blood from the periphery, creating a steal syndrome, and increases the oxygen supply to vital organs, minimizing blood loss, and allowing additional time for surgical repair.

Conclusions.—With these encouraging data, there is hope that "pressure support" will be the "resuscitation" considered necessary for a patient's optimum survival.

▶ In this selection, the authors provide a comprehensive review of the literature regarding the use of arginine vasopressin in shock. There seems to be definite merit (considering the maintenance of perfusion by way of arginine vasopressin administration) in the fact that hemorrhaging patients might not require as many fluid and blood product infusions. The ultimate goal is effective vasoconstriction and robust maintenance of perfusion pressure to vital organs for these patients, and this must be pursued actively. Compared with adrenergic agents, arginine vasopressin is more responsive to vascular hyporeactivity in conditions of acidosis. The question regarding the dose and timing of administration remains unknown. The authors' recommendation is to consider studying/using a low-dose arginine vasopressin infusion early in resuscitation, before fluids, and definitely before the onset of the decompensatory phase of hemorrhagic shock. They purport that this will likely aid in maintaining perfusion pressure early and lead to calculated amounts of fluid, blood product, and pressor administration, which will hopefully lead to decreased secondary complications of massive fluid infusions.

D. W. Mozingo, MD

A standardized rapid sequence intubation protocol facilitates airway management in critically injured patients
Ballow SL, Kaups KL, Anderson S, et al (Univ of California, San Francisco-Fresno)
J Trauma Acute Care Surg 73:1401-1405, 2012

Background.—In the emergency department (ED) of a teaching hospital, rapid sequence intubation (RSI) is performed by physicians with a wide range of experience. A variety of medications have been used for RSI, with potential for inadequate or excessive dosing as well as complications including hypotension and the need for redosing. We hypothesized that the use of a standardized RSI medication protocol has facilitated endotracheal intubation requiring less medication redosing and less medication-related hypotension.

Methods.—An RSI medication protocol (ketamine 2 mg/kg intravenously administered and rocuronium 1 mg/kg intravenously administered, or succinylcholine 1.5 mg/kg intravenously administered) was implemented for all trauma patients undergoing ED intubation at a Level I trauma center. We retrospectively reviewed patients for the 1-year period before (PRE) and after (KET) the protocol was instituted. Data collected included age, sex,

Injury Severity Score (ISS), Abbreviated Injury Scale (AIS) score of the head/face, AIS score of the chest, RSI drugs, need for redosing, time to intubation, indication for RSI, and number of RSI attempts.

Results.—During the study period, 439 patients met inclusion criteria; 266 without protocol (PRE) and 173 with protocol (KET). Patients were severely injured with a mean ISS of 24 and median AIS score of the head/face of 3. Dosing in the KET group was appropriate with a mean dose of 1.9-mg/kg ketamine administered. Compliance after KET introduction approached 90%. Fifteen patients in the PRE group required redosing of medication versus three in the KET group ($p < 0.05$, χ^2). For patients younger than 14 years, (26 in PRE and 10 in KET), 2 patients in the PRE group required redosing and none in the KET group (not significant). In all patients, mean time from drug administration to intubation decreased from 4 minutes to 3 minutes.

Conclusion.—A standardized medication protocol simplifies RSI and allows efficient airway management of critically injured trauma patients in the ED of a teaching hospital. Incorporation of ketamine avoids potential complications of other commonly used RSI medications.

Level of Evidence.—Therapeutic study, level IV.

▶ The concept behind protocol-driven approaches is that routine clinical care is enhanced when interdisciplinary teams of health professionals use evidence-based protocols to complement their clinical judgment, thereby reducing unnecessary variations in practice. The rapid sequence intubation protocol described in the selection is a guideline with the intent to streamline intubation of trauma patients with the goal of having mediations readily available, reduce errors in dosing of medications, and achieve safe and efficient intubation. Many prospective trials have found that strategies using protocolized treatment by health care professionals can not only reduce variation and cost of medicine but also improve morbidity and mortality of critically ill patients. The use of a rapid sequence intubation protocol for intubation of trauma patients in the emergency department results in an increased efficiency and success. Having a single simple protocol that is appropriate for patients of all ages and types of injuries facilitates correct dosing and ease of drug administration. The use of ketamine as an induction agent is effective in both pediatric and adult trauma patients, including those with traumatic brain injury.

D. W. Mozingo, MD

Admission rapid thrombelastography predicts development of pulmonary embolism in trauma patients
Cotton BA, Minei KM, Radwan ZA, et al (The Univ of Texas Health Science Ctr, Houston)
J Trauma Acute Care Surg 72:1470-1477, 2012

Background.—Injury leads to dramatic disturbances in coagulation with increased risk of bleeding followed by a hypercoagulable state.

A comprehensive assessment of these coagulation abnormalities can be measured and described by thrombelastography. The purpose of this study was to identify whether admission rapid-thrombelastography (r-TEG) could identify patients at risk of developing pulmonary embolism (PE) during their hospital stay.

Methods.—Patients admitted between September 2009 to February 2011 who met criteria for our highest-level trauma activation and were transported directly from the scene were included in the study. PE defined as clinically suspected and computed tomography angiography confirmed PE. We evaluated r-TEG values with particular attention to the maximal amplitude (mA) parameter that is indicative of overall clot strength. Demographics, vital signs, injury severity, and r-TEG values were then evaluated. In addition to r-TEG values, gender and injury severity score (ISS) were chosen a priori for developing a multiple logistic regression model predicting development of PE.

Results.—r-TEG was obtained on 2,070 consecutive trauma activations. Of these, 2.5% (53) developed PE, 97.5% (2,017) did not develop PE. Patients in the PE group were older (median age, 41 vs. 33 years, $p = 0.012$) and more likely to be white (69% vs. 54%, $p = 0.036$). None of the patients in the PE group sustained penetrating injury (0% vs. 25% in the no-PE group, $p < 0.001$). The PE group also had admission higher mA values (66 vs. 63, $p = 0.050$) and higher ISS (median, 31 vs. 19, $p = 0.002$). When controlling for gender, race, age, and ISS, elevated mA at admission was an independent predictor of PE with an odds ratio of 3.5 for mA > 65 and 5.8 for mA > 72.

Conclusion.—Admission r-TEG mA values can identify patients with an increased risk of in-hospital PE. Further studies are needed to determine whether alternative anticoagulation strategies should be used for these high-risk patients.

Level of Evidence.—Prognostic study, level III.

▶ Despite increased aggressiveness in initiating chemoprophylaxis for venous thromboembolism (VTE) and more liberal use of vena cava filters, the incidence of pulmonary embolism (PE) in trauma patients continues to increase. Fortunately, there has been a simultaneous reduction in PE-related mortality. The source of these trends, both the increasing incidence and decreasing lethality, is likely the increased use of helical computed tomography. Despite this, postinjury PE remains a considerable burden, carrying with it an increased risk of mortality. In fact, the incidence of PE directly causing or contributing to death in hospitalized patients has remained at approximately 15% for the last 40 years. Admission rapid-thrombelastography using elevated maximal amplitude (mA) values, can identify patients with an increased risk of in-hospital PE. Compared with previous studies stratifying risk factors and those proposing algorithms for VTE prophylaxis, an admission mA value of greater than 65 mm portends a risk that exceeds those for high-risk factors, such as pelvic and lower extremity fractures, spinal cord injury, and severe head injury. Additionally, mA values exceeding 72 mm predict those patients noted to be at very high risk for PE.

82 / Surgery

Further studies are needed to determine whether alternative or more aggressive anticoagulation strategies should be used for these high-risk and very high-risk patients.

D. W. Mozingo, MD

Hydroxyethyl Starch or Saline for Fluid Resuscitation in Intensive Care
Myburgh JA, for the CHEST Investigators, Australian and New Zealand Intensive Care Society Clinical Trials Group (George Inst for Global Health, Sydney, New South Wales, Australia; et al)
N Engl J Med 367:1901-1911, 2012

Background.—The safety and efficacy of hydroxyethyl starch (HES) for fluid resuscitation have not been fully evaluated, and adverse effects of HES on survival and renal function have been reported.

Methods.—We randomly assigned 7000 patients who had been admitted to an intensive care unit (ICU) in a 1:1 ratio to receive either 6% HES with a molecular weight of 130 kD and a molar substitution ratio of 0.4 (130/0.4, Voluven) in 0.9% sodium chloride or 0.9% sodium chloride (saline) for all fluid resuscitation until ICU discharge, death, or 90 days after randomization. The primary outcome was death within 90 days. Secondary outcomes included acute kidney injury and failure and treatment with renal-replacement therapy.

Results.—A total of 597 of 3315 patients (18.0%) in the HES group and 566 of 3336 (17.0%) in the saline group died (relative risk in the HES group, 1.06; 95% confidence interval [CI], 0.96 to 1.18; P = 0.26). There was no significant difference in mortality in six predefined subgroups. Renal-replacement therapy was used in 235 of 3352 patients (7.0%) in the HES group and 196 of 3375 (5.8%) in the saline group (relative risk, 1.21; 95% CI, 1.00 to 1.45; P = 0.04). In the HES and saline groups, renal injury occurred in 34.6% and 38.0% of patients, respectively (P = 0.005), and renal failure occurred in 10.4% and 9.2% of patients, respectively (P = 0.12). HES was associated with significantly more adverse events (5.3% vs. 2.8%, P < 0.001).

Conclusions.—In patients in the ICU, there was no significant difference in 90-day mortality between patients resuscitated with 6% HES (130/0.4) or saline. However, more patients who received resuscitation with HES were treated with renal-replacement therapy. (Funded by the National Health and Medical Research Council of Australia and others; CHEST ClinicalTrials.gov number, NCT00935168.)

▶ In this article, one of the main reasons the authors cited for conducting this study was to determine whether currently used hydroxyethyl starch solutions increased the risk of acute kidney injury in intensive care unit (ICU) patients. They demonstrated that resuscitation with hydroxyethyl starch resulted in a 21% relative increase in the number of patients treated with renal-replacement therapy. Criteria for the initiation of renal replacement therapy were not controlled by the protocol, and therapy was initiated at the discretion of the attending physicians. The clinicians were unaware of study group assignments, making it unlikely that the difference was caused by variations in thresholds for initiating therapy. The RIFLE (risk, injury to kidney, failure, loss of kidney function, end-stage kidney disease) score is a composite endpoint measure that combines effects on serum creatinine levels and urine output. In this study, the use of hydroxyethyl starch had opposite effects on the 2 components of this score, as compared with saline. Their post hoc analysis showed that treatment with hydroxyethyl starch was associated with increased urine output in patients with less severe acute kidney injury, which may have been caused by increased intravascular volume or through a diuretic effect. Conversely, serum creatinine levels were consistently higher in the hydroxyethyl starch group, suggesting a progressive reduction in creatinine clearance and more severe acute kidney injury. Fig 3 in the original article demonstrates this finding. This study failed to identify any clinical benefit related to the use of hydroxyethyl starch for resuscitation in ICU patients compared with saline.

D. W. Mozingo, MD

Acute kidney injury is associated with increased in-hospital mortality in mechanically ventilated children with trauma

Prodhan P, McCage LS, Stroud MH, et al (Univ of Arkansas Med Sciences, Little Rock; Univ of Texas Med Branch at Galveston)
J Trauma Acute Care Surg 73:832-837, 2012

Background.—Acute kidney injury (AKI) is associated with significant morbidity and mortality in patients with critical illness; however, its impact on children with trauma is not fully unexplored. We hypothesized that AKI is associated with increased in-hospital mortality.

Methods.—A retrospective review of consecutive mechanically ventilated patients aged 0 years to 20 years from 2004 to 2007 with trauma hospitalized at our institution was performed. Univariate and multivariate analyses were performed to identify whether AKI was a risk factor for hospital mortality.

Results.—Eighty-eight patients met inclusion/exclusion criteria. The study cohort included 58 (66%) males with mean (SD) age of 11.6 (5.5) years (median, 13.25; range, 0.083−19.42 years) and mean (SD) Pediatric Expanded Logical Organ Dysfunction score of 24 (11) (median, 22; range 2−51). Mean pediatric intensive care unit length of stay (median, 11; range, 4−43) and duration of mechanical ventilation (median, 9; range, 3−34), was 13.5 (8.2) days and 11.2 (7.2) days, respectively. The mean (SD) Injury Severity Score for the cohort was 28 (14). Pediatric RIFLE identified those at risk (R), those with injury (I), or those with failure (F) in 30 (51%), 10 (17%), and 12 (21%) patients, respectively. There was a 10% (3 of 30 patients) mortality rate in those at risk, 30% (3 of 10 patients) in those with injury, and 33% (4 of 12 patients) in those with failure. AKI (injury and failure groups) was significantly associated with increased in-hospital mortality.

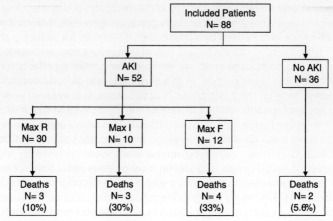

FIGURE 1.—Number of deaths in study cohort according to pRIFLE criteria based groups. (Reprinted from Prodhan P, McCage LS, Stroud MH, et al. Acute kidney injury is associated with increased in-hospital mortality in mechanically ventilated children with trauma. *J Trauma Acute Care Surg.* 2012;73:832-837, with permission from Lippincott Williams & Wilkins.)

TABLE 1.—pRIFLE Criteria

	eCCL	UOP
Risk	eCCL decreased by 25%	<0.5 mL/kg/h for 8 h
Injury	eCCL decreased by 50%	<0.5 mL/kg/h for 16 h
Failure	eCCL decreased by 75% or eCCL <35mL/min/1.73 m^2	<0.5 mL/kg/h for 24 h or anuric for 12 h

Conclusion.—Development of AKI (injury or failure) is a significant risk factor associated with in-hospital mortality. Our study highlights the need to consider both urine output as well as creatinine-based components of the pRIFLE criteria to define AKI.

Level of Evidence.—Prognostic and epidemiological study, level II (Fig 1, Table 1).

▶ In this article the authors report that acute kidney injury is associated with increased in-hospital mortality, intensive care unit days, and hospital stay in pediatric patients with critical illness trauma. A novel finding in their study not previously reported is the importance of the urinary output criteria in defining acute kidney injury in their study patients. Also, in two-thirds of the study patients, the maximum pediatric RIFLE (risk, injury to kidney, failure, loss of kidney function, end-stage kidney disease) criteria were achieved early in the hospital course (within the first 48 hours after admission). Pediatric RIFLE criteria facilitate identification of patients with critical illness who are at risk for acute kidney injury, which may allow for earlier initiation of both preventive and therapeutic renal protective strategies. As evidenced by this investigation, particular attention should be paid to the pediatric RIFLE urinary output criteria for patients with trauma because this identified a large number of patients with acute kidney injury who would have otherwise been missed when using only the creatinine clearance criteria. Table 1 and Fig 1 define the pediatric RIFLE criteria and categorize patient outcomes, respectively.

D. W. Mozingo, MD

Venous thromboembolism after trauma: A never event?
Thorson CM, Ryan ML, Van Haren RM, et al (Univ of Miami Miller School of Medicine, FL)
Crit Care Med 40:2967-2973, 2012

Objective.—Rates of venous thromboembolism as high as 58% have been reported after trauma, but there is no widely accepted screening protocol. If Medicare adds venous thromboembolism to the list of "preventable complications," they will no longer reimburse for treatment, which could have devastating effects on many urban centers. We hypothesized that prescreening with a risk assessment profile followed by routine surveillance with venous duplex ultrasound that could identify asymptomatic venous thromboembolism in trauma patients.

Design.—Prospective, observational trial with waiver of consent.

Setting.—Level I trauma center intensive care unit.

Patients.—At admission, 534 patients were prescreened with a risk assessment profile.

Interventions.—Patients (n = 106) with risk assessment profile scores >10 were considered high risk and received routine screening venous duplex ultrasound within 24 hrs and weekly thereafter.

Results.—In prescreened high-risk patients, 20 asymptomatic deep vein thrombosis were detected with venous duplex ultrasound (19%). An additional ten venous thromboembolisms occurred, including six symptomatic deep vein thrombosis and four pulmonary emboli, resulting in an overall venous thromboembolism rate of 28%. The most common risk factors discriminating venous thromboembolism vs. no venous thromboembolism were femoral central venous catheter (23% vs. 8%), operative intervention >2 hrs (77% vs. 46%), complex lower extremity fracture (53% vs. 32%), and pelvic fracture (70% vs. 47%), respectively (all $p < .05$). Risk assessment profile scores were higher in patients with venous thromboembolism (19 ± 6 vs. 14 ± 4, $p = .001$). Risk assessment profile score (odds ratio 1.14) and the combination of pelvic fracture requiring operative intervention >2 hrs (odds ratio 5.75) were independent predictors for development of venous thromboembolism. The rates of venous thromboembolism for no chemical prophylaxis (33%), unfractionated heparin (29%), dalteparin (40%), or inferior vena cava filters (20%) were not statistically different ($p = .764$).

Conclusions.—Medicare's inclusion of venous thromboembolism after trauma as a "never event" should be questioned. In trauma patients, high-risk assessment profile score and pelvic fracture with prolonged operative

TABLE 2.—Demographics in Venous Thromboembolism Versus No Venous Thromboembolism

	No Venous Thromboembolism (n = 76)	Venous Thromboembolism (n = 30)	p
Age	47 ± 20	45 ± 19	.615
Gender, n (%) male	21 (28%)	7 (23%)	.651
Mechanism, n (%) blunt	61 (80%)	23 (77%)	.681
Emergent operative intervention, n (%)	23 (77%)	57 (75%)	.857
Injury Severity Score	30 ± 13	28 ± 11	.558
Outcomes			
Hospital length of stay, days	27 (43)	48 (39)	.088
Intensive care unit length of stay, days	17 (28)	20 (33)	.443
Mortality, n (%)	14 (18%)	1 (3%)	.062

Data are mean ± SD or median (interquartile range).

intervention are independent predictors for venous thromboembolism development, despite thromboprophylaxis. Although routine venous duplex ultrasound screening may not be cost-effective for all trauma patients, pre-screening using risk assessment profile yielded a cohort of patients with a high prevalence of venous thromboembolism. In such high-risk patients, routine venous duplex ultrasound and/or more aggressive prophylactic regimens may be beneficial (Table 2).

▶ The objectives of this study were to prospectively prescreen trauma patients with a risk assessment profile, to use surveillance venous Doppler ultrasound to screen for the occurrence of venous thromboembolism, and to identify risk factors for venous thromboembolism in this population. The authors hypothesized that prescreening would identify a cohort at highest risk for venous thromboembolism. They found that the performance of serial venous Doppler ultrasounds on patients with high-risk assessment profile scores identified a population at significant risk for venous thromboembolism. Two factors—risk assessment profile score and combination of pelvic fracture with prolonged operative intervention—were independently predictive for the development of venous thromboembolism after trauma. Table 2 demonstrates the influence of combinations of these risk factors on the development of venous thromboembolism. Development of venous thromboembolism is a complex multifactorial process, and more research is needed to elucidate additional markers of hypercoagulability and risk factors for venous thromboembolism development. Nonetheless, the inclusion of venous thromboembolism after trauma as a never event should be questioned.

D. W. Mozingo, MD

Surrogate and patient discrepancy regarding consent for critical care research

Newman JT, Smart A, Reese TR, et al (Univ of Colorado School of Medicine, Aurora; et al)
Crit Care Med 40:2590-2594, 2012

Objective.—Critically ill patients frequently display impaired decision-making capacity due to their underlying illness and the use of sedating medications. Healthcare providers often rely on surrogates to make decisions for medical care and participation in clinical research. However, the accuracy of surrogate decisions for a variety of critical care research studies is poorly understood.

Design.—Cross-sectional observational study.

Setting.—Academic medical center.

Patients.—Medical intensive care unit patients and their designated surrogates.

Intervention.—Patients were asked whether they would consent to participate in hypothetical research studies of increasing complexity, and surrogates independently indicated whether they would consent to enroll the patient in the same scenarios.

Results.—Overall, 69 medical intensive care unit patients were enrolled into the study. The majority of surrogates were either the spouse (58%) or parent (22%) of the patient. The percentage of patients that would agree to participate in a research study and the percentage of surrogates that would agree to have the patient enrolled into a research study both declined as the risk of the study increased ($p < .001$ for both analyses). In addition, the overall discrepancy, the false-negative rates, and the false-positive rates between patient and surrogates were greater as the risk of the study increased ($p < .001$, $p < .001$, and $p = .049$, respectively). κ values for all seven scenarios demonstrated less-than-moderate agreement (range 0.03–0.41).

Conclusions.—There are significant discrepancies in the willingness to participate in various types of clinical research proposals between critically ill patients and their surrogate decision makers. The results of this study

TABLE 4.—Predictive Values of Surrogate Decision Making with 95% Confidence Intervals

	Positive Predictive Value of Surrogate	Negative Predictive Value of Surrogate
Collection of medical information	96% (91–100%)	100%
Collection of urine	80% (70–90%)	0%
Collection of blood	76% (65–87%)	29% (18–40%)
Computed tomography scan	72% (61–83%)	65% (54–76%)
Muscle biopsy	45% (33–57%)	65% (54–76%)
Bronchoalveolar lavage while intubated	61% (50–72%)	64% (53–75)%
Clinical trial	50% (38–62%)	56% (44–68%)

raise concerns about the use of surrogate consent for inclusion of critically ill patients into research protocols (Table 4).

▶ Surrogates are commonly approached to make medical decisions for critically ill patients who have impaired decisional capacity. This study found that surrogates often make inaccurate decisions regarding the enrollment of patients in a variety of hypothetical critical care research studies. The authors also identified that the discrepancy between the patient and surrogate increased in association with the perceived risk of the research study. Obtaining informed consent, particularly using surrogates, is complex and involves many factors that make it difficult to develop simple or straightforward improvements in the process. In this study, for example, if surrogates were relied on to enroll patients in studies involving a muscle biopsy, the patient's wishes would have been violated nearly one-fourth of the time. The contributing factors and values that influence surrogate consent decisions remain poorly understood. Using the decision of the patient as the gold standard and decision of the surrogate as the diagnostic test, the positive and negative predictive values for each of the 7 scenarios evaluated in this study are displayed in Table 4, which is included in this selection.

D. W. Mozingo, MD

Systemic inflammation worsens outcomes in emergency surgical patients
Becher RD, Hoth JJ, Miller PR, et al (Wake Forest Univ School of Medicine, Winston-Salem, NC)
J Trauma Acute Care Surg 72:1140-1149, 2012

Background.—Acute care surgeons are uniquely aware of the importance of systemic inflammatory response and its influence on postoperative outcomes; concepts like damage control have evolved from this experience. For surgeons whose practice is mostly elective, the significance of such systemic inflammation may be underappreciated. This study sought to determine the influence of preoperative systemic inflammation on postoperative outcome in patients requiring emergent colon surgery.

Methods.—Emergent colorectal operations were identified in the American College of Surgeons National Surgical Quality Improvement Program 2008 dataset. Four groups were defined by the presence and magnitude of the inflammatory response before operation: no inflammation, systemic inflammatory response syndrome (SIRS), sepsis, or severe sepsis/septic shock. Thirty-day survival was analyzed by Kaplan-Meier method.

Results.—A total of 3,305 patients were identified. Thirty-day survival was significantly different ($p < 0.0001$) among the four groups; increasing magnitudes of preoperative inflammation had increasing probability of mortality ($p < 0.0001$). Hazard ratios indicated that, compared with patients without preoperative systemic inflammation, the relative risk of death from SIRS was 1.9 ($p < 0.0001$), from sepsis was 2.5 ($p < 0.0001$), and from severe sepsis/septic shock was 6.7 ($p < 0.0001$). Operative time

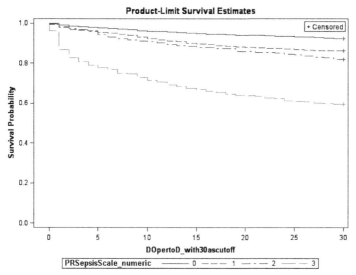

FIGURE.—Kaplan-Meier survival probability curves by degree of preoperative inflammation. Survival probability on vertical axis; days from operation to death on horizontal axis. 0, no inflammation; 1, systemic inflammatory response syndrome (SIRS); 2, sepsis; 3, severe sepsis and/or septic shock. (Reprinted from Becher RD, Hoth JJ, Miller PR, et al. Systemic inflammation worsens outcomes in emergency surgical patients. *J Trauma Acute Care Surg.* 2012;72:1140-1149, with permission from Lippincott Williams & Wilkins.)

of <150 minutes was associated with decreased risk of morbidity (odds ratio = 0.64; $p < 0.0001$).

Conclusions.—Upregulation of the systemic inflammatory response is the primary contributor to death in emergency surgical patients. In SIRS or sepsis patients, operations < 2.5 hours are associated with fewer postoperative complications. These results further reinforce the concept of timely surgical intervention and suggest a potential role for damage control operations in emergency general surgery (Fig).

▶ The authors of this selection aim to define and quantify the risks of mortality associated with increasing severity of preoperative systemic inflammation in patients requiring emergent colorectal surgery and to identify the operating time associated with the lowest risk of postoperative complications in this patient population. The hypothesis was that increasing degrees of preoperative inflammation would be associated with increasing levels of mortality and that shorter operating times would be associated with decreased morbidity and mortality. Their results definitively establish that preoperative systemic inflammation is a key predictor of mortality in emergency surgical patients and that increasing degrees of preoperative inflammation are associated with increasing levels of mortality. The figure is included showing this finding. In patients with systemic inflammatory response syndrome and sepsis, operations lasting longer than 2.5 hours are associated with greater postoperative morbidity but not mortality. These results further reinforce the concept of timely surgical intervention and potentially suggest a role for damage control operations in emergency surgical patients.

D. W. Mozingo, MD

Predictors of critical care-related complications in colectomy patients using the National Surgical Quality Improvement Program: Exploring frailty and aggressive laparoscopic approaches
Obeid NM, Azuh O, Reddy S, et al (Henry Ford Hosp, Detroit, MI; Cottage Health System, Santa Barbara, CA; et al)
J Trauma Acute Care Surg 72:878-883, 2012

Background.—Colectomy patients experience a broad set of adverse outcomes. Complications requiring critical care support are common in this group. We hypothesized that as frailty increases, the risk of Clavien class IV and V complications will increase in colectomy patients.

Methods.—Using the National Surgical Quality Improvement Program (NSQIP) participant use files for 2005-2009, we identified patients who underwent laparoscopic and open colectomies by Current Procedural Terminology code. Using the Clavien classification for postoperative complications, we identified NSQIP data points most consistent with Clavien class IV requiring intensive care unit (ICU) care or class V complications (death). We used a modified frailty index with 11 variables based on mapping the Canadian Study of Health and Aging Frailty Index and existing NSQIP variables. Logistic regression was performed to acuity adjust the findings.

Results.—A total of 58,448 colectomies were identified. As frailty index increased from 0 to 0.55, the proportion of those experiencing Clavien class IV or V complications increased from 3.2% at baseline to 56.3%. Variables

---

TABLE 4.—Frailty Index as a Predictor of Postoperative Complications

Frailty Index	N	Emergency Case	All Postoperative Complications	All Wound Infections	Clavien Class IV or V Complication	Mortality (Clavien V)
0	22,630	2,675 (11.8%)	4,492 (19.8%)	3,718 (16.4%)	718 (3.2%)	164 (0.7%)
0.09	18,258	2,711 (14.8%)	4,507 (24.7%)	3,673 (20.1%)	1,382 (7.6%)	491 (2.7%)
0.18	10,059	2,265 (22.5%)	3,266 (32.5%)	2,628 (26.1%)	1,474 (14.7%)	690 (6.9%)
0.27	4,464	1,558 (34.9%)	1,871 (41.9%)	1,432 (32.1%)	1,143 (25.6%)	633 (14.2%)
0.36	1,899	828 (43.6%)	933 (49.1%)	720 (37.9%)	643 (33.9%)	371 (19.5%)
0.45	769	442 (57.5%)	440 (57.2%)	324 (42.1%)	344 (44.7%)	217 (28.2%)
0.55	272	185 (68%)	149 (54.8%)	105 (38.6%)	153 (56.3%)	105 (38.6%)
0.64	81	54 (66.7%)	50 (61.7%)	37 (45.7%)	48 (59.3%)	35 (43.2%)
0.73	12	11 (91.7%)	8 (66.7%)	5 (41.7%)	6 (50%)	3 (25%)
0.82	3	2 (66.7%)	1 (33.3%)	0	2 (66.7%)	2 (66.7%)
0.91	1	1 (100%)	0	0	0	0
Total	58,448	10,732	15,717 (26.9%)	12,462	5,913 (10.1%)	2,711 (4.6%)
p		<0.001	<0.001	<0.001	<0.001	<0.001

Percentages indicate proportion within frailty index group.

found to be significant by logistic regression (odds ratio) were frailty index (14.4; $p = 0.001$), open procedure (2.35; $p < 0.001$), and American Society of Anesthesiologists class 4 (3.2; $p = 0.038$) or 5 (7.1; $p = 0.001$) while emergency operation and wound classification 3 or 4 were not.

Conclusions.—Complications requiring ICU care represent a significant morbidity in the colectomy patient population. Frailty index seems to be an important predictor of ICU-level complications and death, and laparoscopy seems to be protective (Table 4).

▶ Studies to predict postoperative morbidity and mortality increasingly have included frailty as a variable. Much effort has been concentrated on developing a standardized measure for a patient's physiologic reserve, which can then serve as a predictor of postoperative complications. Several reports have found an association between frailty and increased morbidity and prolonged postoperative recovery. The authors of this selection hypothesized that use of a modified frailty index in colectomy patients would be predictive of intensive care unit—level complications and postoperative mortality. This retrospective study was performed using the National Surgical Quality Improvement Program dataset. The variables for the frailty index included (1) nonindependent functional status; (2) history of diabetes mellitus; (3) history of either chronic obstructive pulmonary disease or pneumonia; (4) history of congestive heart failure; (5) history of myocardial infarction; (6) history of percutaneous coronary intervention, cardiac surgery, or angina; (7) hypertension requiring the use of medications; (8) peripheral vascular disease or rest pain; (9) impaired sensorium; (10) transient ischemic attack or cerebrovascular accident without residual deficit; and (11) cerebrovascular accident with deficit. The frailty index was then calculated as the proportion of the total number of variables present in the patient's medical history from the 11 total items measured. Table 4 shows the impact of increasing frailty on serious complications. The authors also identified that increasing frailty, American Society of Anesthesiologists class of 4 or 5, and an open colectomy approach resulted in increased patient mortality. They identified a significant trend of increasing frailty in influencing the outcome of colectomy with respect to Clavien IV and V complications. The acuity of these complications and the associated increased length of stay infer a prolonged recovery course and may have serious clinical implications.

D. W. Mozingo, MD

Early albumin use improves mortality in difficult to resuscitate burn patients
Park SH, Hemmila MR, Wahl WL (Univ of Michigan Health System, Ann Arbor)
J Trauma Acute Care Surg 73:1294-1297, 2012

Background.—The optimal resuscitation algorithm remains elusive for patients with a large burn injury. Recent reports from the military support that larger burns that do not respond well to ongoing lactated Ringer's solution resuscitation may improve with the use of 5% albumin and vasopressors. We hypothesized that the use of 5% albumin and vasopressors,

TABLE 2.—Outcomes and Complications

Variable	Preprotocol	Postprotocol	p
n	98	61	
Mortality, n (%)	26 (26)	5 (10)	<0.01
No. ventilator days, mean ± SD	20 ± 30	10 ± 11	<0.05
PaO$_2$/FIO$_2$ ratio at 24 h, mean ± SD	247 ± 112	289 ± 06	<0.05
Admission PaO$_2$/FIO$_2$ <200, n (%)	27 (38)	13 (30)	NS
VAP, n (%)	40 (41)	12 (19)	<0.01
Length of stay, mean ± SD, d	29 ± 30	32 ± 35	NS
Length of stay per % TBS burn, mean ± SD, d	0.8 ± 0.7	0.9 ± 0.6	NS
ACS, n (%)	10 (10)	2 (3)	0.056
ACS exploratory laparotomy, n (%)	6 (6)	0	<0.05
Any escharotomy, n (%)	21 (21)	10 (16)	NS
Hemodialysis, n (%)	5 (5)	2 (4)	NS

as needed, would decrease complications of fluid resuscitation and burn mortality.

Methods.—Fluid needs during the first 24 hours after burn injury, complications, and demographics were collected from all patients 12 years and older with burn size 20% or more of total body surface area admitted from 2003 to 2010. In March 2007, we changed our resuscitation to include the use of 5% albumin in the first 24 hours if the estimated fluid needs at 12 hours after burn would lead to a fluid volume of 6 mL/kg per percent burn at 24 hours. The patients treated before this change (Preprotocol) were compared with those treated after the guideline change (Postprotocol).

Results.—The two groups were well matched for age, burn size, and inhalation injury. Ventilator days and mortality were decreased in the Postprotocol group. There was a trend toward less intravenous fluid use in the Postprotocol group where the use of albumin was higher. There was significantly less vasopressor infusion in the Postprotocol group. There was no statistical difference in the number of escharotomies performed or overall incidence of abdominal compartment syndrome, but no patient required open laparotomy in the Postprotocol group.

Conclusion.—An algorithm incorporating albumin use in the first 24 hours after burn injury was associated with the use of less vasopressor agents and lower mortality. Early albumin use was also associated with a shorter duration of mechanical ventilation in burn patients sustaining burns 20% or more total body surface area.

Level of Evidence.—Therapeutic study, level IV (Table 2).

▶ Initial fluid resuscitation remains a difficult challenge for patients with large surface area burns. Since the introduction of intravenous fluid resuscitation for burn injuries, the rate and type of fluids have been debated. In this article, the authors initiated albumin infusion by protocol at 12 hours postburn when fluid administration was predicted to exceed 6 mL/kg per percentage of total burn surface area. Although this study reflects the outcomes of only 1 burn center with a limited number of large burns, there were significant improvements in important outcomes, including mortality, mechanical ventilator use, ventilator-associated pneumonia rates, and need for open laparotomy for treatment of abdominal compartment syndrome. Table 2 highlights these findings. The relatively small number of patients in the study may have made detection of differences in overall fluid use and abdominal compartment syndrome difficult to obtain; however, the trends were in a favorable direction. The use of 5% albumin and vasopressors as needed for patients deemed difficult to resuscitate seems beneficial, but further study in a larger patient population could define the advantages of this approach.

D. W. Mozingo, MD

A novel sponge-based wound stasis dressing to treat lethal noncompressible hemorrhage
Mueller GR, Pineda TJ, Xie HX, et al (Oregon Med Laser Ctr, Portland; Oregon Biomedical Engineering Inst, Portland; et al)
J Trauma Acute Care Surg 73:S134-S139, 2012

Background.—Noncompressible hemorrhage is the leading cause of preventable death caused by hemorrhage on the battlefield. Currently, there are no hemostatic agents with the ability to control noncompressible hemorrhage. A wound stasis dressing based upon rapidly expanding cellulose minisponges (MS) was developed and tested in a lethal noncompressible model in swine, by fully transecting subclavian artery and vein. MS were compared with conventional hemostasis dressings, Combat Gauze (CG), in a randomized comparison.

Methods.—Sixteen 40-kg swine underwent transection of the subclavian artery and vein through a 4.5-cm aperture. After 30-second free bleeding, randomly selected MS or CG (n = 8 per group) were administered by an independent medical officer. The wound cavity was filled with either MS + no external pressure or one CG + one KERLIX gauze with 3 minutes of external pressure. One reapplication was allowed for CG. Mean arterial pressure was maintained at 60 mm Hg with 500-mL Hextend and lactated Ringer's solution intravenously administered up to a maximum of 10-L until study termination at 1 hour.

Results.—Mean pretreatment blood loss was similar for MS (719 mL) and CG (702 mL). Primary end points, namely, hemostasis at 4 minutes (MS, 75%; CG, 25%; $p = 0.13$), hemostasis at 60 minutes (MS, 100%; CG, 25%; $p = 0.007$), and survival at 60 minutes (MS, 100%; CG, 37.5%; $p = 0.026$), were improved with MS as were secondary end points, namely, total blood loss (MS, 118 mL; CG 1,242 mL; $p = 0.021$) and length of application time (MS, 25 seconds; CG, 420 seconds; $p = 0.004$).

Conclusion.—The use of MS is a novel approach for the rapid, simple treatment of severe noncompressible hemorrhage, which provided statistically significant improvement in hemostasis and survival 60 minutes after injury and a large reduction in blood loss, resuscitation fluid requirement, and medic treatment time compared with conventional hemorrhage control dressings in a swine model.

▶ Lethal hemorrhage from large vessel battlefield injuries continues to beset military medicine. In addition, this problem occurs all too frequently in urban areas with individuals shot multiple times with large-caliber weapons. Immediate treatment with compression or tourniquets can be lifesaving, but often the anatomical site of the injury does not lend itself to this form of therapy. The use of rapidly expanding cellulose minisponges is a novel mechanism to stop hemorrhage when compression may not work. This animal study used a lethal subclavian injury model in swine and demonstrated significantly better hemorrhage control compared with standard compression dressings. The authors have also demonstrated a new application device for these minisponges that could be applied to humans in battlefield conditions.

It would be interesting to understand the longer term consequences of these cellulose sponges remaining in place in organs such as the liver, for example. However, clearly, these are for short-term, life-saving events. The authors should be complimented for this novel approach.

J. M. Daly, MD

5 Wound Healing

Primary Versus Secondary Closure of Cutaneous Abscesses in the Emergency Department: A Randomized Controlled Trial
Singer AJ, Taira BR, Chale S, et al (Stony Brook Univ, NY; et al)
Acad Emerg Med 20:27-32, 2013

Objectives.—Cutaneous abscesses have traditionally been treated with incision and drainage (I&D) and left to heal by secondary closure. The objective was to compare the healing rates of cutaneous abscesses following I&D after primary or secondary closure.

Methods.—This was a randomized, controlled, trial, balanced by center, with blocked randomization created by a random-number generator. One urban and one suburban academic emergency department (ED) participated. Subjects were randomized to primary or secondary wound closure following I&D of the abscess. Main outcome measures were the percentage of healed wounds (wound was completely closed by visual inspection; a 40% difference in wound healing was sought) and overall failure rate (need for additional intervention including suture removal, additional drainage, antibiotics, or admission within 7 days after drainage).

Results.—Fifty-six adult patients with simple localized cutaneous abscesses were included; 29 were randomized to primary closure, and 27 were randomized to secondary closure. Healing rates at 7 days were similar between the primary and secondary closure groups (69.6%, 95% confidence interval [CI] = 49.1% to 84.4% vs. 59.3%, 95% CI = 40.7% to 75.5%; difference 10.3%, 95% CI = −15.8% to 34.1%). Overall failure rates at 7 days were also similar between the primary and secondary closure groups (30.4%, 95% CI = 15.6% to 50.9% vs. 28.6%, 95% CI = 15.2% to 47.1%; difference 1.8%, 95% CI = −24.2% to 28.8%).

Conclusions.—The rates of wound healing and treatment failure following I&D of simple abscesses in the ED are similar after primary or secondary closure. The authors did not detect a difference of at least 40% in healing rates between primary and secondary closure.

▶ For centuries, the treatment of cutaneous abscesses has been to perform drainage and then allow the wound to close secondarily. A variety of irrigation solutions and packing materials have been touted to accelerate the healing process. Few have recommended primary closure after drainage. This prospective, randomized trial proposed to study this very question. Interestingly, patients randomly assigned to primary closure after drainage of cutaneous abscesses did as well as those in whom secondary closure was used. Failure rates at 7 days were quite high—30% vs 51% in the primary closure vs secondary closure groups, respectively. The authors suggested a difference of 40% in wound healing rates and complications when they designed the study and included only a total of 56 patients. Thus, the study was underpowered to detect a smaller difference and should have included a greater number of patients perhaps using more institutions. It is a positive thing that both urban and suburban hospitals were study centers. Given these results, it would be important to repeat the study using more hospitals to provide certainty as to future treatment of cutaneous abscesses.

J. M. Daly, MD

Wound Healing after Open Appendectomies in Adult Patients: A Prospective, Randomised Trial Comparing Two Methods of Wound Closure
Kotaluoto S, Pauniaho S-L, Helminen M, et al (Tampere Univ Hosp, Finland; Tampere Univ and Univ Hosp, Finland; Pirkanmaa Hosp District, Tampere, Finland)
World J Surg 36:2305-2310, 2012

Background.—The skin is closed in open appendectomy traditionally with few interrupted nonabsorbable sutures. The use of this old method is based on a suggestion that this technique decreases wound infections. In pediatric surgery, skin closure with running intradermal absorbable sutures has been found to be as safe as nonabsorbable sutures, even in complicated cases. Our purpose was to compare the safety of classic interrupted nonabsorbable skin closure to continuous intradermal absorbable sutures in appendectomy wounds in adult patients.

Methods.—A total of 206 adult patients with clinically suspected appendicitis were allocated to the study and prospectively randomized into two groups of wound closure: the interrupted nonabsorbable (NA) suture and the intradermal continuous absorbable (A) suture group. Primary wound healing was controlled on the first postoperative day, at 1 week clinically and after 2 weeks by means of a telephone interview. Follow-up data were obtained from 185 patients (90 in group NA and 95 in group A).

Results.—Continuous absorbable intradermal suturing was as safe as nonabsorbable sutures in regard to wound infections.

Conclusion.—Continuous, absorbable sutures can be used safely even in complicated appendicectomies without increasing the risk of wound infection. Considering the benefits of absorbable suturing, we recommend this method in all open appendectomies.

▶ Appendectomy for acute appendicitis results in a clean contaminated or contaminated wound. Thus, many forms of wound closure have been used to obviate the risk of postoperative wound infection. This prospective, randomized trial evaluated continuous absorbable suture closure vs interrupted nonabsorbable suture as a technique of skin/wound closure. Evaluation of wound complications was done at 1 week clinically (nurse, resident, attending physician) and by telephone interview. It is presumed that all wound infectious complications would present themselves by at least 2 weeks, although some declare themselves after this period. No significant differences in wound infectious and other complications were noted comparing the 2 groups. As the authors noted, the use of continuous absorbable suture technique is easier on the patient. Given the results of this trial, continuous nonabsorbable suture technique should become the gold standard after uncomplicated appendectomy.

J. M. Daly, MD

Exercise Speeds Cutaneous Wound Healing in High-Fat Diet-Induced Obese Mice

Pence BD, Dipietro LA, Woods JA (Univ of Illinois at Urbana-Champaign; Univ of Illinois at Chicago)
Med Sci Sports Exerc 44:1846-1854, 2012

Purpose.—Obesity has been shown to impair cutaneous wound healing, which is associated with increased wound inflammation. Exercise is known to decrease obesity-associated inflammation and has been shown to speed cutaneous wound healing in aged mice. Therefore, we investigated whether treadmill exercise could speed cutaneous wound healing in obese, high-fat diet-fed mice.

Methods.—We fed female C57Bl/6J mice a high-fat diet (45% calories from fat) for 16 wk to induce a state of obesity and insulin resistance. Mice then ran on a treadmill for 3 d before excisional wounding. On day 4, mice were wounded 1 h after exercise. Mice then exercised for 5 d after wounding, and healing was assessed by photoplanimetry for 10 d.

Results.—As described previously, obesity impaired wound healing, with significantly larger wound sizes measured from days 3 to day 10 after wounding ($P < 0.05$). Exercise did not improve healing in lean mice fed a normal chow diet. However, wound size was significantly smaller in exercised obese mice compared with their lean counterparts ($P < 0.05$ at day 1, day 4, and day 5 after wound). Surprisingly, we were unable to detect any differences in gene or protein expression of proinflammatory cytokines interleukin-1β and tumor necrosis factor-α or the anti-inflammatory cytokine interleukin-10 in the wounds. Likewise, there were no differences in gene expression of chemokines monocyte chemoattractant protein-1 and keratinocyte chemoattractant or of growth factor platelet-derived growth factor in wounds of exercise and sedentary mice.

Conclusion.—This suggests an effect of exercise independent of alterations in inflammation. Future work should focus on early events after wounding, including exercise effects on hemostasis and myofibroblast function.

▶ Obesity and obesity-related diabetes markedly impairs wound healing in animal models and in humans. Many have advocated strict blood glucose control as a means of improving the healing process, but often the improvement is minimal. In this current study, the authors created an animal model to simulate the human condition. The diet used created both obesity and insulin resistance. The animals were put on a treadmill for periods during the 3 days leading up to wounding and for 5 days thereafter. Wound healing improved in the exercised animals compared with nonexercised controls.

It is hard to translate these studies directly to humans because obesity often is associated with a lack of exercise and with marked elevations in blood glucose levels that are associated with altered inflammatory processes. Thus, it may be difficult to actively exercise obese humans to a similar degree as in this current animal study. Nevertheless, the results are interesting for future reference.

J. M. Daly, MD

Negative pressure wound therapy in the prevention of wound infection in high risk abdominal wound closures
Vargo D (Univ of Utah School of Medicine, Salt Lake City)
Am J Surg 204:1021-1024, 2012

Background.—Wound infections continue to be an issue in abdominal surgery. Tissue perfusion may be a contributing factor. Negative pressure application may have promise in decreasing wound complication.

Method.—A retrospective review of prospectively collected data in patients with high-risk abdominal wounds was undertaken. Comorbidities, risk factors for infection, wound classification, and wound outcomes were all evaluated. The primary outcome measure was wound infection rate. Secondary outcomes included device safety and overall surgical site complication rate.

Results.—Thirty patients were identified who had skin flaps in whom negative pressure was used. Negative pressure was applied for an average of 5.6 days (range, 5–7 days). No patient developed ischemia or necrosis of the skin flaps. No wound infections were identified. The overall wound complication rate was 3%. The comparable historical control wound complication rate was 20%, and χ^2 analysis showed a statistically significant decrease in the infection rate with negative-pressure wound therapy ($P < .05$).

Conclusions.—Negative-pressure wound therapy applied to a closed, high-risk surgical wound is safe, with no evidence of skin necrosis and decreased wound infection rate.

▶ Application of negative pressure has made a major difference in the surgical management of major wounds. Generally, its use has resulted in earlier closure times and rates, decreased wound infections, and faster return of patients to pre-wound activities. This study was a retrospective review of prospectively collected data on a small number (N = 30) of patients that were then compared with historical controls. The treated patients had skin flaps to which negative pressure was applied postoperatively. Clearly, this therapy is safe because no evidence of flap necrosis was noted. However, comparing the complication rates in the treated group to previously treated historical controls is fraught with difficulties and usually leads to overall optimistic conclusions. Thus, the reader should conclude that the use of negative pressure therapy for skin flaps is safe, but he or she should not draw further conclusions until prospective randomized trials are properly conducted.

J. M. Daly, MD

EPO reverses defective wound repair in hypercholesterolaemic mice by increasing functional angiogenesis
Elsherbiny A, Högger DC, Borozadi MK, et al (Univ Hosp Zurich, Switzerland)
J Plast Reconstr Aesthet Surg 65:1559-1568, 2012

This study aims to elucidate the effect of erythropoietin (EPO) on the microcirculation during wound healing in mice genetically depleted of apolipoprotein E ($ApoE^{-/-}$). The skinfold chamber in mice was used for intravital microscopy, whereby an incisional wound was created within the chamber. Animals received Recormon® 1000 U kg^{-1} body weight (BW) intra-peritoneally (i.p.) at day 1, 3, 5, 7, 9 and 11 post-wounding at a concentration of 100 U ml^{-1} ($n = 42$). Normal healing and vehicle-treated wild type animals (WT) served as controls. The microcirculation of the wound was analysed quantitatively in vivo using epi-illumination intravital fluorescence microscopy. Microtomography (micro-CT) analysis of casted wound microvessels was performed allowing three-dimensional (3D) histomorphometric analysis. Tissue samples were examined *ex vivo* for wound scoring and for expression analysis of EPO-Receptor (Epo-R) and endothelial nitric oxide synthase (eNOS). Upon EPO treatment, the total wound score in $ApoE^{-/-}$ mice was increased by 23% on day 3, by 26% on day 7 and by 18% on day 13 when compared to untreated $ApoE^{-/-}$ mice (all $P < 0.05$ vs. vehicle). Improved wound healing was accompanied with a significant increase of functional angiogenetic density and angiogenetic red blood cell perfusion on days 5, 7, 9 and 11 post-wounding. 3D histomorphometric analysis revealed an increase of vessel thickness (1.7-fold), vessel volume (2.4-fold) and vessel surface (1.7-fold) (all $P < 0.05$ vs. vehicle). In addition, improved wound healing was associated with enhanced Epo-R expression (4.6-fold on day 3 and 13.5-fold on day 7) and eNOS expression (2.4-fold on day 7) (all $P < 0.05$ vs. vehicle). Our data demonstrate that repetitive systemic EPO treatment reverses microvascular dysfunction during wound healing in hypercholesterolaemic mice by inducing new vessel formation and by providing the wound with more oxygen.

▶ Both hypercholesterolemia and diabetes adversely affect wound healing to the point that life and limb are in jeopardy. Attempts to increase oxygen delivery to the wound have taken the form of increasing angiogenesis using vascular growth factors, such as epidermal growth factor, increasing oxygen concentrations in the blood directly, and increasing oxygen delivery, using factors such as erythropoietin (EPO). This experimental study in mice used intravital microscopy to assess vessel ingrowth after incisions were made. Use of EPO did enhance vessel ingrowth as well as wound healing in this model. EPO has side effects in humans and much further study would be required to translate these results to the clinical situation. Nevertheless, it is interesting to suggest that treatment with EPO might enhance healing in patients with hypercholesterolemia and impaired healing.

J. M. Daly, MD

Nonsteroidal Anti-inflammatory Drugs and Anastomotic Dehiscence in Bowel Surgery: Systematic Review and Meta-Analysis of Randomized, Controlled Trials

Burton TP, Mittal A, Soop M (The Univ of Auckland, New Zealand)
Dis Colon Rectum 56:126-134, 2013

Background.—Nonsteroidal anti-inflammatory drugs are a key component of contemporary perioperative analgesia. Recent experimental and observational clinical data suggest an associated increased incidence of anastomotic dehiscence in bowel surgery.

Objective.—The aim of this study was to conduct a systematic review and meta-analysis of anastomotic dehiscence in randomized, controlled trials of perioperative nonsteroidal anti-inflammatory drugs.

Data Sources.—Published and unpublished trials in any language reported 1990 or later were identified by searching electronic databases, bibliographies, and relevant conference proceedings.

Study Selection.—Trials of adults undergoing bowel surgery randomly assigned to perioperative nonsteroidal anti-inflammatory drugs or control were included. The number of patients with a bowel anastomosis and the incidence of anastomotic dehiscence had to be reported or be available from authors for the study to be included.

Intervention.—At least 1 dose of a nonsteroidal anti-inflammatory drug was given perioperatively within 48 hours of surgery.

Main Outcome Measures.—The primary outcome measured was 30-day incidence of anastomotic dehiscence as defined by authors.

Results.—Six trials comprising 480 patients having a bowel anastomosis met inclusion criteria. In 4 studies, anastomotic dehiscence rates were higher in the intervention groups. Overall rates were 14/272 participants (5.1%) in intervention arms vs 5/208 (2.4%) in control arms. Peto OR was 2.16 (95% CI 0.85, 5.53; $p = 0.11$), and there was no heterogeneity between studies (I^2 statistic 0%).

Limitations.—Sizes of available trials were small, preventing firm conclusions and subset analysis of drugs of different cyclooxygenase specificity. A precise and consistent definition of anastomotic dehiscence was not used across trials.

Conclusions.—A statistically significant difference in incidence of anastomotic dehiscence was not demonstrated. However, the Peto OR of 2.16 (0.85, 5.53) and lack of heterogeneity between trials suggest that this finding may be due to a lack of power of the available data rather than a lack of effect.

▶ It has become very common for patients to receive nonsteroidal anti-inflammatory medications for pain postoperatively. Although use of these drugs may result in perioperative bleeding, they do not result in postoperative ileus, which is associated with use of morphine-derived medications. The anti-inflammatory nature of these medications, however, may result in the inhibition of wound healing in the early postoperative period, leading to major morbidity.

The authors performed a meta-analysis (N = 480 patients), but unfortunately, found only 4 studies that met their criteria for inclusion. Each of the studies was small, used different nonsteroidal drugs, and did not always define precisely what was meant by anastomotic leak. As noted, 4 of 6 studies showed a numerically higher anastomotic dehiscence rate, but the complication rates were not statistically different.

Despite the lack of statistically significant differences, this meta-analysis points out some potential problems with the early use of nonsteroidal anti-inflammatory medications in the perioperative period. Perhaps the authors should look to encompass and review all clinical studies in which these drugs were used in postoperative patients to evaluate potential problems with wound healing.

J. M. Daly, MD

Evidence-based decisions for local and systemic wound care
Brölmann FE, Ubbink DT, Nelson EA, et al (Academic Med Centre, Amsterdam, The Netherlands; Univ of Leeds, UK; et al)
Br J Surg 99:1172-1183, 2012

Background.—Decisions on local and systemic wound treatment vary among surgeons and are frequently based on expert opinion. The aim of this meta-review was to compile best available evidence from systematic reviews in order to formulate conclusions to support evidence-based decisions in clinical practice.

Methods.—All Cochrane systematic reviews (CSRs), published by the Cochrane Wounds and Peripheral Vascular Diseases Groups, and that investigated therapeutic and preventive interventions, were searched in the Cochrane Database up to June 2011. Two investigators independently categorized each intervention into five levels of evidence of effect, based on size and homogeneity, and the effect size of the outcomes.

Results.—After screening 149 CSRs, 44 relevant reviews were included. These contained 109 evidence-based conclusions: 30 on venous ulcers, 30 on acute wounds, 15 on pressure ulcers, 14 on diabetic ulcers, 12 on arterial ulcers and eight on miscellaneous chronic wounds. Strong conclusions could be drawn regarding the effectiveness of: therapeutic ultrasonography, mattresses, cleansing methods, closure of surgical wounds, honey, antibiotic prophylaxis, compression, lidocaine—prilocaine cream, skin grafting, antiseptics, pentoxifylline, debridement, hyperbaric oxygen therapy, granulocyte colony-stimulating factors, prostanoids and spinal cord stimulation.

Conclusion.—For some wound care interventions, robust evidence exists upon which clinical decisions should be based.

▶ Meta-analysis is a proven statistical method that helps to determine the relevance of scientific information on which to draw conclusions. The strength of such analysis can be the large number of clinical trials used in the information database, but problems can arise from trials with small numbers of patients, inappropriate trial methodologies, and disparate types of patients, treatments, and follow-up. In this review, the authors tried to separate the types of skin ulcers into different groups and then evaluate the types of treatment used in their management. They found that strong evidence exists that would dictate protocols for treatment. It would be valuable if the conclusions of this article were to be published as a separate entity outlining the appropriate management principles for the variety of skin ulcers that were studied. This would provide firm guidance to the practicing surgeon regarding evidence-based decisions of care.

J. M. Daly, MD

Surgical Staples Compared With Subcuticular Suture for Skin Closure After Cesarean Delivery: A Randomized Controlled Trial
Figueroa D, Jauk VC, Szychowski JM, et al (Univ of Alabama at Birmingham)
Obstet Gynecol 121:33-38, 2013

Objective.—To compare the risk of cesarean wound disruption or infection after closure with surgical staples compared with subcuticular suture.

Methods.—Women with viable pregnancies at 24 weeks of gestation or greater undergoing scheduled or unscheduled cesarean delivery were randomized to wound closure with surgical staples or absorbable suture. Staples were removed at postoperative days 3—4 for low transverse incisions and days 7—10 for vertical incisions. Standardized wound evaluations were performed at discharge (days 3—4) and 4—6 weeks postoperatively. The primary outcome was a composite of wound disruption or infection within 4—6 weeks. Secondary outcomes included operative time, highest pain score on analog scale, cosmesis score, and patient scar satisfaction score. Analyses were by intent to treat.

Results.—Of 398 patients, 198 were randomized to staples and 200 to suture (but four received staples). Baseline characteristics including body mass index, prior cesarean delivery, labor, and type of skin incision were similar by group. The primary outcome incidence at hospital discharge was 7.1% for staples and 0.5% for suture ($P < .001$, relative risk 14.1, 95% confidence interval [CI] 1.9—106). Of 350 (87.9%) with follow-up at 4—6 weeks, the cumulative risk of the primary outcome at 4—6 weeks was 14.5% for staples and 5.9% for suture ($P = .008$, relative risk 2.5, 95% CI 1.2—5.0). Operative time was longer with suture closure (median time of 58 versus 48 minutes; $P < .001$). Pain scores at 72—96 hours and at

6 weeks, cosmesis score, and patient satisfaction score did not differ by group.

Conclusion.—Staples closure compared with suture is associated with significantly increased composite wound morbidity after cesarean delivery.

Clinical Trial Registration.—ClinicalTrials.gov, www.clinicaltrials.gov, NCT01008449.

Level of Evidence.—I.

▶ Many methods of wound closure have been studied over the years. Clearly, use of skin staples has often become the mainstay of skin closures because of the rapidity with which closure can be accomplished with this approach. This prospective, randomized trial evaluated the use of skin staples vs use of absorbable sutures for women undergoing cesarean sections. One might wonder about the wisdom of removing the skin staples at postoperative day 3 or 4. However, it is assumed that the authors chose these dates because of the poor cosmetic effects when these staples remain longer. Nevertheless, removal of skin staples at day 3 or 4 resulted in wound disruptions in 7% of patients, clearly inferior to the results with absorbable sutures. It is important to note that the study evaluations continued for 4 to 6 weeks because the wound disruption rate increased to 14.5% with staples compared with 5.9% using the suture technique. The study demonstrates the wisdom of using a more prolonged period of observation time in humans when evaluating wound healing. It also suggests that a longer period should elapse before temporary closure devices (eg, staples, sutures) are removed from postoperative wounds.

J. M. Daly, MD

Low-energy extracorporeal shock wave therapy enhances skin wound healing in diabetic mice: A critical role of endothelial nitric oxide synthase
Hayashi D, Kawakami K, Ito K, et al (Tohoku Univ Graduate School of Medicine, Sendai, Japan)
Wound Repair Regen 20:887-895, 2012

Low-energy extracorporeal shock wave (LE-ESW) treatment has been shown to accelerate wound repair; however, the mechanisms of treatment remain unclear. In the present study, we addressed the role of endothelial nitric oxide synthase (eNOS). A single LE-ESW treatment accelerated the healing of wounds in diabetic mice caused by the injection of streptozotocin. This accelerated healing was accompanied by the increased expression of eNOS and vascular endothelial growth factor (VEGF) and the generation of new vessels at the wound tissues. These results raised the possibility that eNOS may be involved in the beneficial effects of LE-ESW treatment. To address this possibility, we compared the effects of this treatment between mice with a genetic disruption of eNOS knockout (eNOS-KO mice) and wild-type (WT) control mice. Interestingly, the LE-ESW-induced acceleration of wound closure and the increase in VEGF expression and neovascularization was significantly attenuated in eNOS-KO mice compared with WT mice. Considered collectively, these results showed that eNOS was induced at the wound tissues by LE-ESW treatment and played a critical role in the therapeutic effects of this treatment by accelerating the wound healing by promoting VEGF expression and neovascularization.

▶ Numerous methods of external applied energy have been studied in an effort to improve wound healing. This interesting study evaluated low-energy extracorporeal shock wave (LE-ESW) treatment as a means to accelerate wound repair. The model chosen was wounds in diabetic mice because it is well-known that healing is delayed in this animal model, similar to that of diabetic humans. The authors first noted that the LE-ESW groups had improvement in healing and that there was an increased expression of endothelial nitric oxide synthase (eNOS). They carried the experiments further showing that this benefit was ameliorated in eNOS knockout mice, strongly supporting their hypothesis that eNOS is critical to the beneficial effects of LE-ESW. It will be important to determine in humans if eNOS is the critical factor in the healing process after LE-ESW. It will also be important to study LE-ESW in a variety of wound-healing settings to determine the full range of its efficacy.

J. M. Daly, MD

Does treatment of split-thickness skin grafts with negative-pressure wound therapy improve tissue markers of wound healing in a porcine experimental model?
Ward C, Ciraulo D, Coulter M, et al (Maine Med Ctr, Portland; et al)
J Trauma Acute Care Surg 73:447-451, 2012

Background.—Negative-pressure wound therapy (NPWT) has been used for to treat wounds for more than 15 years and, more recently, has been used to secure split-thickness skin grafts. There are some data to support this use of NPWT, but the actual mechanism by which NPWT speeds healing or improves skin graft take is not entirely known. The purpose of this project was to assess whether NPWT improved angiogenesis, wound healing, or graft survival when compared with traditional bolster dressings securing split-thickness skin grafts in a porcine model.

Methods.—We performed two split-thickness skin grafts on each of eight 30 kg Yorkshire pigs. We took graft biopsies on postoperative days 2, 4, 6, 8, and 10 and submitted the samples for immunohistochemical staining, as well as standard hematoxylin and eosin staining. We measured the degree of vascular ingrowth via immunohistochemical staining for von Willenbrand's factor to better identify blood vessel epithelium. We determined the mean cross-sectional area of blood vessels present for each representative specimen, and then compared the bolster and NPWT samples. We also assessed each graft for incorporation and survival at postoperative day 10.

Results.—Our analysis of the data revealed that there was no statistically significant difference in the degree of vascular ingrowth as measured by mean cross-sectional capillary area ($p = 023$). We did not note any difference in graft survival or apparent incorporation on a macroscopic level, although standard hematoxylin and eosin staining indicated that microscopically, there seemed to be better subjective graft incorporation in the NPWT samples and a nonsignificant trend toward improved graft survival in the NPWT group.

Conclusion.—We were unable to demonstrate a significant difference in vessel ingrowth when comparing NPWT and traditional bolster methods for split-thickness skin graft fixation. More studies are needed to elucidate the manner by which NPWT exerts its effects and the true clinical magnitude of these effects.

▶ The use of negative pressure to accelerate the healing of wounds has become commonplace with the subjective assessment that this treatment improves wound-healing outcomes; therefore, this animal study is important. The authors used 8 pigs that had undergone 2 split-thickness skin grafts per animal with 1 graft serving as a control for the negative-pressure treated graft. In their initial analysis, the authors anticipated a large difference in histologic variables and, thus, chose only 8 animals to study. As they stated in their discussion, 26 more animals should have been studied to have adequate power to detect a difference. In addition, in the control grafts, 2 skin grafts did not take, further limiting the number of histologic observations. Yet, the study was made important because it examined a generally held belief and attempted to study it experimentally. Further studies such as this one are important to truly identify the mechanisms in which negative-pressure wound therapy *may* be important to improve outcomes in patients.

J. M. Daly, MD

Impact of neoadjuvant chemotherapy on wound complications after breast surgery

Decker MR, Greenblatt DY, Havlena J, et al (Univ of Wisconsin School of Medicine and Public Health, Madison)
Surgery 152:382-388, 2012

Background.—Use of neoadjuvant chemotherapy for breast cancer is increasing. The objective was to examine risk of postoperative wound complications in patients receiving neoadjuvant chemotherapy for breast cancer.

Methods.—Patients undergoing breast surgery from 2005 to 2010 were selected from the American College of Surgeons National Surgical Quality Improvement Program database. Patients were included if preoperative diagnosis suggested malignancy and an axillary procedure was performed. We performed a stepwise multivariable regression analysis of predictors of postoperative wound complications, overall and stratified by type of breast surgery. Our primary variable of interest was receipt of neoadjuvant chemotherapy.

Results.—Of 44,533 patients, 4.5% received neoadjuvant chemotherapy. Wound complications were infrequent with or without neoadjuvant chemotherapy (3.4% vs 3.1%; $P = .4$). Smoking, functional dependence, obesity, diabetes, hypertension, and mastectomy were associated with wound complications. No association with neoadjuvant chemotherapy was seen (odds ratio [OR], 1.01; 95% confidence interval [CI], 0.78–1.32); however, a trend was observed toward increased complications in neoadjuvant patients undergoing mastectomy with immediate reconstruction (OR, 1.58; 95% CI, 0.98–2.58).

Conclusion.—Postoperative wound complications after breast surgery are infrequent and not associated with neoadjuvant chemotherapy. Given the trend toward increased complications in patients undergoing mastectomy with immediate reconstruction, however, neoadjuvant chemotherapy should be among the many factors considered when making multidisciplinary treatment decisions.

▶ The National Surgical Quality Improvement Program database is a very robust entity with more than 300 hospitals entering their data in an effort to be able to examine trends in patient care and patient outcomes. It also allows hospitals to benchmark their results against other institutions. The impact of neoadjuvant chemotherapy and its effects of wound healing are important. Previously, Adriamycin therapy was shown in animal studies to be deleterious to healing. With the advent of breast-conserving therapy, patients with T2 breast cancers now often undergo neoadjuvant chemotherapy in an effort to reduce the size of the tumor, making the patient eligible for breast-conserving surgical therapy. Generally, one waits 30 days for the adverse effects of chemotherapy to dissipate, but certain biologic agents (Avastin) may require more time, perhaps as much as 6 weeks. It is interesting that in cases of patients undergoing mastectomies plus reconstruction, there was a trend toward poor healing in those who had received neoadjuvant chemotherapy. This suggests that more time must elapse before initiating surgery in these patients in order to achieve the optimal result.

J. M. Daly, MD

Systematic review and meta-analysis of wound dressings in the prevention of surgical-site infections in surgical wounds healing by primary intention
Walter CJ, Dumville JC, Sharp CA, et al (Nottingham Univ Hosps NHS Trust, UK; Univ of York, UK; Univ of Adelaide and Royal Adelaide Hosp, South Australia)
Br J Surg 99:1185-1194, 2012

Background.—Postoperative surgical-site infections are a major source of morbidity and cost. This study aimed to identify and present all randomized controlled trial evidence evaluating the effects of dressings on surgical-site infection rates in surgical wounds healing by primary intention; the secondary outcomes included comparisons of pain, scar and acceptability between dressings.

Methods.—Randomized controlled trials comparing alternative wound dressings, or wound dressings with leaving wounds exposed for postoperative management of surgical wounds were included in the review regardless of their language. Databases searched included the Cochrane Wounds Group Specialised Register and Central Register of Controlled Trials, Ovid MEDLINE, Ovid Embase and EBSCO CINAHL from inception to May 2011. Two authors performed study selection, risk of bias assessment and data extraction, including an assessment of surgical contamination according to the surgical procedure. Where levels of clinical and statistical heterogeneity permitted, data were pooled for meta-analysis.

Results.—Sixteen controlled trials with 2594 participants examining a range of wound contamination levels were included. They were all unclear or at high risk of bias. There was no evidence that any dressing significantly reduced surgical-site infection rates compared with any other dressing or leaving the wound exposed. Furthermore, no significant differences in pain, scarring or acceptability were seen between the dressings.

Conclusion.—No difference in surgical-site infection rates was demonstrated between surgical wounds covered with different dressings and those left uncovered. No difference was seen in pain, scar or acceptability between dressings.

▶ There is considerable interest in reducing the potential for surgical-site infections. Several methods have been studied, such as the use of antibiotic irrigation, antiseptics to prepare the skin, methods of removing hair and the timing of such, drapes impregnated with antibacterial medications, and so on. The reason for this interest is the major morbidity to the patient and the substantial cost to the hospital when a surgical-site infection occurs. Many studies have been done at the behest of commercial entities; some have been underpowered and some have inherent biases. Thus, this large meta-analysis is interesting because the authors included 16 randomized, controlled trials with more than 2500 patients. Importantly, no major differences either in infection rates, cosmetic results, or pain were observed when comparing different types of dressings. Thus, it appears that the type of dressing used has little influence on the potential for resultant infectious complications. Further work should be carried out to find other approaches. In addition, better surgical trials are needed to provide definitive results.

J. M. Daly, MD

Diabetes-Impaired Wound Healing Is Improved by Matrix Therapy With Heparan Sulfate Glycosaminoglycan Mimetic OTR4120 in Rats
Tong M, Tuk B, Shang P, et al (Univ Med Ctr, Rotterdam, the Netherlands)
Diabetes 61:2633-2641, 2012

Wound healing in diabetes is frequently impaired, and its treatment remains a challenge. We tested a therapeutic strategy of potentiating intrinsic tissue regeneration by restoring the wound cellular environment using a heparan sulfate glycosaminoglycan mimetic, OTR4120. The effect of OTR4120 on healing of diabetic ulcers was investigated. Experimental diabetes was induced by intraperitoneal injection of streptozotocin. Seven weeks after induction of diabetes, rats were ulcerated by clamping a pair of magnet disks on the dorsal skin for 16 h. After magnet removal, OTR4120 was administered via an intramuscular injection weekly for up to 4 weeks. To examine the effect of OTR4120 treatment on wound healing, the degree of ulceration, inflammation, angiogenesis, and collagen synthesis were evaluated. We found that OTR4120 treatment significantly reduced the degree of ulceration and the time of healing. These effects were associated with reduced neutrophil infiltration and macrophage accumulation and enhanced angiogenesis. OTR4120 treatment also increased the collagen content with an increase of collagen type I biosynthesis and reduction of collagen type III biosynthesis. Moreover, restoration of the ulcer biomechanical strength was significantly enhanced after OTR4120 treatment. This study shows that matrix therapy with OTR4120 improves diabetes-impaired wound healing.

▶ Diabetes-impaired wound healing is the bane of patients and surgeons alike. Many attempts have been made to correct the deficiencies in healing created by a lack of angiogenesis, fibroblast proliferation, inflammatory reaction, deficient matrix formation, and collagen synthesis in the wounds of diabetic subjects. Investigators have provided growth factors, increased local oxygen concentrations, and attempted to improve each and all of the aforementioned deficiencies with varying degrees of success. This experiment using an ulceration model in rats provided a heparin sulfate glycosaminoglycan mimetic, OTR4120. Compared with controls, the treated group showed improved wound healing using a number of parameters, including improvement in angiogenesis. It will certainly require a great deal more study, ultimately in humans, to determine if this aminoglycan and others like it can improve healing in ulcers and other types of wounds. It will probably turn out that a multifactorial approach will be necessary providing several growth factors and matrix enhancers in order to maximize healing in the diabetic population.

J. M. Daly, MD

6 Transplantation

Introduction

Organ transplantation is the optimal therapy for many people with organ failure. However, the applicability to the population in need is limited by the lack of available organs. Traditionally, organs have been obtained from two sources: brain dead individuals and live directed donors. Because of the organ shortage, analysis of existing systems and an expansion of the donor pool has become a necessity. The first four articles in this section address some of the issues associated with deceased organ donation. As most organs for transplantation come from deceased individuals, article 1 analyzes the geographic differences in the death rate (trauma and cerebrovascular deaths accounting for most donor deaths) within the United States. The authors propose that the heterogeneity in the distribution of US deaths should be addressed in the national allocation policy. It is suggested that an inefficiency of organ utilization occurs from the mismatch of demand for organs (waitlist geographic distribution) and the availability of organs. The second article by Malinoski et al addresses institutional resources and donation process issues. It is presupposed that organ donation will be more efficient and with better results in settings with good management of trauma victims. Comparison of facilities meeting American College of Surgeons (ACS) trauma criteria were compared to those without the ACS trauma expertise. Surprisingly, irrespective of compliance with ACS trauma qualifications, donor numbers were equivalent. However, when a center had catastrophic brain injury guidelines in place, the numbers of organ donors was found to be significantly increased. Whether the resources required for optimal care of the injured patient coincides with that required for organ donation remains to be seen. However, these two articles suggest that the mismatch between potential donor availability/allocation and donor hospital's resource commitment to care for the donor is significant and may be an important element limiting organ transplantation.

The next two articles address issues associated with donation expansion to include those individuals that die after circulatory cessation (DCD). Article 3 recounts the experience from the United Kingdom quantifying a common sense observation, that the hurry up retrieval in the DCD event is associated with more surgical damage to the organs. Compared with organ retrieval from neurologic dead donors, kidneys were damaged almost twice as frequently (11.4 vs 6.8%, p < 0.001) with DCD, leading to an increased frequency of organ discard. With so few organs available for transplantation, there is a need to understand process variables and work to control them. This article highlights the technical and procedural differences associated with different types of organ donation. Article 4 by Fondevila addresses the outcomes of transplantation from the donor with an uncontrolled circulatory arrest. Liver transplantation with Maastricht 2 donors (circulatory death after resuscitation efforts failed after an unexpected arrest) had an inferior patient and graft survival compared to those retrieved from neurologic donors (Fig 4). These four articles emphasize that the expansion of the deceased donor population will have problems requiring special understanding of a multitude of differences found in the care of individuals with catastrophic injuries. In the field of live organ donation, the issues are more regulatory at the present time, with both CMS and UNOS/OPTN placing compliance stipulations upon the transplanting centers. However, there appears to be a slow resurgence of live liver donation. Article 5 makes an increasingly obvious observation: the more liver that is removed from an individual, the greater the likelihood that a complication will occur. Outcomes were compared from groups after right hepatectomy for either benign disease or organ donation. More liver was resected for donation and the complications were greater. The authors suggest that this observation may be an inherent limitation of the donation process and imply that the community should work to find less morbid liver donation procedures.

The next two articles deal with a few of the conundrums that the transplant community must confront from the perspective of patient heterogeneity. Most people believe that children with end-stage organ disease should be treated preferentially with organ transplantation. Levine's report (6) analyzes the outcomes after kidney transplantation for adolescents receiving the ideal deceased donor organ. Using national data, they found that adolescent kidney transplantation had an inferior graft survival compared to all other age groups, except those over 70. The reason is not clear from the OPTN data, but most prior literature cites compliance with drug regimens as a major factor. They proposed that the current allocation system results in significant loss of excellent kidneys and that perhaps a reevaluation of the policy that allocates the nation's most ideal organs to individuals with an inferior long-term outcome should be entertained. The other group that constitutes a significant percentage of individuals with organ failure is the elderly.

Article 7 summarizes many of the issues of transplanting individuals with advanced age, including outcomes of immunosuppression, infection and malignancies, numbers of people that could be treated with organ transplantation, and organ quality and availability. As long as society has limited numbers of organs, the elderly will continue to have psychologically limited access. However, a more fundamental question as to whether a significant survival and quality of life benefit is associated with organ transplantation in whatever population affected. There will most certainly be an increased debate about recipient worthiness as the disparity in numbers waiting continues to outstrip the numbers of organs that are available for transplantation.

Article 8 analyzes the single center liver transplantation outcomes for hepatocellular carcinoma over a 20-year period. Despite changes in diagnosis and therapies, recurrent hepatocellular carcinoma has not been common, although the HCCa indication has increased in frequency. As national MELD scores increase in order to receive a liver transplant, there is a significant risk that oncologic control will be lost during the ensuing time necessary to gain priority and that the excellent results after liver transplantation will begin to decline. Monitoring of HCCa recurrence after liver transplantation will need to become part of the liver transplantation metric. Host immunologic response to the transplanted organ is fundamental of transplantation science. The liver has long been known to be an organ with certain immunologic privilege. The role of donor specific antibody (DSA) in liver transplantation has been controversial. It has been common practice of liver transplantation to ignore whether or not a recipient has DSA before accepting a liver for transplantation. Article 9 describes clinical and histologic findings of the liver of transplant recipients with and without DSA. Consistent with other reports and practice, the main clinical outcomes (survival and rejection episodes) were not adversely affected by DSA. However, the hallmark of antibody mediated rejection, C4d deposition, is commonly found in the liver of recipients with DSA, but also in other inflammatory conditions such as HCV and autoimmune hepatitis. In the event of diffuse deposition and DSA, the authors suggest that antibody rejection may be operative, but further study needs to be done. Despite the longstanding practice of liver transplantation, there is still uncertainty regarding some of the most fundamental practices within the discipline. Pancreas transplantation has had many technical issues that influence outcomes. Article 10 provides a historic overview of the many technical and immunosuppressive changes that have led us to our current practice. Clinical outcomes have dramatically improved, but this must be balanced by the observation that distribution of simultaneous kidney-pancreas, pancreas after kidney, pancreas alone and retransplantation has varied considerably over the decades. Morbidity of the procedure continues to be significant and pushes for advancements to better achieve glycemic control in the type 1 diabetic. The morbidity of whole organ pancreas transplantation has spurred many to continue to strive for euglycemia through cell-based therapies. Article 11 addresses the role of induction immunotherapy upon islet survival. Lymphocyte depletion in combination with TNF blockade resulted in islet durability similar to that of whole organ pancreas. But why anti-TNF — a therapy that has not been necessary in whole organ transplants? Significant information regarding non-alloimmunity therapies about islet transplantation has been gained from the autoislet transplantation after total pancreatectomy. The numbers of autoislets necessary to achieve euglycemia is lower than with alloislets. Whether this is the consequence of differences in islet damage from antemortem events or immunologic events remains to be discerned. Article 12 describes many of the variables associated with outcomes after total pancreatectomy and autoislet transplantation and lessons that could be learned through autotransplantation. Optimal therapy for glycemic control remains to be defined between the therapeutic options of exogenous insulin through various devices, cell or organ-based therapies.

Outcomes after transplantation in the US are released into the public domain through the Scientific Registry of Transplant Recipients. These results are currently used for a number of diverse purposes including patient and physician education regarding which center to access for care and by insurer and oversight agencies regarding center suitability for participation in payment networks. Article 13 analyzes the national data base for outcomes after heart transplantation. Not surprisingly, the authors demonstrate that numbers of procedures alone is not the sole predictor of outcomes. Effective risk adjustment and reporting remains a significant challenge with public release of outcome information with implications that are profound for the specific transplant center. Organ transplantation is a treatment that can be applied to a number of unique clinical indications and has expanded over the years. Diffuse mesenteric thrombosis is one such condition that was once a contraindication to liver transplantation and is now one where multivisceral transplantation might be applicable. Article 14 reports on a single-center experience reporting satisfactory patient and graft survival, but the discussion must be more about the reasons by which some people are deemed not to be candidates. In some respects multivisceral transplantation presents improved opportunities than other methods designed to address technical challenges. The challenge is to balance benefit and risk. Another combination that has proven quite controversial has been the combination of a liver and kidney transplant. As liver allocation in the US favors those with impaired renal function, it is quite tempting to simultaneously transplant a liver and a kidney. As native kidney function may improve, it is difficult to discern the most efficacious use of the combined organs. Article 15 assesses survivors of combined liver/kidneys with renal scans. Unfortunately, the timing of the renal scan was not clearly defined in the article, and it is not clear whether recovery of native renal function had stabilized. However, it is clear that return of native renal function played a major role in the recipient's long-term renal function. While it is certain that multiple organs can be successfully transplanted into the same individual, clear indications remain to be delineated.

While surgical and organ preservation innovation has been fundamental to the growth of organ transplantation, immunosuppressive therapies are the foundation upon which the entire discipline resides. However, while the numbers of agents has expanded, the mandatory use of glucocorticoids is one therapy that most transplant patients have repeatedly requested be eliminated. Chronic steroid has a variety of untoward physical and psychological effects and article 16 reports that liver recipients on high dose chronic steroids have a significantly lower mental and physical score on a battery of quality of life testing (SF-36, Beck anxiety inventory, the center for epidemiologic studies depression scale, CES-D) irrespective of other immunosuppressive drugs. These sorts of studies will become much more important as outcomes improve and long-term strategies must embrace a variety of immunosuppressive chemotherapies in order to maintain organ function. As organ transplantation continues to expand, the necessity to deliver therapies that are associated with higher function and quality of life is paramount.

In article 17, the impact of two induction therapies upon circulating lymphocyte populations was compared. Depleting therapy with alemtuzumab resulted in marked differences in circulating lymphocytes compared to basiliximab, especially in the β-cell populations. Certain phenotypes of lymphocytes were associated with increased likelihood of a rejection-free course, raising the prospect that it might be possible to engineer a lymphocyte repertoire that will be slow to respond to a transplanted organ. In this vein, there is an increasing drift away from chemo immunosuppression and towards cell-based therapy to enhance immunosuppression. Regulatory T cells and autologous mesenchymal stem cells are gaining favor as immunomodulators. Article 18 describes outcomes after kidney transplantation by infusing autologous stem cells just prior to kidney reperfusion (and at two weeks post) followed by monotherapy calcineurin inhibitor. Rejection episodes were less frequent and more easily treated with cell-based infusion than with standard IL-2 receptor inhibition. There will be a wide spectrum of therapies that are performed in the near future to maximize outcome benefit and minimize drug toxicities. This article speaks to a significant model change in the treatment of people with organ transplantation.

The final two articles address the infectious/microbiota consequences of transplantation. The routine use of anti-CMV therapies has been associated with concerns about drug resistance. A comparative study (Article 19) of prophylactic valganciclovir vs CMV monitoring and preemptive therapy observed that prophylactic dosing was associated with a lower risk of failure and subsequent drug resistance to the antiviral treatment. While not an expected outcome, this study emphasizes the importance of observation and hypothesis testing. The final article (20) followed the composition of the microbiome of the transplanted bowel. The authors describe a change of composition of the microbiota that was considered to be predictive of the immunologic condition of the transplanted gut. If true, this shift may prove useful in understanding not only the graft status, but it may also help understand the interface between the host and the microbiome.

Organ transplantation continues to evolve in the social, regulatory, and scientific arenas. In 2012, the availability of suitable organs for recipients continued as the most vexing problem for the community. There is much work to be done to better meet the needs of society. However, immunologic and physiologic barriers still exist in order to allow for a more reliable and cost efficient therapy for those with organ failure.

Timothy L. Pruett, MD

Investigating Geographic Variation in Mortality in the Context of Organ Donation

Sheehy E, O'Connor KJ, Luskin RS, et al (New England Organ Bank, Waltham, MA; LifeCtr Northwest, Bellevue, WA; et al)
Am J Transplant 12:1598-1602, 2012

Organ procurement organizations (OPOs) report a nearly fourfold difference in donor availability as measured by eligible deaths per million population (PMP) based on hospital referrals. We analyzed whether mortality data help explain geographic variation in organ supply as measured by the number of eligible deaths for organ donation. Using the 2007 National Center for Health Statistics' mortality data, we analyzed deaths occurring in acute care hospitals, aged ≤ 70 years from cerebrovascular accidents and trauma. These deaths were mapped at the county level and compared to eligible deaths reported by OPOs. In 2007, there were 2 428 343 deaths reported in the United States with 42 339 in-hospital deaths ≤ 70 years from cerebrovascular accidents (CVA) or trauma that were correlated with eligible deaths PMP ($r^2 = 0.79$.) Analysis revealed a broad range in the death rate across OPOs: trauma deaths: 44−118 PMP; deaths from CVA: 34−118 PMP; and combined CVA and trauma: 91−229 PMP. Mortality data demonstrate that deaths by neurologic criteria of people who are likely to be suitable deceased donors are not evenly distributed across the nation. These deaths are correlated with eligible deaths for organ donation. Regional availability of organs is affected by deaths which should be accounted for in the organ allocation system.

▶ The authors use data from the National Center for Health Statistics to point out the obvious: Deaths in the United States do not occur in a homogeneous fashion. Just as the population density is inhomogeneous, deaths occur sporadically. The difficulty with this analysis is that it gives little insight into areas of opportunity to more promptly identify and treat the individual with catastrophic brain injury. In the unfortunate percentage of individuals who are not successfully treated, organ donation may prove to be one of the outcomes. An intriguing method employed by the authors was to match the total numbers of deaths with those reported to the organ procurement organizations (OPOs). Of the 2.43 million deaths, 42 339 were identified by the OPOs as potential donors with trauma, cerebrovascular accidents, and less than 70 years old. What about the other 2.39 million deaths? How many deaths were of a similar category and were lost to donation through an inability to stabilize or because of system limitations or process issues? There is significant potential to improve the organ donation system, but without analyzing the system's limitations, one will never gain insights.

T. Pruett, MD

Impact of Compliance with the American College of Surgeons Trauma Center Verification Requirements on Organ Donation-Related Outcomes

Malinoski DJ, Patel MS, Lush S, et al (Cedars-Sinai Med Ctr, Los Angeles, CA; Univ of California Irvine, Orange)

J Am Coll Surg 215:186-192, 2012

Background.—In order to maximize organ donation opportunities, the American College of Surgeons (ACS) requires verified trauma centers to have a relationship with an organ procurement organization (OPO), a policy for notification of the OPO, a process to review organ donation rates, and a protocol for declaring neurologic death. We hypothesized that meeting the ACS requirements will be associated with improved donation outcomes.

Study Design.—Twenty-four ACS-verified Level I and Level II trauma centers were surveyed for the following registry data points from 2004 to 2008: admissions, ICU admissions, patients with a head Abbreviated Injury Score ≥ 5, deaths, and organ donors. Centers were also queried for the presence of the ACS requirements as well as other process measures and characteristics. The main outcomes measure was the number of organ donors per center normalized for patient volume and injury severity. The relationship between center characteristics and outcomes was determined.

Results.—Twenty-one centers (88%) completed the survey and referred 2,626 trauma patients to the OPO during the study period, 1,008 were eligible to donate, and 699 became organ donors. Compliance with the 4 ACS requirements was not associated with increased organ donation outcomes. However, having catastrophic brain injury guidelines (CBIGs) and the presence of a trauma surgeon on a donor council were associated with significantly more organ donors per 1,000 trauma admissions (6.3 vs 4.2 and 6.0 vs 4.2, respectively, $p < 0.05$).

Conclusions.—Although the ACS trauma center organ donation-related requirements were not associated with improved organ donor outcomes, involvement of trauma surgeons on donor councils and CBIGs were and should be encouraged. Additionally, incorporation of quantitative organ donation measures into the verification process should be considered.

▶ As noted in the critique of Investigating Geographic Variation in Mortality in the Context of Organ Donation by E. Sheehy et al, heterogeneity of organ availability and distribution is considerable within the United States. The skill of the treating center to recognize potential donors, as well as a move toward donation, has been a source of discussion. This article assesses differences between the American College of Surgeons level 1 and 2 trauma center vs others regarding organ donation. The premise would be that such centers would preferentially get referrals, have the skill to identify neurologic death, and have practice algorithms to sustain the donor until organ donation became feasible. However, a survey of trauma center results vs all others did not show that the dedicated resources of a level 1/2 center resulted in increased organ donations. It is worth pointing out that the presence of brain injury guidelines and participation of the trauma members on a donation council did impact donation availability.

People die. Processes to effectively facilitate organ donation do not directly correlate with those resources necessary to care for the injured patient. This article reinforces that observation, but it suggests some of the key elements necessary to move beyond just counting potential donors and quantitate processes necessary to achieve organ donation. The first premise of all systems must be to sustain life and protect the injured. The vast majority of our resources are rightly pushed toward this end. However, after death has occurred, different resources are necessary to maximize the ability of those waiting for an organ to receive the gift of an organ.

T. Pruett, MD

Kidney Damage During Organ Recovery in Donation After Circulatory Death Donors: Data From UK National Transplant Database

Ausania F, White SA, Pocock P, et al (Freeman Hosp, Newcastle Upon Tyne, UK; NHS Blood and Transplant (NHSBT), Bristol, UK)
Am J Transplant 12:932-936, 2012

During the last 10 years, kidneys recovered/ transplanted from donors after circulatory death (DCD) have significantly increased. To optimize their use, there has been an urgent need to minimize both warm and cold ischemia, which often necessitates more rapid removal. To compare the rates of kidney injury during procurement from DCD and donors after brain death (DBD) organ donors. A total of 13 260 kidney procurements were performed in the United Kingdom over a 10-year period (2000–2010). Injuries occurred in 903 procedures (7.1%). Twelve thousand three hundred seventy-two (93.3%) kidneys were recovered from DBD donors and 888 (6.7%) from DCD donors. The rates of kidney injury were significantly higher when recovered from DCD donors (11.4% vs. 6.8%, $p < 0.001$). Capsular, ureteric and vascular injuries were all significantly more frequent ($p = 0.002$, $p < 0.001$ and $p = 0.017$, respectively). Discard because of injury was more common after DCD donation ($p = 0.002$). Multivariate analysis demonstrated procurement injuries were significantly associated with DCD donors ($p = 0.035$) and increased donor age (<0.001) and donor body mass index (BMI; 0.001), donor male gender ($p = 0.001$) and no liver donation (0.009). We conclude that procurement from DCD donors leads to higher rates of injury to the kidney and are more likely to be discarded.

▶ Since the 2006 Institute of Medicine report on organ donation, there has been a concerted effort in the United States to increase the retrieval and utilization of organs from donors after circulatory death (DCD). In many respects, these organs have proven functional for recipients, but retrieval has significant process hurdles. The legal aspects of donor death and damage to the organs during the warm, waiting time have been extensively detailed. The present article addresses a very specific question: Does the DCD process affect the efficiency of surgical retrieval? The answer is affirmative. An outcome review of DCD kidneys demonstrated significantly more retrieval damage to the organs and accompanying discard. This finding would not be unexpected considering the "hurry-up" nature of the DCD retrieval process. The study implies that a different surgical technique, or at least care, be taken for the DCD retrieval contrasted to the conventional neuro-logically deceased donor.

T. Pruett, MD

Applicability and Results of Maastricht Type 2 Donation After Cardiac Death Liver Transplantation
Fondevila C, Hessheimer AJ, Flores E, et al (Univ of Barcelona, Spain)
Am J Transplant 12:162-170, 2012

Maastricht type 2 donation after cardiac death (DCD) donors suffer sudden and unexpected cardiac arrest, typically outside the hospital; they have significant potential to expand the donor pool. Herein, we analyze the results of transplanted livers and all potential donors treated under our type 2 DCD protocol. Cardiac arrest was witnessed; potential donors arrived at the hospital after attempts at resuscitation had failed. Death was declared based on the absence of cardiorespiratory activity during a 5-min no-touch period. Femoral vessels were cannulated to establish normo-thermic extracorporeal membrane oxygenation, which was maintained until organ recovery. From April 2002 to December 2010, there were 400 potential donors; 34 liver transplants were performed (9%). Among recipients, median age, model for end stage liver disease and cold and reperfusion warm ischemic times were 55 years (49−60), 19 (14−21) and 380 (325−430) and 30 min (26−35), respectively. Overall, 236 (59%) and 130 (32%) livers were turned down due to absolute and relative contraindications to donate, respectively. One-year recipient and graft survivals were 82% and 70%, respectively (median follow-up 24 months). The applicability of type 2 DCD liver transplant was <10%; however, with better preservation technology and expanded transplant criteria, we may be able to improve this figure significantly.

▶ The conventional donation after cardiac death (DCD) donor in the United States is an individual having life support withdrawn in a controlled hospital setting, referred to as a Maastricht 3 donor. Because DCD donors appear to function reasonably, expansion of the donor pool to other types of death has been proposed. The Maastricht convention describes individuals with a witnessed cardiac arrest and unsuccessful resuscitation as type 2 deaths. Many European organ-retrieval efforts more aggressively use organs from "uncontrolled" deaths. This article describes the Barcelona experience with liver donation associated with Maastricht 2 donors. Overall, recipients of such livers had satisfactory, but lesser, outcomes than would have been expected with a conventional organ donor. However, the startling factor was that less than 10% of livers from the potential donors were used. Of 400 Maastricht 2 donors, only 34 liver transplants were performed. This article highlights the increasing cost/effort associated with obtaining increasingly inferior grafts for the purposes of organ transplantation. It is necessary to identify the balance between effort/cost and benefit for those on the wait list. It is not feasible to expend more and more resources on fewer possible donors.

T. Pruett, MD

"Inherent Limitations" in Donors: Control Matched Study of Consequences Following a Right Hepatectomy for Living Donation and Benign Liver Lesions

Belghiti J, Liddo G, Raut V, et al (Beaujon Hospital—Assistance Publique Hôpitaux de Paris—100 Bd du Général Leclerc, France)
Ann Surg 255:528-533, 2012

Objective.—The aim of this study was to identify "inherent limitations" in healthy donors who are responsible for donor morbidity after right hepatectomy (RH) for adult-to-adult living donor liver transplantation (ALDLT).

Background.—Right hepatectomy for ALDLT remains a challenging procedure without significant improvement in morbidity over time. This suggests some "inherent limitations" in healthy individuals, which are beyond the recent improvements in the donor evaluation and selection process and refinements in surgical technique during the learning curve.

Methods.—To identify response of RH in ALDLT, we prospectively studied 32 patients requiring an RH for benign liver lesions (BL), matched with 32 living donors (LD) operated by same team. All patients underwent liver volume evaluation by computed tomographic (CT) volumetry preoperatively and 1 week after RH, postoperative complications graded with Clavien's system.

Results.—The comparison (LD vs BL) showed that remnant liver volume (RLV) on preoperative CT volumetry was higher in the BL group (450 ± 150 vs 646 ± 200 mL, $P < 0.001$) representing $31\% \pm 7\%$ in LD group versus $36\% \pm 7\%$ of the total liver volume in BL group ($P = 0.03$). On postoperative day 7, the RLV was similar in the 2 groups (866 ± 162 vs 941 ± 153 mL) resulting from a significantly higher regeneration rate in the LD group (89% vs 55%, $P = 0.009$). Overall complications rate was lower in the BL group (46% vs 21%, $P = 0.035$).

Conclusions.—Right hepatectomy in LDLT induces a more severe deprivation of liver volume than in BL, which induce an accelerated regeneration. Accelerated regeneration could represent "inherent limitation" in healthy donors that makes them more vulnerable for postoperative complications.

▶ The prior studies have stressed the lack of organ availability as one of the major challenges to contemporary organ transplantation.[1-4] However, live donors represent another source of organs for those with chronic organ failure. In caring for the live donor, it is incumbent upon the center/system to effectively assess the risk for the healthy donor. Live liver donation is still in process of evolution. The article by Belghiti et al describes a single, very experienced center outcome with right hepatectomy for organ donation or benign liver disease. The authors demonstrate that a right hepatectomy for disease is not the same as a right hepatectomy for donation. The remnant liver volume is significantly greater after therapeutic operation vs donation. Not too surprisingly, the complication rate after resection is directly proportional to the amount of liver resected. This was shown in this article, where the overall complication rate was significantly lower in resection for benign disease contrasted with donation. With a larger resection of liver, there is an increasing likelihood that the liver donor will suffer some sort of adverse outcome. The precise risk has not yet been discerned, but the calculation is one that should be taken by each center that performs live liver donation and transplantation.

T. Pruett, MD

References

1. Sheehy E, O'Connor KJ, Luskin RS, et al. Investigating geographic variation in mortality in the context of organ donation. *Am J Transplant.* 2012 Jun;12(6): 1598-1602.
2. Malinoski DJ, Patel MS, Lush S, et al. Impact of compliance with the American College of Surgeons trauma center verification requirements on organ donation-related outcomes. *J Am Coll Surg.* 2012 Aug;215(2):186-192.
3. Ausania F, White SA, Pocock P, Manas DM. Kidney damage during organ recovery in donation after circulatory death donors: data from UK National Transplant Database. *Am J Transplant.* 2012 Apr;12(4):932-936.
4. Fondevila C, Hessheimer AJ, Flores E, et al. Applicability and results of Maastricht type 2 donation after cardiac death liver transplantation. *Am J Transplant.* 2012 Jan;12(1):162-170.

Inferior Allograft Outcomes in Adolescent Recipients of Renal Transplants From Ideal Deceased Donors
Levine MH, Reese PP, Wood A, et al (Univ of Pennsylvania, Philadelphia; et al)
Ann Surg 255:556-564, 2012

Objective.—To measure the impact of the Share-35 policy on the allocation of ideal deceased donor kidneys and to examine the impact of age on outcomes after kidney transplantation using ideal donor kidneys.

Background.—In the United States, through Share-35, transplant candidates aged 18 years or younger receive priority for the highest-quality deceased donor kidneys. Adolescent (15—18 years) kidney transplant recipients (KTRs), however, may be more susceptible to allograft loss due to elevated rates of acute rejection and a possible increased risk of primary renal disease recurrence.

Methods.—We used registry data to perform a retrospective cohort study of 39,136 KTRs from January 1, 1994, to December 31, 2008. Ideal donors were defined as 2 to 34 years old with creatinine <1.5 mg/dL and absence of hypertension, diabetes, and hepatitis C.

Results.—After Share-35, the percentage of ideal donor kidneys allocated to pediatric recipients increased from 7% to 16%. In multivariable Cox regression, compared with adolescent KTRs, all age strata except recipients older than 70 years had a lower risk of allograft failure ($P < 0.01$ for each comparison); results were similar after excluding KTRs with diseases at high risk of recurrence. Adolescent recipients had higher mortality rates than KTRs younger than 14 years, similar mortality compared with that of KTRs older than 18 and younger than 40 years, and lower mortality than KTRs older than 40 years.

Conclusions.—The allocation of "ideal donors" to adolescent recipients may not maximize graft utility. Reevaluation of pediatric allocation priority may offer opportunities to optimize ideal renal allograft survival.

▶ The current US allocation system preferentially identifies the pediatric age group for individuals to receive the best organs from deceased donors. This article formalizes a discussion that has been taking place for years. Adolescent organ recipients are often not compliant with the medical regimen necessary to maintain graft function, so why give preference to these patients? The authors queried the national Organ Procurement and Transplantation Network's database and found that under the current system, adolescents receive a substantial amount of kidneys from ideal donors. However, when assessing short-term functional outcomes, kidney function in adolescents was inferior to all age groups except for those over 70 years old. The authors appropriately raise the question whether this is an appropriate use of the nation's organ supply. It feels right to preferentially give the youngest recipient a chance for a better life, but does it benefit the population? Unless we find a renewable source of organs, optimization of outcomes will have to be balanced against what is perceived as the right thing.

T. Pruett, MD

Solid-Organ Transplantation in Older Adults: Current Status and Future Research

Abecassis M, Bridges ND, Clancy CJ, et al (Northwestern Univ Feinberg School of Medicine, Chicago, IL; Natl Inst of Allergy and Infectious Diseases, Bethesda, MD; Univ of Pittsburgh, PA; et al)
Am J Transplant 12:2608-2622, 2012

An increasing number of patients older than 65 years are referred for and have access to organ transplantation, and an increasing number of older adults are donating organs. Although short-term outcomes are similar in older versus younger transplant recipients, older donor or recipient age is associated with inferior long-term outcomes. However, age is often a proxy for other factors that might predict poor outcomes more strongly and better identify patients at risk for adverse events. Approaches to transplantation in older adults vary across programs, but despite recent gains in access and the increased use of marginal organs, older patients remain less likely than other groups to receive a transplant, and those who do are highly selected. Moreover, few studies have addressed geriatric issues in transplant patient selection or management, or the implications on health span and disability when patients age to late life *with* a transplanted organ. This paper summarizes a recent trans-disciplinary workshop held by ASP, in collaboration with NHLBI, NIA, NIAID, NIDDK and AGS, to address issues related to kidney, liver, lung, or heart transplantation in older adults and to propose a research agenda in these areas.

▶ It is hardly earth-shattering news that the elderly are more prone to chronic organ disease. Where organ transplantation fits into their care has been a source of discussion for years. The elderly have been defined as anyone between the ages of 45 and 70 and older. But this is certainly not an absolute range. Many long-term survival and successful transplants have occurred with elderly individuals. However, we do not have sufficient transplant organs for those with potentially significant years to live; why give precious organs to those with most of their lives behind them? This question will continue to vex the allocation system and resources required to care for those with chronic organ failure. This article is an excellent summary of our current practice—what we know and that which is still ill defined. Not surprisingly, older individuals will not live as long as younger people. However, the effect of assessment and intervention on life expectancy and quality is not clear. Additionally, the quality of the organ required to improve the life of the older individual remains to be quantified. There is certainly a large population of individuals with organ failure over the age of 65 (approximately half of all end-stage renal disease patients in the United States). The modality to best care for these individuals remains to be elucidated.

T. Pruett, MD

Liver Transplantation for Hepatocellular Carcinoma: Long-Term Results Suggest Excellent Outcomes
Doyle MBM, Vachharajani N, Maynard E, et al (Washington Univ School of Medicine, St Louis, MO)
J Am Coll Surg 215:19-28, 2012

Background.—Selected 5-year survival results after liver transplantation for hepatocellular carcinoma (HCC) have been reported to be 70%. Our hypothesis was that liver transplantation is effective for long-term cancer control for HCC.

Study Design.—A 20-year retrospective review of a prospectively collected database was carried out. Demographic data and patient survival were calculated.

Results.—There were 1,422 liver transplantations performed between January 1990 and April 2011. Of these, 264 had HCC and 157 (59%) were pretreated with transarterial chemoembolization. Recipient age was 55.9 (±7.9) years and 208 (79%) of patients were male. The underlying disease was hepatitis C virus in 155 (58.7%), hepatitis B virus in 16 (6%), alcohol in 21 (8%), and miscellaneous in the remaining 72 cases. The mean number of tumors was 1.8 (± 1.7) and the mean largest tumor diameter was 2.3 (± 1.3) cm in the explanted liver. One, 5, and 10-year patient survival was 88.5%, 69.1%, and 40.5%, respectively; disease-specific survival was 99.1%, 94.4% and 87.9%; and disease-free survival was 86.0%, 64.6%, and 40.1%. One, 5, and 10-year graft survival was 87.3%, 68.0%, and 41.8%. Nine (3.4%) patients required retransplantation; 75 patients (28.4%) have died, but only 10 of 75 (13.3%) died of recurrent HCC (3.7% of all HCC patients receiving a transplant) and 6 (8%) died of recurrent viral hepatitis. An additional 9 recipients developed recurrence (total HCC recurrence, n = 19 [7%]), 4 of whom died of causes other than HCC. The remaining 5 are disease-free posttreatment (mean 5.5 years after orthotopic liver transplantation).

Conclusions.—Orthotopic liver transplantation offers an effective treatment strategy for HCC in the setting of cirrhosis, even in the setting of hepatitis C virus. Hepatocellular carcinoma recurrence is uncommon in properly selected patients and disease-specific long-term survival approaches 90%.

▶ The current liver allocation scheme in the United States gives preferential allocation points to individuals with hepatocellular carcinoma within certain size and number. In the mid-1990s, it was observed that patients with T2 lesions and cirrhosis have a better survival with transplantation than other forms of treatment. However, long-term outcomes have been somewhat more controversial, although most feel that liver transplantation is the optimal treatment for those individuals with disease confined to the liver. This single-center report revisits the issue of survival after liver transplant. Importantly, there were more deaths from viral hepatitis effect on the allograft than recurrent cancer. Although there are many other issues to address regarding management strategies for individuals with hepatocellular carcinoma and cirrhosis, this treatment is still the optimal form of treatment.

T. Pruett, MD

Re-examination of the Lymphocytotoxic Crossmatch in Liver Transplantation: Can C4d Stains Help in Monitoring?
Lunz J, Ruppert KM, Cajaiba MM, et al (Univ of Pittsburgh Med Ctr, PA; Univ of Pittsburgh Graduate School of Public Health, PA; et al)
Am J Transplant 12:171-182, 2012

C4d-assisted recognition of antibody-mediated rejection (AMR) in formalin-fixed paraffin-embedded tissues (FFPE) from donor-specific antibody-positive (DSA+) renal allograft recipients prompted study of DSA+ liver allograft recipients as measured by lymphocytotoxic crossmatch (XM) and/or Luminex. XM results did not influence patient or allograft survival, or cellular rejection rates, but XM+ recipients received significantly more prophylactic steroids. Endothelial C4d staining strongly correlates with XM+ (<3 weeks posttransplantation) and DSA+ status and cellular rejection, but not with worse Banff grading or treatment response. Diffuse

C4d staining, XM+, DSA+ and ABO− incompatibility status, histopathology and clinical−serologic profile helped establish an isolated AMR diagnosis in 5 of 100 (5%) XM+ and one ABO-incompatible, recipients. C4d staining later after transplantation was associated with rejection and nonrejection-related causes of allograft dysfunction in DSA− and DSA+ recipients, some of whom had good outcomes without additional therapy. Liver allograft FFPE C4d staining: (a) can help classify liver allograft dysfunction; (b) substantiates antibody contribution to rejection; (c) probably represents nonalloantibody insults and/or complete absorption in DSA− recipients and (d) alone, is an imperfect AMR marker needing correlation with routine histopathology, clinical and serologic profiles. Further study in late biopsies and other tissue markers of liver AMR with simultaneous DSA measurements are needed.

▶ Antibodies that are directed against the transplanted organ have traditionally been a clinical barrier to be avoided. However, in recent years, attempts to diminish alloantibodies have been made. The liver has held a special place within the scope of transplanted organs as not requiring donor-recipient antibody-antigen compatibility for successful outcomes. It is now common to assess for complement activation within the transplanted organ in the diagnosis and assessment of antibody-mediated rejection of virtually all organs. This article describes a single-center review of C4d deposition within the transplanted liver and its correlation with circulating donor-specific antibody (DSA) before the transplant. Although evidence of complement activation correlated with DSA, increased rejection episodes, steroid use, and patient and graft survival were not statistically altered. The role of preexisting immunologic recognition of a donor liver is not a contraindication but does appear to use different pathways to achieve immunologic balance over the long term. Strategies to gain graft acceptance in the face of immunologic barriers can be tempered through understanding the relative resistance of the liver to damage.

T. Pruett, MD

Evolution of Pancreas Transplantation: Long-Term Results and Perspectives From a High-Volume Center
Öllinger R, Margreiter C, Bösmüller C, et al (Med Univ Innsbruck, Tyrol, Austria)
Ann Surg 256:780-787, 2012

Objective.—To describe the evolution of pancreas transplantation from 1979 to 2011. The aim was to examine factors influencing long-term patient and graft survival, surgical methods, and risk factors influencing organ performance after transplantation.

Background.—Pancreas transplantation has become the therapy of choice for patients suffering insulin-dependent diabetes and end stage renal failure.

Methods.—Retrospective analysis of 509 consecutive pancreas transplants (442 simultaneous pancreas and kidney [SPK], 20 pancreas transplanted alone [PTA], and 47 pancreas transplanted after kidney [PAK]), performed at the University Hospital Innsbruck. The data were statistically analyzed using the Kaplan-Meier method and log-rank test.

Results.—After overcoming initial immunological and technical problems between 1979 and 1988 (5-year pancreas graft survival rate, 29.7%), pancreas transplantation evolved during the second decade (1989–1996; 5-year pancreas graft survival rate, 42.2%). Technical changes, optimized immunosuppression, careful pretransplant evaluation, and improved graft monitoring have become standard in the last decade and result in excellent 5-year patient (94.3%), kidney (89.4%), and pancreas (81.5%) graft survival. Five-year graft survival was superior in SPK (68.8%) compared with PAK (62.5%) and PTA (16.4%). SPK retransplantation can be carried out safely with 5-year patient (87.5%) and pancreas graft (75.0%) survival. Overall 5-year patient survival after loss of the first pancreas graft is significantly better in patients who underwent retransplantation (89.4% vs. 67.9%, $P = 0.001$). Long-term pancreas graft survival is independent of donor body mass index, sex, and cause of death, anastomosis time and the number of human leukocyte antigen (HLA) mismatches, recipient age, body mass index, sex, current panel reactive antibodies, and waiting time. Significant risk factors for reduced graft survival are cold ischemia time and donor age.

Conclusions.—During the last 32 years, many problems in pancreas transplantation have been overcome and it may currently represent the therapeutic gold standard for some patients with diabetes and end stage renal failure.

▶ Pancreas transplantation for glucose control has been controversial but extraordinarily popular with recipients of the grafts. There have been many technical challenges to overcome to achieve predictable euglycemia. This article gives a nice review, highlighting the improvements in patient and graft survival that have accompanied refinements in management, technical, and immunosuppressive regimens. It is commendable that cardiac deaths in the current era occurred at a rate of only 1.1%. Even infectious deaths are infrequent at 2.8%. These results could only happen with extraordinary attention to the surgical details associated with the retrieval, preparation, and implantation of the transplanted pancreas. The precise role for pancreas transplantation within the spectrum of therapies for diabetes remains to be discerned. However, the risk/benefit calculation is markedly improved when the risk is diminished as much as is currently being described.

T. Pruett, MD

Potent Induction Immunotherapy Promotes Long-Term Insulin Independence After Islet Transplantation in Type 1 Diabetes
Bellin MD, Barton FB, Heitman A, et al (Univ of Minnesota, Minneapolis; The Emmes Corporation, Rockville, MD; et al)
Am J Transplant 12:1576-1583, 2012

The seemingly inexorable decline in insulin independence after islet transplant alone (ITA) has raised concern about its clinical utility. We hypothesized that induction immunosuppression therapy determines durability of insulin independence. We analyzed the proportion of insulin-independent patients following final islet infusion in four groups of ITA recipients according to induction immunotherapy: University of Minnesota recipients given FcR nonbinding anti-CD3 antibody alone or T cell depleting antibodies (TCDAb) and TNF-a inhibition (TNF-α-i) (group 1; n = 29); recipients reported to the Collaborative Islet Transplant Registry (CITR) given TCDAb+TNF-α-i (group 2; n = 20); CITR recipients given TCDAb without TNF-α-i (group 3; n = 43); and CITR recipients given IL-2 receptor antibodies (IL-2RAb) alone (group 4; n = 177). Results were compared with outcomes in pancreas transplant alone (PTA) recipients reported to the Scientific Registry of Transplant Recipients (group 5; n = 677). The 5-year insulin independence rates in group 1 (50%) and group 2 (50%) were comparable to outcomes in PTA (group 5: 52%; p>>0.05) but significantly higher than in group 3 (0%; $p = 0.001$) and group 4 (20%; $p = 0.02$). Induction immunosuppression was significantly associated with 5-year insulin independence ($p = 0.03$), regardless of maintenance immunosuppression or other factors. These findings support potential for long-term insulin independence after ITA using potent induction therapy, with anti-CD3 Ab or TCDAb+TNF-α-i.

▶ Islet transplantation has held the promise of achieving glycemic control of the diabetic without the morbidities. It appears to be a form of therapy that is finally coming into its own. Alloislet transplantation has faced many hurdles, including a combination of technical, immunologic, and drug toxicity. This article highlights outcomes after islet transplantation proportional to immunosuppressive induction regimens. The authors demonstrated that insulin independence could be achieved at the same frequency as with pancreas transplantation alone when the combination of lymphocyte depleting and anti-tumor necrosis factor (TNF) antibodies were given as induction. The importance of negating the TNF effect on the transplanted islet was demonstrated in the group receiving no anti-TNF, in which there were no long-term (5-year) insulin-independent recipients. Nonlymphocyte-depleting therapy with interleuken-2 receptor blockade proved an inferior form of induction. The role of cell-based therapy for diabetes remains to be seen, but sustainable results, such as those demonstrated in this article, are essential in order for the discussions to move forward. As with the article Evolution of Pancreas Transplantation: Long-Term Results and Perspectives From a High-Volume Center by R. Öllinger et al, risk/benefit will need to be assessed to finally discern where optimal therapies reside. However, it now appears that there are competing therapies to achieve similar clinical benefit.

T. Pruett, MD

Total Pancreatectomy and Islet Autotransplantation for Chronic Pancreatitis
Sutherland DE, Radosevich DM, Bellin MD, et al (Univ of Minnesota, Minneapolis)
J Am Coll Surg 214:409-424, 2012

Background.—Total pancreatectomy (TP) with intraportal islet auto-transplantation (IAT) can relieve pain and preserve β-cell mass in patients with chronic pancreatitis (CP) when other therapies fail. We report on a >30-year single-center series.

Study Design.—Four hundred and nine patients (including 53 children, 5 to 18 years) with CP underwent TP-IAT from February 1977 to September 2011 (etiology: idiopathic, 41%; Sphincter of Oddi dysfunction/biliary, 9%; genetic, 14%; divisum, 17%; alcohol, 7%; and other, 12%; mean age was 35.3 years, 74% were female; 21% has earlier operations, including 9% Puestow procedure, 6% Whipple, 7% distal pancreatectomy, and 2% other). Islet function was classified as insulin independent for those on no insulin; partial, if known C-peptide positive or euglycemic on once-daily insulin; and insulin dependent if on standard basal–bolus diabetic regimen. A 36-item Short Form (SF-36) survey for quality of life was completed by patients before and in serial follow-up since 2007, with an integrated survey that was added in 2008.

Results.—Actuarial patient survival post TP-IAT was 96% in adults and 98% in children (1 year) and 89% and 98% (5 years). Complications requiring relaparotomy occurred in 15.9% and bleeding (9.5%) was the most common complication. IAT function was achieved in 90% (C-peptide >0.6 ng/mL). At 3 years, 30% were insulin independent (25% in adults, 55% in children) and 33% had partial function. Mean hemoglobin A1c was <7.0% in 82%. Earlier pancreas surgery lowered islet yield (2,712 vs 4,077/kg; $p = 0.003$). Islet yield (<2,500/kg [36%]; 2,501 to 5,000/kg [39%]; >5,000/kg [24%]) correlated with degree of function with insulin independent rates at 3 years of 12%, 22%, and 72%, and rates of partial function 33%, 62%, and 24%. All patients had pain before TP-IAT and nearly all were on daily narcotics. After TP-IAT, 85% had pain improvement. By 2 years, 59% had ceased narcotics. All children were on narcotics before, 39% at follow-up; pain improved in 94%; and 67% became pain-free. In the SF-36 survey, there was significant improvement from baseline in all dimensions, including the Physical and Mental Component Summaries ($p < 0.01$), whether on narcotics or not.

Conclusions.—TP can ameliorate pain and improve quality of life in otherwise refractory CP patients, even if narcotic withdrawal is delayed or incomplete because of earlier long-term use. IAT preserves meaningful islet function in most patients and substantial islet function in more than two thirds of patients, with insulin independence occurring in one quarter of adults and half the children.

▶ Autotransplantation of islets is not associated with the immunologic barriers of the allopancreas or islet. To this end, insights can be gleaned. This article describes the outcomes of 409 autoislets over a 30-year period. There are too many variables to make sweeping claims, but insulin independence is achieved with far fewer autoislets than required in allotransplantation. Durability of insulin independence is pretty good, but not predictably so. Are these immunologic or technical reasons? The answers may finally bring reliable insights into the disparate and sometimes conflicting discourse about optimal cell-based or organ-based therapy for the diabetic individual.

T. Pruett, MD

Institutional Factors Beyond Procedural Volume Significantly Impact Center Variability in Outcomes After Orthotopic Heart Transplantation
Kilic A, Weiss ES, Yuh DD, et al (The Johns Hopkins Hosp, Baltimore, MD; Yale School of Medicine, New Haven, CT)
Ann Surg 256:616-623, 2012

Objective.—To evaluate the contribution of institutional volume and other unmeasured institutional factors beyond volume to the between-center variability in outcomes after orthotopic heart transplantation (OHT).

Background.—It is unclear if institutional factors beyond volume have a significant impact on OHT outcomes.

Methods.—The United Network for Organ Sharing registry was used to identify OHTs performed between 2000 and 2010. Separate mixed-effect logistic regression models were constructed, with the primary endpoint being post-OHT mortality. Model A included only individual centers, model B added validated recipient and donor risk indices as well as the year of transplantation, and model C added institutional volume as a continuous variable to model B. The reduction in between-center variability in mortality between models B and C was used to define the contribution of institutional volume. Kaplan-Meier survival curves were also compared after stratifying patients into equal-size tertiles based on center volume.

Results.—A total of 119 centers performed OHT in 19,156 patients. After adjusting for transplantation year and differences in recipient and donor risk, decreasing center volume was associated with an increased risk of 1-year mortality ($P < 0.001$). However, procedural volume only accounted for 16.7% of the variability in mortality between centers, and significant between-center variability persisted after adjusting for institutional volume ($P < 0.001$). In Kaplan-Meier analysis, there was significant variability in 1-year survival between centers within each volume category: low-volume (66.7%–96.6%), intermediate volume (80.7%–97.3%), and high-volume (83.8%–93.9%). These trends were also observed with 5-year mortality.

Conclusions.—This large-cohort analysis demonstrates that although institutional volume is a significant predictor of post-OHT outcomes, there are other unmeasured institutional factors that contribute substantially to the between center variability in outcomes. Institutional volume should therefore not be the sole indicator of "center quality" in OHT.

▶ The ability of centers to offer organ replacement (transplantation) therapies is entirely dependent on their recouping of the costs associated with providing those therapies. The two major drivers of access to payments for the care provided are (1) risk-adjusted outcomes provided by the Scientific Registry of Transplant Recipients and (2) numbers of procedures performed. The Centers for Medicare and Medicaid Services and most private insurers rely on these values. However, the capriciousness of the system is pointed out in this article. Although center volume was positively correlated with survival after heart transplantation, it accounted for less than 20% of the predictive outcomes. The article raises a good point relating to availability and access to transplant care in the United States. The payers are determining where care can be provided under the guise of improved and expert care. This article and others press the issue stating the obvious: Excellent care can be provided in many locations, and volume alone is not the major determinant. By demanding that certain volumes be achieved, the payers (private and public) drive many providers out of business and restrict availability. This may be acceptable public policy, but there should be an open discussion about the intent and repercussions to our delivery system.

T. Pruett, MD

Multivisceral Transplantation for Diffuse Portomesenteric Thrombosis
Vianna RM, Mangus RS, Kubal C, et al (Indiana Univ School of Medicine, Indianapolis)
Ann Surg 255:1144-1150, 2012

Objective.—To evaluate the clinical outcomes of multivisceral transplantation (MVT) in the setting of diffuse thrombosis of the portomesenteric venous system.

Background.—Liver transplantation (LT) in the face of cirrhosis and diffuse portomesenteric thrombosis (PMT) is controversial and contraindicated in many transplant centers. LT using alternative techniques such as portocaval hemitransposition fails to eliminate complications of portal hypertension. MVT replaces the liver and the thrombosed portomesenteric system.

Methods.—A database of intestinal transplant patients was maintained with prospective analysis of outcomes. The diagnosis of diffuse PMT was established with dual-phase abdominal computed tomography or magnetic resonance imaging with venous reconstruction.

Results.—Twenty-five patients with grade IV PMT received 25 MVT. Eleven patients underwent simultaneous cadaveric kidney transplantation. Biopsy proven acute cellular rejection was noted in 5 recipients, which was treated successfully. With a median follow-up of 2.8 years, patient and graft survival were 80%, 72%, and 72% at 1, 3, and 5 years, respectively. To date, all survivors have good graft function without any signs of residual/recurrent features of portal hypertension.

Conclusions.—MVT can be considered as an option for the treatment of patients with diffuse PMT. MVT is the only procedure that completely reverses portal hypertension and addresses the primary disease while achieving superior survival results in comparison to the alternative options.

▶ Complex problems sometimes require complex solutions. The problem of total mesenteric thrombosis can preclude successful liver transplantation, but it is also one that undergoes significant remodeling over time. This makes one query when the substantial operative endeavor of combined liver—bowel transplantation is necessary for optimal outcomes. This article is a recounting of the longitudinal experience of a single program. The results are good with 1-year and 5-year patient-to-graft survival of 80% and 72%, respectively. The authors describe that in 6 patients it was possible to gain sufficient portal flow to allow a liver-alone transplant. It is likely that an additional percentage of patients could be treated with a solitary liver transplant. The question that remains is how to assess when enough flow is enough and when a multivisceral transplant is truly optimal.

T. Pruett, MD

Outcomes and Native Renal Recovery Following Simultaneous Liver—Kidney Transplantation

Levitsky J, Baker T, Ahya SN, et al (Northwestern Univ, Chicago, IL; et al)
Am J Transplant 12:2949-2957, 2012

With the increase in patients having impaired renal function at liver transplant due to MELD, accurate predictors of posttransplant native renal recovery are needed to select candidates for simultaneous liver—kidney transplantation (SLK). Current UNOS guidelines rely on specific clinical criteria for SLK allocation. To examine these guidelines and other variables predicting nonrecovery, we analyzed 155 SLK recipients, focusing on a subset (n = 78) that had post-SLK native GFR (nGFR) determined by radionuclide renal scans. The 77 patients not having renal scans received a higher number of extended criteria donor organs and had worse posttransplant survival. Of the 78 renal scan patients, 31 met and 47 did not meet pre-SLK UNOS criteria. The UNOS criteria were more predictive than our institutional criteria for all nGFR recovery thresholds (20—40 mL/min), although at the most conservative cut-off (nGFR $\leq$ 20) it had low sensitivity (55.3%), specificity (75%), PPV (67.6%) and NPV (63.8%) for predicting post-SLK nonrecovery. On multivariate analysis, the only predictor of native renal nonrecovery (nGFR $\leq$ 20) was abnormal pre-SLK renal imaging (OR

3.85, CI 1.22–12.5). Our data support the need to refine SLK selection utilizing more definitive biomarkers and predictors of native renal recovery than current clinical criteria.

▶ This article is an extension of the article review by Vianna et al, Multivisceral transplantation for diffuse portomesenteric thrombosis.[1] The authors analyzed their experience with renograms in combined liver–kidney recipients in order to discern the return of native renal function and ultimate utility of the combined organ transplant. Renograms for recipients with indications consistent with those from a consensus conference were compared with those for recipients meeting institutional criteria alone. Failure of return of native renal function was best predicted by the consensus conference indications. The use of combined organs from older donors resulted in lesser outcomes than the standard criteria donor. Because the retrospective nature of the analysis and the scans were not homogeneously applied to the population, there are significant limitations in the reliability of the observations.

T. Pruett, MD

Reference

1. Vianna RM, Mangus RS, Kubal C, et al. Multivisceral transplantation for diffuse portomesenteric thrombosis. *Ann Surg.* 2012 Jun;255(6):1144-1150.

Reduction in Corticosteroids Is Associated with Better Health-Related Quality of Life after Liver Transplantation

Zaydfudim V, Feurer ID, Landman MP, et al (Vanderbilt Univ Med Ctr, Nashville, TN)
J Am Coll Surg 214:164-173, 2012

Background.—Corticosteroid use during post-transplant immunosuppression contributes to documented long-term complications in liver transplant recipients. However, the effects of steroids on post-transplant physical and mental health-related quality of life (HRQOL) have not been established. We aimed to test the association between steroid-based immunosuppression and post-transplant HRQOL in liver transplant recipients.

Study Design.—We performed a retrospective analysis of prospective, longitudinal HRQOL measured using the Short Form 36 Health Survey physical and mental component summary scores, Beck Anxiety Inventory, and Center for Epidemiologic Studies Depression Scale. Steroid use (none, low [<10 mg/d], high [≥10 mg/d]) and temporally associated acute rejection (within previous 6 weeks, previous 7 to 12 weeks, and never or >12 weeks before HRQOL measurement) were determined at every post-transplant HRQOL data point. Linear mixed-effects models tested the effects of contemporaneous steroid use and dosing on post-transplant HRQOL.

Results.—The sample included 186 adult liver transplant recipients (mean age 54 ± 8 years, 70% male) with pre- and at least 1 post-transplant

HRQOL data point. Individual follow-up posttransplant averaged 21 ± 18 months (range 1 to 74 months). After controlling for pretransplant HRQOL, time post-transplant, pre-transplant diagnosis group, and temporally associated episodes of rejection, post-transplant high-dose steroid use (≥10 mg/d) was associated with lower physical component summary ($p < 0.001$) and mental component summary ($p = 0.049$) scores and increased Beck Anxiety Inventory ($p = 0.015$) scores. Low-dose steroid use (<10 mg/d) was not associated with post-transplant HRQOL in any model (all $p \geq 0.28$).

Conclusions.—High-dose steroid use for post-transplant immunosuppression in liver transplant recipients was associated with reduced physical and mental HRQOL, and increased symptoms of anxiety. There was an association between better HRQOL and steroid reduction to <10 mg/d in liver transplant recipients during a broad follow-up period.

▶ Although not overwhelming, there are a number of immunosuppressive drugs available for posttransplant therapy. The drugs are usually used in some form of combination and have reduced rejection episodes to low levels. For years, steroids (glucocorticoids) have been a cornerstone of immunosuppressive regimens; however, side effects are often complicating and limiting. This article asserts that liver recipients who remain on steroids have an impaired quality of life as compared with individuals who could have steroids removed. Although there are serious limitations to this article (small numbers, inexact definitions, no clear association of medication to quality-of-life issues, and other perioperative complications), it is yet another bit of information that demonstrates that side effects can have a significant impact on life. It is a goal of transplantation to gain long-term benefit from functional organs but with the least morbidity and complications.

T. Pruett, MD

An Analysis of Lymphocyte Phenotype After Steroid Avoidance With Either Alemtuzumab or Basiliximab Induction in Renal Transplantation

Cherukuri A, Salama AD, Carter C, et al (Univ of Leeds, UK; Royal Free Hosp, London, UK; et al)
Am J Transplant 12:919-931, 2012

Several studies have analyzed the phenotype of repopulated T-lymphocytes following alemtuzumab induction; however there has been less scrutiny of the reconstituted B-cell compartment. In the context of a randomized controlled trial (RCT) comparing alemtuzumab induction with tacrolimus monotherapy against basiliximab induction with tacrolimus and mycophenolate mofetil (MMF) therapy in renal transplantation, we analyzed the peripheral B- and T-lymphocyte phenotypes of patients at a mean of 25 +/− 2 months after transplantation. We examined the relationship between peripheral lymphocyte phenotype and graft function. Patients who received alemtuzumab had significantly higher numbers of

B cells including näive, transitional and regulatory subsets. In contrast, the CD4+ T-cell compartment was dominated by amemory cell phenotype. Following either basiliximab or alemtuzumab induction, patients with lower numbers of B cells or B subsets had significantly worse graft function. For alemtuzumab, there was also a correlation between these subsets the stability of graft function and the presence of HLA-specific antibodies. These results demonstrate that a significant expansion of regulatory type B cells is associated with superior graft function and that this pattern is more common after alemtuzumab induction. This phenomenon requires further prospective study to see whether this phenotype could be used to customize immunotherapy.

▶ After organ transplantation, immunologic and physiologic changes occur. In this article, the authors followed lymphocyte characteristics 2 years after transplantation after either interleukin-2 (IL-2) receptor or alemtuzumab induction therapy. The clinical outcomes are not statistically different, although trends are suggestive that depletion may trend toward less rejection episodes. IL-2 receptor inhibition occurs with a nondepleting antibody, and the depleting antibody is associated with marked early reductions and long-term reconstitution of circulating lymphocytes. There is much to be learned from the kinetics of reconstitution, especially with the observation that regulatory B cells occur late. These sorts of observational studies are fraught with conflicting hypotheses to explain the observations. However, the mechanisms by which particular cells appear/reappear remains to be elucidated.

T. Pruett, MD

Induction Therapy With Autologous Mesenchymal Stem Cells in Living-Related Kidney Transplants: A Randomized Controlled Trial

Tan J, Wu W, Xu X, et al (Xiamen Univ, Fuzhou, China; Univ of Miami Miller School of Medicine, FL; et al)
JAMA 307:1169-1177, 2012

Context.—Antibody-based induction therapy plus calcineurin inhibitors (CNIs) reduce acute rejection rates in kidney recipients; however, opportunistic infections and toxic CNI effects remain challenging. Reportedly, mesenchymal stem cells (MSCs) have successfully treated graft-vs-host disease.

Objective.—To assess autologous MSCs as replacement of antibody induction for patients with end-stage renal disease who undergo ABO-compatible, cross-match–negative kidney transplants from a living-related donor.

Design, Setting, and Patients.—One hundred fifty-nine patients were enrolled in this single-site, prospective, open-label, randomized study from February 2008-May 2009, when recruitment was completed.

Intervention.—Patients were inoculated with marrow-derived autologous MSC ($1-2\times10^6$/kg) at kidney reperfusion and two weeks later. Fifty-three patients received standard-dose and 52 patients received low-dose CNIs (80% of standard); 51 patients in the control group received anti–IL-2 receptor antibody plus standard-dose CNIs.

Main Outcome Measures.—The primary measure was 1-year incidence of acute rejection and renal function (estimated glomerular filtration rate [eGFR]); the secondary measure was patient and graft survival and incidence of adverse events.

Results.—Patient and graft survival at 13 to 30 months was similar in all groups. After 6 months, 4 of 53 patients (7.5%) in the autologous MSC plus standard-dose CNI group (95% CI, 0.4%-14.7%; P =.04) and 4 of 52 patients (7.7%) in the low-dose group (95% CI, 0.5%-14.9%; P =.046) compared with 11 of 51 controls (21.6%; 95% CI, 10.5%-32.6%) had biopsy-confirmed acute rejection. None of the patients in either autologous MSC group had glucocorticoid-resistant rejection, whereas 4 patients (7.8%) in the control group did (95% CI, 0.6%-15.1%; overall P =.02). Renal function recovered faster among both MSC groups showing increased eGFR levels during the first month after surgery than the control group. Patients receiving standard-dose CNI had a mean difference of 6.2 mL/min per 1.73 m^2 (95% CI, 0.4-11.9; P =.04) and those in the low-dose CNI of 10.0 mL/min per 1.73 m^2 (95% CI, 3.8-16.2; P =.002). Also, during the 1-year followup, combined analysis of MSC-treated groups revealed significantly decreased risk of opportunistic infections than the control group (hazard ratio, 0.42; 95% CI, 0.20-0.85, P =.02).

Conclusion.—Among patients undergoing renal transplant, the use of autologous MSCs compared with anti-IL-2 receptor antibody induction therapy resulted in lower incidence of acute rejection, decreased risk of opportunistic infection, and better estimated renal function at 1 year.

Trial Registration.—clinicaltrials.gov Identifier: NCT00658073.

▶ Successful immunologic adaptation to a transplanted organ up until very recently has depended on the use of immunosuppressive drugs. However, the target of these drugs is host cells. The idea that cellular manipulation can influence outcomes with much less or even no immunosuppressive drugs is an intriguing notion. This article reports 1 of several attempts at cellular manipulation. The administration of autologous mesenchymal stem cells was associated with similar/reduced rejection episodes with better function and less immunosuppression associated infections contrasted to a "control" group. Although there can always be arguments about appropriate controls and endpoints, this and other reports represent the appearance of the inexorable march toward the use of cellular manipulations to achieve clinical acceptance of the transplanted organ. The use of autologous cell–based immunotherapy in this report is encouraging, and the lessons will be useful in learning whether the effects are direct or indirect on the immune system.

T. Pruett, MD

High Incidence of Anticytomegalovirus Drug Resistance Among D+R−
Kidney Transplant Recipients Receiving Preemptive Therapy

Couzi L, Helou S, Bachelet T, et al (Centre Hospitalier Universitaire de Bordeaux, France; et al)
Am J Transplant 12:202-209, 2012

Anti-cytomegalovirus (CMV) prophylaxis is recommended in D+R− kidney transplant recipients (KTR), but is associated with a theoretical increased risk of developing anti-CMV drug resistance. This hypothesis was retested in this study by comparing 32 D+R− KTR who received 3 months prophylaxis (valganciclovir) with 80 D+R− KTR who received preemptive treatment. The incidence of CMV infections was higher in the preemptive group than in the prophylactic group (60% vs. 34%, respectively; $p = 0.02$). Treatment failure (i.e. a positive DNAemia 8 weeks after the initiation of anti-CMV treatment) was more frequent in the preemptive group (31% vs. 3% in the prophylactic group; $p = 0.001$). Similarly, anti-CMV drug resistance (*UL97* or *UL54* mutations) was also more frequent in the preemptive group (16% vs. 3% in the prophylactic group; $p = 0.05$). Antiviral treatment failures were associated with anti-CMV drug resistance ($p = 0.0001$). Patients with a CMV load over 5.25 $\log_{10}$ copies/mL displayed the highest risk of developing anti-CMV drug resistance (OR = 16.91, $p = 0.0008$). Finally, the 1-year estimated glomerular filtration rate was reduced in patients with anti-CMV drug resistance ($p = 0.02$). In summary, preemptive therapy in D+R− KTR with high CMV loads and antiviral treatment failure was associated with a high incidence of anti-CMV drug resistance.

▶ The development of cytomegalovirus (CMV) after organ transplantation has been a major complication for the transplant recipient. A number of advances have greatly reduced the impact of this virus on the clinical well-being of the recipient. However, an efficient and efficacious strategy for the use of antivirals is still being debated. One approach is to give prophylactic antivirals to all at risk, and the other is to closely monitor recipients and treat preemptively when the virus is detectable. It has been assumed that universal prophylaxis would be associated with more viral resistance, but a less frequent CMV could be missed through clinical vagaries.

This study is from a single center that sought to address the issues through randomization of patients at risk—those kidney recipients without prior CMV exposure (R−) who were transplanted with a kidney from a donor with prior CMV (D+). Over a 23-month period, 32 of 172 individuals were D + /R− and randomized between prophylactic vs preemptive therapy. The results were surprising in 1 area: the percentage of patients who had resistant mutations was statistically higher ($P < .05$) and treatment failures were more frequent ($P < .001$) in the preemptive therapy group. This single center study is hampered by relatively small numbers of patients. The issues surrounding optimization of disease minimization and patient benefit are not solely virologic. Short-term and longer-term follow-up of these and other patients will help clarify issues surrounding the consequences of immunosuppression postorgan transplantation.

T. Pruett, MD

Characterization of the Ileal Microbiota in Rejecting and Nonrejecting Recipients of Small Bowel Transplants
Oh PL, Martínez I, Sun Y, et al (Univ of Nebraska-Lincoln; Univ of Nebraska Med Ctr, Omaha)
Am J Transplant 12:753-762, 2012

Small bowel transplantation can be a life-preserving procedure for patients with irreversible intestinal failure. Allograft rejection remains a major source of morbidity and mortality and its accurate diagnosis and treatment are critical. In this study, we used pyrosequencing of 16S ribosomal RNA gene tags to compare the composition of the ileal microbiota present during nonrejection, prerejection and active rejection states in small bowel transplant patients. During episodes of rejection, the proportions of phylum Firmicutes ($p < 0.001$) and the order Lactobacillales ($p < 0.01$) were significantly decreased, while those of the phylum Proteobacteria, especially the family Enterobacteriaceae, were significantly increased ($p < 0.005$). Receiver-operating characteristic analysis revealed that relative proportions of several bacterial taxa in ileal effluents and especially Firmicutes, could be used to discriminate between nonrejection and active rejection. In conclusion, the findings obtained during this study suggest that small bowel transplant rejection is associated with changes in the microbial populations in ileal effluents and support microbiota profiling as a potential diagnostic biomarker of rejection. Future studies should investigate if the dysbiosis that we observed is a cause or a consequence of the rejection process.

▶ The role and composition of the gut flora are becoming of increasing interest in understanding the consequence of many diseases. Investigation of the changes induced in the microbiota of the transplanted bowel as a function of immunologic and infectious results was a study that needed to be done. This article demonstrated that the proportion of bacteria in the gut microbiota changes dramatically over time and is coincident with immunologic events. The variables that may drive changes in flora include not only antimicrobial agents but also other drugs (including fungal products used in immunosuppression tacrolimus and cyclosporin-A), compositional changes in enteric fluid (bile salt replacement), or cytokines or host cells in the enteric fluids. The results of this article are intriguing, but the factors associated with observed variations in the gut microbiota need further elucidation prior to concluding that microbiota changes can be used as an immunologic monitoring tool.

T. Pruett, MD

7   Surgical Infections

Introduction

Infections continue to be a major source of patient morbidity after surgical procedures. It is amazing that standardization of process has not reduced the frequency of surgical site infections (SSIs) to a very low rate. To this end, the continued focus upon these untoward events will continue to raise the level of awareness. The publicity surrounding the release of National Surgical Quality Improvement Program (NSQIP, administered by the Am College of Surgeons) results has changed the dynamic within hospitals and operating theaters as well as the relationship with private and public insurers. This year's papers selection will predominantly focus upon the infection data and how the surgical community is addressing the vagaries of surgical infections as well as some of the anticipated changes.

In most hospitals, it is rare that the people collecting and reporting information about SSIs are directly involved with the performance of the procedures. To that end, there is always a question about the reliability of the information. Most hospital infection control personnel follow the trends of SSIs through a variety of direct observations, chart surveillance, survey of hospital staff, and pharmacy review. To the extent that different systems report and document different events, the rates of what is called SSI will vary between institutions. Programs such as NSQIP are trying to standardize definitions so that more meaningful information will be made to the public.

The extent of variance induced by some of these variables is demonstrated in the first article selection (1). The authors in this article assessed hospital identification of SSI using surgeon notification, bacterial culture results, antibiotic prescription, and discharge diagnosis. The identification rate increased from 18% when a surgeon notification was required to make the diagnosis to over 86% when laboratory results, prescribing patterns, and discharge diagnoses were included. However, the true rate or accuracy of SSI could be under-recognized, because the authors only focused on in-hospital events or overestimated by reason of suboptimal microbiologic collection or prescribing practices that were more preventative than therapeutic. With the dramatically decreasing length of stays in the United States, many SSIs don't develop during the hospitalization period. Newer techniques will be necessary to track outcomes of in- and out-patients. However, because much of the NSQIP data is only about in-patient events, there is little motivation for hospital systems to fund surveillance of the diverse out-patient environment.

One of the problems with risk stratification falls to the reliability and inclusiveness of codes for all the variables that influence clinical outcomes. Article 2 discusses a simple factor that is not risk adjusted in NSQIP reporting; that is, the indication for colorectal surgery. Using the national database, it was found that the risk of SSI varied almost 100% between benign lesion resection and rectal carcinoma and was stratified in-between with the diagnosis of inflammatory bowel disease, diverticular disease, and others. A caution must be issued for use of risk adjusted data until one understands how to query and discern methodologies. Too many administrators and insurers assume that risk adjustment accounts for all variables, and they do not understand the vagaries of clinical medicine.

Most surgeons are aware of the fundamental elements of SSI prevention: appropriate and timely administration of antimicrobial agents, minimize trauma to the wound (avoid razor shaving), and maintain body temperature and perfusion during the procedure. Despite knowing these elements, monitoring and feedback of compliance with these variables has not been commonplace in US hospitals. A team from Toronto took on the task of establishing the audit and feedback loop and then set out to measure the acceptance from the operative teams. This was associated with a significant reduction in the SSI rate but was met with variable amounts of enthusiasm by members of the operative team. The article (3) reemphasizes the importance of team dynamics when implementing strategies to reduce SSI. The task of implementation of culture change is the theme of article 4. The team from Johns' Hopkins discusses their implementation of the Comprehensive Unit-Based Safety Program. Specific attention to details associated with performance of colorectal cases was associated with a 33% reduction in SSI during the implementation period. This is a laudatory outcome, but one must wonder if it will be sustained after the process novelty wears off. Durability of changed outcomes is the end that is to be achieved.

Surgical practice is strongly influenced by tradition as well as science. The next series of papers address some practices, which have assumed an aura of dogma in some surgical practices. Preparation of the individual for a surgical procedure is highly ritualized and repetitive. Surprisingly, the type of antiseptic utilized can engender considerable passion by practitioners. Article 5 defends the routine use of povidone-iodine-alcohol as the patient skin preparation. The study methodology utilized observation of the numbers of SSI and correlated this event to semiquantitative culture of residual bacteria on the skin. The study rate of SSI was 4.4% and numbers of residual resident skin bacteria were not associated with the subsequent development of SSI. The purpose of the skin prep is to minimize the inoculum size from cut skin during the time when the wound is open — not just at the time of incision. Surprisingly, the authors did not address the time interval from skin preparation until wound closure as a variable.

Barrier devices between wound and open abdomen have been debated for years. Article 6 reports the results of a meta-analysis of wound protectors. With 1,993 patient results to review, the conclusion was that wound protectors *may* be beneficial. The wound protector literature was rife with potential bias and lent support to the observation that much of clinical practice is still not predicated upon sound evidence. Another time-honored practice has been the inclusion of antimicrobial agents in irrigation solutions.

Article 7 is a report from a single center colorectal service comparing saline vs gentamicin/clindamycin irrigation for its effect upon development of intra-abdominal infections and detection of bacteria before and after irrigation. With antibiotic irrigation, there were fewer SSI, intra-abdominal infections and detectable bacteria after irrigation. The study supports the contention that inhibiting bacterial numbers/proliferation is an effective strategy to reduce infections. This study stated that the patients had procedures for cancer, although the lessons learned through confounding diagnoses mentioned in article 2 should be remembered. Another approach that surgeons have employed to decrease SSI has been to impregnate materials to be left in the wound with antiseptics. This practice has been controversial as most antiseptic are more injurious to mammalian cells than bacteria at any given concentration. Article 8 reports the results of a meta-analysis of studies using Triclosan-impregnated sutures. The compilation of seven randomized controlled trials concluded that the addition of Triclosan did not statistically reduce the risk of infection but, equally important, it did not increase the risk of wound dehiscence. Article 9 reports the effect of silver-impregnated synthetic membranes for treatment of chronic wounds and burns. The use of silver nanoparticles provide wound antiseptic in a manner that is less cytotoxic to mammalian cells. Using a murine model, the investigators demonstrated that bacterial burden was significantly reduced, leading to the hope that topical antiseptics will be possible for therapy in conditions requiring barrier dressing.

The surgical repair of a hernia in the presence of bacterial contamination requires a series of decisions for wound closure. Article 10 assessed NSQIP data to discern outcomes from ventral hernia repair in clean or clean-contaminated procedures. Not surprisingly, those procedures requiring mesh for closure in the face of bacterial contamination had a higher risk of surgical infection. Slightly more than 10% of all ventral hernias were classified as clean-contaminated or contaminated with significantly more infectious complications in the bacterially contaminated wound. The report, however, is limited because the data base cannot differentiate between biologic and synthetic mesh, contamination through enteral contents or chronic infection from skin infection or appropriateness of the preoperative antibiotics. Closure of a contaminated hernia can sometimes be done through primary repair, abdominal wall release procedures and at other times requires mesh irrespective of closure manipulations. Many of the variables that influence the optimal clinical choice were absent from this report.

Since the Iraq war, routine use of negative pressure wound therapy has increasingly found a place in surgical wound care. While the benefit of negative pressure has been demonstrated for open wounds, extension to closed wounds has been untested. Article 11 presents results of a randomized controlled study of negative pressure dressings for the primary closed at-risk surgical wound. Unfortunately, there was no demonstrable benefit for the use of negative pressure devices in high risk wounds, either for reduction in infection or dehiscence.

Surgical teaching has stressed that efficiency in surgical technique will yield better results. This tenet was explored using the NSQIP database, with time of procedure being the surrogate for efficient performance of autologous saphenous vein femoral popliteal bypass procedures. Not surprisingly, the incidence of SSI and deep infections was inversely related to the length of the procedure. The discussion is interesting in the assignment of causality. The authors discuss the limitations of their risk adjustment and comments in the discussion are clearly in response to reviewer's critiques. However, in this pay-for-performance world, this type of analysis stressing the relative value of quickness of the procedure can have dramatic effects upon a surgeon's performance without necessarily achieving the desired end. Understanding the risk adjustment methodology and manner in which data is collected remains to be refined. An example of methodology and outcomes is observed in article 13. Over 48,000 mastectomies were analyzed from the NSQIP database. A comparison of SSI risk was made between those with immediate reconstruction vs no reconstruction. Immediate reconstruction was associated with a statistically increased rate of SSI (3.5% vs. 2.5% with appropriate confidence intervals). The authors noted that there were several independent SSI risk factors as well that influenced the risk, including operative time, body mass index, alcohol use, and others. The authors concluded that despite the statistically increased risk of SSI, the actual risk per individual was so close as to be clinically insignificant. However, what does this mean for the independent observer? The authors do not state the total risk for SSI if one include staged breast reconstruction, nor do they include the patient satisfaction from mastectomy without reconstruction. Before one can use these simple outcome formulas, one must understand the desired outcomes for the disease being treated.

Returning to process issues that should be assessed by a surgical service, the next report (article 14) addresses intraoperative temperature management in the trauma setting. A single-center observational study demonstrated a striking relationship between temperature management and risk for developing SSI. This is consistent with some (but not all) of the literature derived from the colorectal procedures and should lead to quality measures for operating room performance. However, is temperature maintenance really the end that one should measure? The population of trauma victims that got hypothermic was not the same as those who were more normothermic (more shotgun wounds, more transfusions). One cannot really criticize the goal of maintaining physiologic homeostasis, however, whether normothermia is truly the end goal or a surrogate remains to be clarified.

Process improvement initiatives have had varying success in achievement of desired ends. Article 15 touts the benefit of bundled efforts to reduce rates of SSI at a single institution after colorectal surgery. The results were impressive with SSI reduction from 9.8% to 4.0%. The methodology was intriguing for what was not included in the groups that addressed the pre-, intra- and post-operative care. Discussion of bowel preparation was not identified as being important for reduction of SSI. While current thoughts have changed the opinion regarding gross fecal contamination of the surgical wound, older surgical literature is replete with the virtues of removal of gross fecal material and the oral or intravenous administration of appropriate antimicrobial agents. Additionally, the fact that changing gloves prior to closure implies that the groups were still concerned with contaminating bacteria. It was not specified that administered antibiotics were effective against aerobic and anaerobic enteric bacteria, but they were given on time. Despite noting in the text that temperature control is important for reduction of SSI after colorectal procedures, maintenance of patient temperature was not in their operative bundle. This paper highlights that the process of focusing the staff attention upon an end, SSI reduction can lead to behavior change and desirable outcomes. However, on analysis, no single variable was associated with the desired change, and there were many putative important variables that were not assessed. The crux of all process improvements will be in the sustainability of outcomes when staff attention is diverted to other projects. The effectiveness or appropriateness of antimicrobial agents is rarely measured on quality dashboards. Article 16 uses the Australian database of over 20,000 procedures to assess differences in SSI depending upon use of β-lactam antibiotic or vancomycin prophylaxis in clean ortho or cardiac procedures. It was demonstrated that the risk of methicillin-resistant staphylococcus aureus SSI was reduced with vancomycin administration, but that the overall rate of SSI was significantly increased. Appropriate timing of vancomycin was only 23%, which makes one wonder how they assessed timing, either from start of administration or the end of infusion. Vancomycin has a longer administration time that would delay infusion completion until well into the procedure. In this database, there was no reason given for the choice of antimicrobial (such as colonization with MRSA or β-lactam allergy), however, this type of analysis should make one pause when drawing a conclusion about stressing only one component (timing of administration, in this case) of an otherwise complex variable.

One of the common conditions requiring surgical attention is acute infection in a chronic wound. The next series of articles address some issues associated with their diagnosis and treatment of infections within the chronic wound. Often, these require debridement and deep tissue biopsy for effective control and diagnosis. Article 17 assesses the existing literature regarding the diagnosis of infection within a chronic wound. The accuracy of the diagnosis ultimately is linked to deep quantitative culture, but clinical signs and symptoms are necessary to precipitate a surgical procedure. An analysis of multiple articles concluded that of all the signs and symptoms, only localized pain had a significant positive correlation with infection within the chronic wound. Article 18 is an example of how the Infectious Diseases Society of America takes these issues for the practice guideline on diabetic foot infections. The importance of accurate diagnosis is stressed as optimal therapy extends from simple antibiotics to surgical debridement to amputation. Most of the recommendations regarding surgical therapies are strong, but lack significant literature justification. Preservation of extremity function mandates accurate and timely diagnosis, appropriate antimicrobials, judicious surgical interventions, and subsequent soft tissue protection.

Soft tissue infections are often the consequence of Staphylococcus aureus. With the concern of antibiotic resistant bacteria, the military reported the prevalence of methicillin resistant SA over a five-year period in article 19. The number of methicillin-resistant Staphylococcus aureus isolates has decreased over the years, despite the growing national recognition that antimicrobial resistance is an increasing problem. This has been true for community and hospital acquired S. aureus infections.

The final article (20) stresses the continuing evolution of the surgical approach to necrotizing pancreatic infections. The authors compared peroral-transgastric necrosectomy to a surgical approach to the necrotic tissue. The surgical goal to minimize the inflammatory response (as measured by cytokine release) is interesting, but the primary goal is to get people better. This article is limited by its selection criteria. Patients were not randomized until almost 2 months into their illness. The timeliness, and not the mode of the intervention, perhaps should have been the measured variable.

The literature pertaining to the prevention and management of surgical infections is increasingly leading to database analysis. The need for clear measures of appropriate variables is vital; however, the root cause or outcome is still not clearly understood. But there is a conflict between evidence-based requirements of our systems and the intrinsic limitations of knowledge and data composition.

Timothy L. Pruett, MD

Evaluation Study of Different Strategies for Detecting Surgical Site Infections Using the Hospital Information System at Lyon University Hospital, France

Gerbier-Colomban S, Bourjault M, Cêtre J-C, et al (Hôpital de la Croix-Rousse, Lyon, France)
Ann Surg 255:896-900, 2012

Objective.—To evaluate different strategies for detecting surgical site infections (SSIs) using different sources (notification by the surgeon, bacteriological results, antibiotic prescription, and discharge diagnosis codes).

Background.—Surveillance plays a role in reducing the risks of SSIs but the performance of case reports by surgeons is insufficient. Indirect methods of SSI detection are an alternative to increase the quality of surveillance.

Methods.—A retrospective cohort study of 446 patients operated consecutively during the first half of 2007 was set up in a 56-bed general surgery unit in Lyon University Hospital, France. Patients were followed up 30 days after intervention. Different methods of detection were established by combining different data sources. The sensitivity and specificity of these methods were calculated by using, as reference method, the manual review of the medical records.

Results.—The sensitivity and specificity of SSI detection were, respectively, 18.4% (*95%* confidence interval [CI]: 7.9—31.6) and 100% for surgeon notification; 63.2% (*95%* CI: 47.3—78.9) and 95.1% (*95%* CI: 92.9—97.1) for detection based on positive cultures; 68.4% (*95%* CI: 52.6—81.6) and 87.5% (*95%* CI: 84.3—90.7) using antibiotic prescription; 26.3% (*95%* CI: 13.2—42.1) and 99.5% (*95%* CI: 98.8—100) using discharge diagnosis codes. By combining the latter 3 sources, the sensitivity increased at 86.8% (*95%* CI: 76.3—97.4) and the specificity was lowered at 85.5% (*95%* CI: 82.1—89.0).

Conclusions.—SSI detection based on the combination of data extracted automatically from the hospital information system performed well. This strategy has been implemented gradually in Lyon University Hospital.

▶ Literature pertaining to discussions of surgical site infections (SSI) is dependent on the methodologies employed for identification. This article reports the disparities from dependence upon surgeon self-reporting, microbiology, chart review, and prescribing practices. Because SSI events are predominantly used as a hospital quality report, the true rate of SSI is not usually reflected in the number, as outpatient records and events are excluded. If one were attempting to assess "true" SSI outcomes for those undergoing surgical procedures, a separate methodology and capture system for the outpatient environment would be necessary. To this end, it behooves the reader of surgical literature to understand not only what is reported but, equally importantly, the cases that are not reported. This article supplies valuable information on the limitations of some of the process metrics within the hospital systems, but it fails to analyze the limitations of restricting interests to hospital events.

T. Pruett, MD

Diagnoses Influence Surgical Site Infections (SSI) in Colorectal Surgery: A Must Consideration for SSI Reporting Programs?
Pendlimari R, Cima RR, Wolff BG, et al (Mayo Clinic College of Medicine, Rochester, MN)
J Am Coll Surg 214:574-581, 2012

Background.—Colorectal surgery is associated with high rates of surgical site infection (SSI). The National Surgery Quality Improvement Program is a validated, risk-adjusted quality-improvement program for surgical patients. Patient stratification and risk adjustment are associated with Current Procedural Terminology codes and primary disease diagnosis is not considered. Our aim was to determine the association between disease diagnosis and SSI rates.

Methods.—Data from all 2009 National Surgery Quality Improvement Program institutions were analyzed. ICD-9 codes were used to differentiate patients into cancer (colon or rectal), ulcerative colitis, regional enteritis, diverticular disease, and others. Diagnosis-specific SSI rates were compared with benign neoplasm, which had the lowest rate (8.9%). Logistic regression was performed adjusting for age, body mass index, American Society of Anesthesiologists classification, wound type, and relative value unit.

Results.—There were 24,673 colorectal procedures, with 1,956 superficial incisional (SSSI), 398 deep incisional (DSSI), and 1,096 organ/space (O/SSSI) infections. Odds ratio (OR) and 95% confidence intervals compared with benign neoplasm diagnosis were computed after adjustment for each diagnosis category. In rectal cancer patients, significantly more SSSI (OR = 1.6; 95% CI, 1.3–2.1; $p < 0.0001$), DSSI (OR = 2.1; 95% CI, 1.3–3.7; $p < 0.006$), and O/SSI (OR = 2.2; 95% CI, 1.6–3.0; $p < 0.0001$) developed. In diverticular patients, more SSSI (OR = 1.6; 95% CI, 1.3–2.0; $p < 0.0001$), but not DSSI or O/SSSI, developed. In ulcerative colitis patients, more DSSI (OR = 2.4; 95% CI, 1.2–4.9; $p < 0.01$), O/SSSI (OR = 2.1; 95% CI, 1.4–3.1; $p = 0.0004$), but fewer SSSIs, developed.

Conclusions.—We found that SSI type is associated with the underlying disease diagnosis. To facilitate colorectal SSI-reduction efforts, the disease process must be considered to design appropriate interventions. In addition, institutional comparisons based on aggregate or stratified SSI rates can be misleading if the colorectal disease mix is not considered.

▶ The National Surgery Quality Improvement Program (NSQIP) dataset is exceptionally valuable because it uses a methodology to risk adjust the reported events. Although risk adjustment is now a commonplace tool for gross performance metrics, the specific, refined elements within the modeling system often leave much to be desired. Often the risk variables are simplified and made dichotomous, when in reality, the clinical problem is more of a continuum. The need for simplification can be deleterious for providers who have a concentrated practice in one portion of the disease spectrum. This article presents one such example. Colorectal surgery is a dichotomous data point in NSQIP risk adjustment. However, the authors demonstrated that within the category of colorectal surgery, there are subsets of diagnoses that have differential risk for development of surgical site infection (SSI). People who undergo colorectal surgical procedures for rectal cancer or inflammatory bowel disease have a different risk for SSI than those with benign colonic neoplasms. As risk-adjusted outcomes are increasingly used for access to care and payment strategies, it is important that the surgical provider understand the processes and limitations of the risk adjustment process and be able to justify outcomes accordingly.

T. Pruett, MD

Surgical Site Infection Prevention: A Qualitative Analysis of an Individualized Audit and Feedback Model
Nessim C, Bensimon CM, Hales B, et al (Univ of Toronto, Ontario, Canada)
J Am Coll Surg 215:850-857, 2012

Background.—Surgical site infection (SSI) adversely affects patient outcomes and health care costs, so prevention of SSI has garnered much attention worldwide. Surgical site infection is recognized as an important quality indicator of patient care and safety. The purpose of this study was to use qualitative research methods to evaluate staff perceptions of the utility and impact of individualized audit and feedback (AF) data on SSI-related process metrics for their individual practice, as well as on overall communication and teamwork as they relate to SSI prevention.

Study Design.—This study was performed in a tertiary care center, based on patients treated in the colorectal and hepatic-pancreatic-biliary surgical oncology services. Eighteen clinicians were interviewed. Analysis of interviews via comparative analysis techniques and coding strategies were used to identify themes.

Results.—The most important finding of this study was that although nearly all participants believed that the individualized AF model was useful in effecting individual practice change as well as improving awareness and accountability around individual roles in preventing SSIs, it was not seen as a means to enable the multidisciplinary teamwork required for sustainable practice changes. Moreover, such teamwork requires a team leader.

Conclusions.—Provision of individualized AF data had a significant impact on promoting individual practice change. Despite this, we concluded that practice change is a shared responsibility, requiring a team leader. So, AF had little bearing on establishing a necessary multidisciplinary team approach to SSI prevention, to create more effective and sustainable practice change among an entire team.

▶ There has been much discussion about the relative benefit of surgical site infection (SSI) outcome reporting to providers. It is often assumed that by simply shedding light on an issue that performance improvements will be achieved. The authors assessed whether the reporting of SSI outcomes to surgical providers affected perceptions for process adherence, teamwork, and communication. Although the outcome reports were perceived as being a valuable component for the quality of surgical performance, the feedback was rarely perceived as enhancing teamwork or communication. In later publications, the need for teams to address SSI reduction initiatives will be proposed as instrumental in improvement strategies. As health care delivery becomes increasingly industrialized, organization units will have to be designed in such a fashion that patient-directed teamwork is integral and not solely task performance (such as the operating theater). Our current structure is not always viewed as fostering teamwork and communication.

T. Pruett, MD

Implementation of a Surgical Comprehensive Unit-Based Safety Program to Reduce Surgical Site Infections

Wick EC, Hobson DB, Bennett JL, et al (Johns Hopkins Univ and Johns Hopkins Hosp, Baltimore, MD)
J Am Coll Surg 215:193-200, 2012

Background.—Surgical site infections (SSI) are a common and costly problem, prolonging hospitalization and increasing readmission. Adherence to well-known infection control process measures has not been associated with substantial reductions in SSI. To date, the global burden of preventable SSI continues to result in patient harm and increased health care costs on a broad scale.

Study Design.—We designed a study to evaluate the association between implementation of a surgery-based comprehensive unit-based safety program (CUSP) and postoperative SSI rates. One year of pre- and post-CUSP intervention SSI rates were collected using the high-risk pilot module of the American College of Surgeons National Surgical Quality Improvement Program (July 2009 to July 2011). The CUSP group met monthly and consisted of a multidisciplinary team of front-line providers (eg, surgeons, nurses, operating room technicians, and anesthesiologists) who were directly involved in the care of colorectal surgery patients. Surgical Care Improvement Project process measure compliance was monitored using standard methods from the Centers for Medicare and Medicaid Services.

Results.—In the 12 months before implementation of the CUSP and interventions, the mean SSI rate was 27.3% (76 of 278 patients). After commencement of interventions, the rate was 18.2% (59 of 324 patients) for the subsequent 12 months—a 33.3% decrease (95% CI, 9–58%; $p < 0.05$). The interventions included standardization of skin preparation; administration of preoperative chlorhexidine showers; selective elimination of mechanical bowel preparation; warming of patients in the preanesthesia area; adoption of enhanced sterile techniques for skin and fascial closure; addressing previously unrecognized lapses in antibiotic prophylaxis. There was no difference in surgical process measure compliance as measured by the Surgical Care Improvement Project during the same time period.

Conclusions.—Formation of small groups of front-line providers to address patient harm using local wisdom and existing evidence can improve patient safety. We demonstrate a surgery-based CUSP intervention that might have markedly decreased SSI in a high-risk population.

▶ Prevention of surgical site infection (SSI) has become an increasingly important metric for payment from the Centers for Medicare and Medicaid. It has been distressing that compliance with Surgical Care Improvement Project (SCIP) practice recommendations has not proven to consistently reduce SSI, because the parameters described in isolation are all commonly thought to be associated with SSI reduction. This article describes the use of small focus groups to address the problem of a high rate (27.3%) of SSI. Through focused efforts, mostly addressing intraoperative issues, the SSI rate was reduced to 18.2%. Compliance with SCIP measures did not vary through the efforts of the small groups. Health care professionals understand the logic behind most of the variables associated with SSI (both SCIP and general culture), so it is not surprising that focused attention resulted in reduction of the rates. However, without clearly identifying a specific variable that was understood to be associated with an untoward outcome, it will prove difficult to sustain the rate reduction after other quality initiatives become necessary.

This article represents something of the Hawthorne effect in experimental models. The subjects modify their behavior when it is recognized that they are being watched. However, precisely how behavior was modified to achieve the desired outcome is not clearly identified.

T. Pruett, MD

No Risk of Surgical Site Infections From Residual Bacteria After Disinfection With Povidone-Iodine-Alcohol in 1014 Cases: A Prospective Observational Study

Tschudin-Sutter S, Frei R, Egli-Gany D, et al (Univ Hosp, Basel, Switzerland)
Ann Surg 255:565-569, 2012

Objective.—We studied the impact of residual bacteria at the incision site after disinfection with polyvinylpyrrolidone (PVP or povidone)-iodine-alcohol and the correlation with postoperative surgical site infections (SSIs).

Background.—Chlorhexidine-based preparations are significantly more effective for catheter insertion care than povidone-iodine solutions to prevent catheter-associated infections, suggesting that the use of PVP-iodine should be reevaluated for disinfection of the surgical site. In the majority of European hospitals PVP-iodine-alcohol is still standard of care to prepare the preoperative site.

Methods.—We consecutively and prospectively enrolled 1005 patients from representative surgical disciplines. Skin cultures to determine skin microbial counts were taken after disinfection with PVP-iodine-alcohol, immediately before incision. Disinfection of the surgical site was performed using standardized procedure under supervision. Criteria for SSI were based on guidelines issued by the Centers for Disease Control including appropriate follow-up of 30 days and 1 year.

Results.—A total of 1014 skin cultures from surgical sites were analyzed from 1005 patients, of which 36 (3.6%) revealed significant colonization of the preoperative site, and 41 SSIs were detected, accounting for an SSI rate of 4.04%; residual bacteria before incision were completely unrelated to the incidence of SSI, even after adjustment for multiple potentially confounding variables.

Conclusions.—A low rate of SSIs of 4.04% was achieved when using PVP-iodine-alcohol for disinfection of the preoperative site. Remaining bacteria after standardized 3-step disinfection did not at all correlate with the development of an SSI. Our data provide clear evidence that PVP-iodine-alcohol is effective for preparation of the preoperative site.

▶ This article reports on one of the mainstay approaches to reduce surgical site infection (SSI): the skin preparation. Standardization of skin preparation was one of the major focus areas in the report in the article Implementation of a surgical comprehensive unit-based safety program to reduce surgical site infections by Wick et al.[1] This article correlates SSI with semiquantitative skin cultures after preparation for surgery. There was no clear correlation between residual bacterial on the skin and subsequent SSI. The overall SSI rates are acceptable, but the most intriguing part of the article is what was not done.

SSI is the consequence of bacteria proliferating in the wound at the time of closure. It would have made more sense to culture the wound at the end of the procedure than immediately after skin preparation. There was no comparison with any other skin preparation technique. Despite the methodologic shortcomings, the study demonstrated that wound infections are more common in cases with intraoperative contamination. The clean rate of 3.1% is probably normative, assuming that there were a significant number of peripheral vascular procedures, and the SSI rates increased in proportion to the numbers of clean-contaminated, contaminated, and dirty wound. This article was so intent on demonstrating that povidone-iodine is an effective skin preparation material that it failed to discuss the important elements of SSI. In light of the previous articles, the differences between environmental control in the operating room and wound contamination through surgical procedure should be compared. The relative contribution of skin preparation and hand washing should be minor in comparison to the inocula from endogenous colonizations.

The surgical teams know the differences and these are probably manifested in overall rate reductions associated with these efforts.

T. Pruett, MD

Reference

1. Wick EC, Hobson DB, Bennett JL, et al. Implementation of a surgical comprehensive unit-based safety program to reduce surgical site infections. *J Am Coll Surg.* 2012 Aug;215(2):193-200.

Systematic Review of the Clinical Effectiveness of Wound-edge Protection Devices in Reducing Surgical Site Infection in Patients Undergoing Open Abdominal Surgery
Gheorghe A, on behalf of the collaborative West Midlands Research Collaborative and ROSSINI Trial Management Group (Univ of Birmingham, UK; et al)
Ann Surg 255:1017-1029, 2012

Objective.—Assess the existing evidence on the clinical effectiveness of wound-edge protection devices (WEPDs) in reducing the surgical site infection (SSI) rate in patients undergoing open abdominal surgery.

Background.—Surgical site infections are a common postoperative complication associated with considerable morbidity, extended hospital stay, increased health care costs, and reduced quality of life. Wound-edge protection devices have been used in surgery to reduce SSI rates for more than 40 years; however, they are yet to be cited in major clinical guidelines addressing SSI management.

Methods.—A review protocol was prespecified. A variety of sources were searched in November 2010 for studies containing primary data on the use of WEPDs in reducing SSI compared with standard care in patients undergoing open abdominal surgery. The outcome of interest was a well-specified, clinically based definition of an SSI. No language or time restrictions were applied. The quality assessment of the studies and the quantitative analyses were performed in line with the principles of the Cochrane Collaboration.

Results.—Twelve studies reporting primary data from 1933 patients were included in the review. The quality assessment found all of them to be at considerable risk of bias. An exploratory meta-analysis was performed to provide a quantitative indication on the effect of WEPDs. The pooled risk ratio under a random effects model was 0.60 (95% confidence interval, 0.41–0.86), indicating a potentially significant benefit from the use of WEPDs. No indications of significant between-study heterogeneity or publication bias, respectively, were identified.

Conclusions.—Evidence to date suggests that WEPDs may be efficient in reducing SSI rates in patients undergoing open abdominal surgery. However, the poor quality of the existing studies and their small sample sizes raise the need for a large, good quality randomized controlled trial to validate this indication.

▶ Part of the surgical wisdom to reduce the risk of surgical site infection (SSI) has been to prevent bacteria from coming into contact with the subcutaneous tissues through the placement of a physical barrier between the operative field and the wound. Wound protectors have many indications and their adherents claim them to be effective in reducing wound contamination. This article is a meta-analysis of the published reports with the use of wound protectors. The analysis suggests that wound protectors may have some benefit in reducing the risk for SSI. If the prior sentence is couched in uncertainty, it is by design. The analysis suggests that the literature carries significant potential for bias in most of the reports and that the need for additional well-controlled studies would be necessary to address the usefulness of wound protectors.

It is unfortunate that the analysis did not discriminate between deep space and superficial SSI. In theory, if they work as proposed, wound protectors should have a significant effect on superficial, but not deep, infections. To the extent that the literature fails to discriminate through the mechanisms of action, a disservice is done to the medical community and improvements will remain distant.

T. Pruett, MD

Effect of Peritoneal Lavage with Clindamycin-Gentamicin Solution on Infections after Elective Colorectal Cancer Surgery

Ruiz-Tovar J, Santos J, Arroyo A, et al (Univ Hosp Elche, Alicante, Spain; et al)
J Am Coll Surg 214:202-207, 2012

Background.—Colorectal surgery may lead to infections because despite meticulous aseptic measures, extravasation of microorganisms from the colon lumen is unavoidable.

Study Design.—A prospective, randomized study was performed between January 2010 and December 2010. Patient inclusion criteria were a diagnosis of colorectal neoplasms and plans to undergo an elective curative operation. Patients were divided into 2 groups: Group 1 (intra-abdominal irrigation with normal saline) and Group 2 (intraperitoneal irrigation with a solution of 240 mg gentamicin and 600 mg clindamycin). The occurrence of wound infections and intra-abdominal abscesses were investigated. After the anastomosis, a microbiologic sample of the peritoneal surface was obtained (sample 1). A second sample was collected after irrigation with normal saline (sample 2). Finally, the peritoneal cavity was irrigated with a gentamicin-clindamycin solution and a third sample was obtained (sample 3).

Results.—There were 103 patients analyzed: 51 in Group 1 and 52 in Group 2. There were no significant differences between the groups in age, sex, comorbidities, or type of colorectal surgery performed. Wound infection rates were 14% in Group 1 and 4% in Group 2 ($p = 0.009$; odds ratio [OR] 4.94; 95% CI 1.27 to 19.19). Intra-abdominal abscess rates were 6% in Group 1 and 0% in Group 2 ($p = 0.014$; OR 2.14; 95% CI 1.13 to 3.57). The culture of sample 1 was positive in 68% of the cases, sample 2 was positive in 59%, and sample 3 in 4%.

Conclusions.—Antibiotic lavage of the peritoneum is associated with a lower incidence of intra-abdominal abscesses and wound infections.

▶ Although wound protectors may keep bacteria from contaminating the subcutaneous space, there are other methods to decrease bacterial contamination within a wound. The current report compares the use of antimicrobial irrigation with saline after colorectal surgery to discern its impact on surgical site infection (SSI). The methodology included taking peritoneal cultures before and after irrigation and the clinical course followed. It is not surprising that in the majority of cases, peritoneal cultures were positive for bacteria prior to irrigation. Saline irrigation did not significantly modify the recovery of bacteria. However, gentamicin and clindamycin irrigation significantly reduced the ability to culture bacteria from the peritoneum at the end of the procedure and was also associated with a significant reduction in superficial and deep wound infections. This study is in contrast to many prior studies of antibiotic irrigation with solutions of single agents (often ineffective against the pathogens associated with intra-abdominal infections). This study reconfirms the premise that reduction in numbers of wound bacteria will lower the risk of SSI; however, toxicity and tolerability remain to be discerned.

T. Pruett, MD

Triclosan-Impregnated Sutures to Decrease Surgical Site Infections: Systematic Review and Meta-Analysis of Randomized Trials

Chang WK, Srinivasa S, Morton R, et al (Univ of Auckland, Otahuhu, New Zealand)
Ann Surg 255:854-859, 2012

Objective.—To determine the efficacy and safety of triclosan-impregnated sutures.

Background.—Surgical-site infections (SSIs) produce considerable morbidity and increase health care costs. A potential strategy to decrease the rates of SSIs may be the use of triclosan-impregnated sutures. These have been endorsed and/or funded by professional and governmental bodies in numerous countries. Laboratory studies and nonsystematic reviews have suggested that these sutures may reduce SSIs but there has been no summative assessment of this intervention with regard to clinical efficacy and safety. Hence, a systematic review and meta-analysis of all randomized controlled trials (RCTs) investigating triclosan-impregnated sutures were conducted.

Methods.—The Cochrane Central Register of Controlled Trials, MEDLINE, EMBASE, Pubmed databases, and trial registries were searched for published and unpublished RCTs. The endpoints of interest were the incidence of SSIs and wound breakdown. A random effects model was used and pooled estimates were reported as odds ratios (ORs) with the corresponding 95% confidence interval (CI).

Results.—Seven RCTs encompassing a total of 836 patients were included in the final analysis. The studies were of moderate quality. Triclosan-impregnated sutures did not statistically significantly reduce the rates of SSIs (OR = 0.77; 95% CI: 0.40−1.51; P = 0.45; I^2 = 24%). There was no difference in the rates of wound breakdown between the 2 groups (OR = 1.07; 95% CI: 0.21−5.43; P = 0.93; I^2 = 44%)

Conclusions.—Triclosan-impregnated sutures do not decrease the rate of SSIs or decrease the rate of wound breakdown. Further high-quality independent studies within the right context are required before routine clinical use can be considered.

▶ Foreign bodies within a wound have been demonstrated to increase the risk of wound infection. Although suture is required (today) for wound closure, it is also a foreign body with potential for increased risk of surgical site infections (SSIs). There has been enthusiasm toward impregnating suture materials with antimicrobial products to prevent local bacterial growth and decrease subsequent wound infections. However, there has also been the concern that these agents will impair human cell function and lead to wound healing problems.

This article reports the results of a meta-analysis of studies using triclosan-impregnated suture. Triclosan is a commonly used antimicrobial agent with broad activity against bacteria and fungi. The good news is that there was not an increased rate of wound dehiscence, but unfortunately the SSI rate was not significantly altered. Although this suture material has some theoretical benefit, at present there is no convincing literature suggesting benefit to its use. It is always problematic when an agent has injurious effects on human cells and bacterial or fungi. However, triclosan-impregnated suture does not appear to have either beneficial or deleterious consequences to wounds.

T. Pruett, MD

Antibacterial Efficacy of Silver-Impregnated Polyelectrolyte Multilayers Immobilized on a Biological Dressing in a Murine Wound Infection Model
Guthrie KM, Agarwal A, Tackes DS, et al (Univ of Wisconsin, Madison)
Ann Surg 256:371-377, 2012

Objective.—To investigate the antibacterial effect of augmenting a biological dressing with polymer films containing silver nanoparticles.

Background.—Biological dressings, such as Biobrane, are commonly used for treating partial-thickness wounds and burn injuries. Biological dressings have several advantages over traditional wound dressings. However, as many as 19% of wounds treated with Biobrane become infected, and, once infected, the Biobrane must be removed and a traditional dressing approach should be employed. Silver is a commonly used antimicrobial in wound care products, but current technology uses cytotoxic concentrations of silver in these dressings. We have developed a novel and facile technology that allows immobilization of bioactive molecules on the surfaces of soft materials, demonstrated here by augmentation of Biobrane with nanoparticulate silver. Surfaces modified with nanometer-thick polyelectrolyte multilayers (PEMs) impregnated with silver nanoparticles have been shown previously to result in in vitro antibacterial activity against *Staphylococcus epidermidis* at loadings of silver that are noncytotoxic.

Methods.—We demonstrated that silver-impregnated PEMs can be nondestructively immobilized onto the surface of Biobrane (Biobrane-Ag) and determined the in vitro antibacterial activity of Biobrane-Ag with *Staphylococcus aureus*. In this study, we used an in vivo wound infection model in mice induced by topical inoculation of *S aureus* onto full-thickness 6-mm diameter wounds. After 72 hours, bacterial quantification was performed.

Results.—Wounds treated with Biobrane-Ag had significantly ($P < 0.001$) fewer colony-forming units than wounds treated with unmodified Biobrane (more than 4 $\log_{10}$ difference).

Conclusions.—The results of our study indicate that immobilizing silver impregnated PEMs on the wound-contact surface of Biobrane significantly reduces bacterial bioburden in full-thickness murine skin wounds. Further research will investigate whether this construct can be considered for human use.

▶ The impregnation of materials with antiseptics is another delivery mechanism to keep bacterial numbers low in the wound. This is particularly important in burn wounds in which covering of the wound with a biologic or synthetic material is often associated with bacterial growth under the coverage. Conceptually, impregnating the undersurface of a membrane placed on a wound would hinder bacterial growth and allow wound repair. This article describes the experimental use of polymer films impregnated with silver nanoparticles that are then transferred to Biobrane. Silver, of course, is a common agent used to diminish burn wound bacterial growth. Using an experimental murine burn model, it was demonstrated that the silver nanoparticles impregnated onto Biobrane reduced bacterial numbers by over 4 logs. Not reported, however, is the durability of the nanoparticles' bacterial inhibition and under what clinical conditions. If durable and nontoxic to the healing wound, this technology may take its place in the therapeutic armamentarium of burn wound care.

T. Pruett, MD

Use of Mesh During Ventral Hernia Repair in Clean-Contaminated and Contaminated Cases: Outcomes of 33,832 Cases

Choi JJ, Palaniappa NC, Dallas KB, et al (Mount Sinai School of Medicine, NY)
Ann Surg 255:176-180, 2012

Objective.—To analyze and compare postoperative occurrences following ventral hernia repairs (VHRs) using mesh in clean-contaminated and contaminated wounds.

Background.—Ventral hernia repairs using mesh is one of the most common surgical procedures performed. However, guidelines and outcomes of repairs in clean-contaminated or grossly contaminated ventral hernias have not been established.

Methods.—Patients who underwent VHR with mesh between the dates January 1, 2005 and April 4, 2010 at all hospitals in the United States participating in the National Surgical Quality Improvement Program (NSQIP) were reviewed. Data from 33,832 patients were analyzed by field contamination level and then compared with data from patients who underwent VHR without mesh. Data were analyzed using the odds ratio test with a 95% confidence interval.

Results.—The odds of having one or more postoperative occurrences were significantly greater in clean-contaminated and contaminated cases using mesh when compared with clean cases, with odds ratios of 3.56 (3.25–3.89) and 5.05 (1.78–12.41), respectively. There was a significantly increased risk of superficial surgical site infections (SSI) (2.53), deep SSI (3.09) and organ/space SSI (6.16), wound disruption (4.41), pneumonia (4.43), and sepsis (4.90) for clean-contaminated cases. Both clean-contaminated and contaminated cases had an increased risk of septic shock (5.82 and 26.74, respectively), and need for ventilator for more than 48 hours (5.59 and 26.76, respectively). In addition, there was a significantly increased odds ratio of complications in patients who underwent VHR with mesh (3.56) to nonmesh (2.52) in clean-contaminated cases.

Conclusion.—There is a significant increase in risk of postoperative occurrences following VHRs using mesh in clean-contaminated and contaminated cases relative to clean cases. We recommend avoiding the use of mesh in any level of contamination.

▶ The repair of ventral hernias in the face of bacterial contamination is more common than most of us like. This article uses National Surgical Quality Improvement Program (NSQIP) data elements to assess outcomes after ventral hernia repair. In those instances with bacterial contamination, the outcome after the use of mesh in the repair of a ventral hernia was associated with higher rates of surgical site infection, dehiscence, sepsis, ventilator days, and other morbidities. However, any surgery in a contaminated field would be associated with more infectious and nonhealing events. The true question resides in how much the use of mesh contributed to the problem. In addition, this report suffers from a lack of clarification of types of mesh. Presently, the use of a biologic mesh is the choice of many clinicians when repair in the face of bacterial contamination is necessary. There are many anecdotal reports of good outcomes in the face of contamination. Whether there truly is a reduction in infectious risks with biologic mesh would have been very beneficial to know. The limitation of the NSQIP database leaves this a conjecture for future study.

T. Pruett, MD

Negative Pressure Wound Therapy for At-Risk Surgical Closures in Patients With Multiple Comorbidities: A Prospective Randomized Controlled Study
Masden D, Goldstein J, Endara M, et al (Georgetown Univ Hosp, Washington, DC)
Ann Surg 255:1043-1047, 2012

Purpose.—The purpose of this study is to evaluate the effect of Negative Pressure Wound Therapy (NPWT) on closed surgical incisions. We performed a prospective randomized controlled clinical trial comparing NPWT to standard dry dressings on surgical incisions.

Methods.—Patients presenting to a high-volume wound center were randomized to receive either a V.A.C. (KCI, San Antonio, TX) or a standard dry dressing over their incision at the conclusion of surgery. These were primarily high-risk patients with multiple comorbidities. The 2 groups were compared, and all incisions were evaluated for infection and dehiscence postoperatively.

Results.—Eighty-one patients were included for analysis. Thirty-seven received dry dressings, and 44 received NPWT. Seventy-four of these underwent lower extremity wound closure. Average follow-up was 113 days. There were no differences in demographic, preoperative, and operative variables between groups; 6.8% of the NPWT group and 13.5% of the dry dressing group developed wound infection, but this was not statistically significant ($P = 0.46$). There was no difference in time to develop infection between the groups. There was no statistical difference in dehiscence between NPWT and dry dressing group (36.4% vs 29.7%; $P = 0.54$) or mean time to dehiscence between the 2 groups ($P = 0.45$). Overall, 35% of the dry dressing group and 40% of the NPWT group had a wound infection, dehiscence, or both. Of these, 9 in the NPWT group (21%) and 8 in the dry dressing group (22%) required reoperation.

Conclusions.—There is a significant rate of postoperative infection and dehiscence in patients with multiple comorbidities. There was no difference in the incidence of infection or dehiscence between the NPWT and dry dressing group. This study is registered with ClinicalTrials.gov. The unique registration number is NCT01366105.

▶ One of the important advances in open wound management has been the routine use of negative pressure wound therapy (NPWT). This has led to significant preservation of soft tissue and reduction of healing time. The current article addresses whether negative pressure is a benefit for the at-risk surgical wound. The study was done through randomization to have either conventional coverage or negative-pressure dressing for patients with closed wounds identified as being at risk for infection or poor healing. The results demonstrated no benefit of NPWT for these wounds. The patients randomized in this study had very high rates of wound infection, dehiscence, or both (35% to 40%). However, it must be queried whether subsets within the group might benefit or whether there was a difference between the heavily contaminated wound or the one with marginal blood supply. There are many reasons a wound could be deemed at risk that were not clearly delineated in this report. The majority of these wounds were lower extremity, and determining whether other types would be beneficially affected would require further study.

T. Pruett, MD

Shorter Duration of Femoral-Popliteal Bypass Is Associated with Decreased Surgical Site Infection and Shorter Hospital Length of Stay

Tan T-W, Kalish JA, Hamburg NM, et al (Boston Univ Med Ctr/Boston Univ School of Medicine, MA)
J Am Coll Surg 215:512-518, 2012

Background.—Duration of femoral-popliteal bypass is based on multiple patient-specific, system-specific, and surgeon-specific factors, and is subject to considerable variability. We hypothesized that shorter operative duration is associated with improved outcomes and might represent a potential quality-improvement measure.

Study Design.—Patients who underwent primary femoral-popliteal bypass with autogenous vein between 2005 and 2009 were identified from the American College of Surgeons NSQIP dataset using ICD-9 codes. Operative duration quartiles (Q) were determined (Q1: ≤149 minutes, Q2: 150 to 192 minutes, Q3: 193 to 248 minutes; and Q4: ≥249 minutes). Perioperative outcomes included mortality, surgical site infection, cardiopulmonary complications, and length of hospital stay. Relevant patient-specific and system-specific confounders, including age, body mass index, smoking, diabetes, end-stage renal disease, indication, American Society of Anesthesiologists' class, type of anesthesia, intraoperative transfusion, nonoperative time in the operating room, and participation of a trainee during the procedure, were adjusted for using multivariable regression.

Results.—There were 2,644 femoral-popliteal bypass procedures in our study. Mean age was 65.9 years and 62% of patients were male. Longer duration of surgery was associated with increased perioperative surgical site infection (Q1: 6.3%; Q2: 9.0%; Q3: 10.1%; and Q4: 13.9%; $p < 0.001$) and longer length of stay (5.4 ± 6.8 days; 6.1 ± 6.7 days; 7.0 ± 11.3 days; 8.1 ± 8.0 days, respectively; $p < 0.001$). In multivariable analysis, longer operative duration was independently associated with higher surgical site infection and longer hospital length of stay. Operative duration of ≥ 260 minutes increased the risk of surgical site infection by 50% compared with operative time of 150 minutes.

Conclusions.—Longer duration of femoral-popliteal bypass with autogenous vein was associated with a significantly higher risk of perioperative surgical site infection and longer hospital length of stay. Surgeon-specific parameters that lead to faster operative time might lead to improved clinical outcomes and more efficient hospital resource use.

▶ Factors associated with surgical site infection (SSI) include a plethora of variables. These variables include environmental factors that can be addressed through operating room routines, inherent differences in patient susceptibility that should be able to be accounted for through appropriate risk stratification, and operator/surgeon differences. This article looks at the single variable of time that it takes a surgeon to perform a single operation (femoral-popliteal bypass) from the National Surgical Quality Improvement Program (NSQIP) database. The time that it took to perform a femoral-popliteal bypass procedure using autologous vein was segregated into 4 quartiles. The SSI rate directly correlated with time to perform the procedure. However, the longer cases also appeared to be the tougher cases, with an increased need for transfusion, a higher body mass index, and individuals that were more likely to have ischemic rest pain. It is unclear whether the quick surgeon performs a better procedure. The use of procedure time as a single variable for the generation of SSI or a surrogate for some other factor (surgeon or patient) remains to be appropriately risk-stratified. There are enough vagaries in the NSQIP database that make the findings suspect.

T. Pruett, MD

Effect of Immediate Reconstruction on Postmastectomy Surgical Site Infection
Nguyen TJ, Costa MA, Vidar EN, et al (Univ of Southern California, Los Angeles, CA)
Ann Surg 256:326-333, 2012

Introduction.—Surgical site infections (SSI) are a source of significant postoperative morbidity and cost. Although immediate breast reconstruction after mastectomy has become routine, the data regarding the incidence of SSI in immediate breast reconstruction is highly variable and series dependent.

Methods.—Using the National Surgical Quality Improvement Program database, all female patients undergoing mastectomy, with or without immediate reconstruction, from 2005 to 2009 were identified. Only "clean" procedures were included. The primary outcome was incidence of SSI within 30 days of operation. Stepwise logistic regression analysis was used to identify risk factors associated with SSI.

Results.—A total of 48,393 mastectomies were performed during the study period, of which 9315 (19.2%) had immediate breast reconstruction. The incidence of SSI was 3.5% (330/9315) (95% CI [confidence interval]: 3.2%—4%) in patients undergoing mastectomy with reconstruction and 2.5% (966/39,078) (95% CI: 2.3%—2.6%) in patients undergoing mastectomy without reconstruction (P < 0.001). Independent risk factors for SSI include increased preoperative body mass index (BMI), heavy alcohol use, ASA (American Society of Anesthesiologists) score greater than 2, flap failure, and operative time of 6 hours or longer.

Conclusions.—Immediate breast reconstruction is associated with a statistically significant increase in risk of SSI in patients undergoing mastectomy (3.5% vs 2.5%). However, this difference was not considered to be clinically significant. In this large series, increased BMI, alcohol use, ASA class greater than 2, flap failure, and prolonged operative time were associated with increased risk of SSI.

▶ There are reports of 48 393 mastectomies in the National Surgical Quality Improvement Program database during the study period; 9315 of these underwent immediate breast reconstruction. It was demonstrated in this article that those patients who underwent immediate breast reconstruction had a significantly increased likelihood of developing surgical site infections (SSI) (3.5% vs 2.5%). Although this number is statistically higher, it is the authors' opinion that the clinical differences are minimal and that women should be given the opportunity for immediate reconstruction. This study demonstrates the importance of the large database and the ease with which small, but real, differences can gain statistical significance. No single paper can discuss all the clinical variables involved in discerning the optimal form of treatment for an individual; however, this type of analysis does make one pause when thinking about how evidence-based medicine will be applied to policy and payment in the future. As learned through prior research, a longer, more complex procedure is associated with a higher risk for SSI. Only when one's primary measurable end is to reduce overall SSI will it become good logic to stage breast reconstructions. What is not discussed in this article is the SSI rate in women undergoing staged reconstructions—does that offset the observed reduction? Is the patient satisfaction similar between the 2 groups? SSI is only one of many outcomes that needs to be balanced going forward.

T. Pruett, MD

The Effects of Intraoperative Hypothermia on Surgical Site Infection: An Analysis of 524 Trauma Laparotomies

Seamon MJ, Wobb J, Gaughan JP, et al (Cooper Univ Hosp, Camden, NJ; Temple Univ School of Medicine, Philadelphia, PA)
Ann Surg 255:789-795, 2012

Objectives.—Our primary study objective was to determine whether intraoperative hypothermia predisposes patients to postoperative surgical site infections (SSI) after trauma laparotomy.

Background.—Although intraoperative normothermia is an important quality performance measure for patients undergoing colorectal surgery, the effects of intraoperative hypothermia on SSI remain unstudied in trauma.

Methods.—A review of all patients (July 2003—June 2008) who survived 4 days or more after urgent trauma laparotomy at a level I trauma center revealed 524 patients. Patient characteristics, along with preoperative and intraoperative care focusing on SSI risk factors, including the depth and duration of intraoperative hypothermia, were evaluated. The primary outcome measure was the diagnosis of SSI within 30 days of surgery. Cut-point analysis of the entire range of lowest intraoperative temperature measurements established the temperature nadir that best predicted SSI development. Single and multiple variable logistic regression determined SSI predictors.

Results.—The mean intraoperative temperature nadir of the study population (n = 524) was 35.2°C ± 1.1°C and 30.5% had at least 1 temperature measurement less than 35°C. Patients who developed SSI (36.1%) had a lower mean intraoperative temperature nadir ($P = 0.009$) and had a greater number of intraoperative temperature measurements <35°C ($P < 0.001$) than those who did not. Cut-point analysis revealed an intraoperative temperature of 35°C as the nadir temperature most predictive of SSI development. Multivariate analysis determined that a single intraoperative temperature measurement less than 35°C independently increased the site infection risk 221% per degree below 35°C (OR: 2.21; 95% CI: 1.24—3.92, $P = 0.007$).

Conclusions.—Just as intraoperative hypothermia is an SSI risk factor in patients undergoing elective colorectal procedures, intraoperative hypothermia less than 35°C adversely affects SSI rates after trauma laparotomy. Our results suggest that intraoperative normothermia should be strictly maintained in patients undergoing operative trauma procedures.

▶ This article extends a growing literature regarding the maintenance of body temperature during surgical procedures and its impact upon subsequent surgical site infection (SSI). To no great surprise, the risk of SSI is associated with a low core body temperature during a surgical procedure. However, the lower temperatures in the trauma victims are also associated with more requirements for blood transfusion, higher bacterial inoculums with colon injuries, more frequent suffering of soft-tissue damage with shotgun injury, and a higher Injury Severity

Score. So, is the increased SSI really associated with the lower temperature or is it the consequence of the greater injury? Which came first, the chicken or the egg?

Certainly, minimization of SSI in the trauma patient is achieved with prompt control of injury, debridement of devitalized tissue, judicious use of antimicrobials to reduce the bacterial inoculum, and good perfusion of the remaining wound. These goals are not helped by hypoperfusion associated with low core temperatures.

T. Pruett, MD

Colorectal Surgery Surgical Site Infection Reduction Program: A National Surgical Quality Improvement Program—Driven Multidisciplinary Single-Institution Experience
Cima R, on behalf of the Colorectal Surgical Site Infection Reduction Team (Mayo Clinic, Rochester, MN)
J Am Coll Surg 216:23-33, 2013

Background.—Surgical site infections (SSI) are a major cause of morbidity in surgical patients and they increase health care costs considerably. Colorectal surgery is consistently associated with high SSI rates. No single intervention has demonstrated efficacy in reducing colorectal SSIs. The American College of Surgeons National Surgical Quality Improvement Program (ACS NSQIP) is a nationally validated system that uses clinically abstracted data on surgical patients and their outcomes to assist participating institutions drive quality improvement.

Study Design.—A multidisciplinary team was assembled to develop a colorectal SSI-reduction bundle at an academic tertiary care medical center. The ACS NSQIP data were used to identify patterns of SSIs during a 2-year period. Multiple interventions across the entire surgical episode of care were developed and implemented in January 2011. Monthly ACS NSQIP data were used to track progress.

Results.—Our ACS NSQIP overall colorectal SSI rate for 2009 and 2010 was 9.8%. One year after implementation of the SSI reduction bundle, we demonstrated a significant decline ($p < 0.05$) in both overall and superficial SSIs, to 4.0% and 1.5%, respectively. Organ space infections declined to 2.6%, which was not a significant change ($p = 0.10$). During the entire analysis period (2009 to 2011), there was no change in our colorectal-specific Surgical Care Improvement Program performance.

Conclusions.—Using our ACS NSQIP colorectal SSI outcomes, a multidisciplinary team designed a colorectal SSI reduction bundle that resulted in a substantial and sustained reduction in SSIs. Our study is not able to identify which specific elements contributed to the reduction.

▶ Reduction of surgical site infection (SSI) after colorectal surgery continues to be a major goal for hospital systems. However, since compliance with individual Surgical Care Improvement Project measures is not associated with the desired reduction, different methodologies have been tried to reduce SSI. After experiencing a high rate of SSI after colorectal procedures, a single institution created teams of providers to address the phases of the surgical process. Because the principles of minimization of SSI are well known, it is not surprising that a concerted team effort to produce reductions worked. The activity of goal-oriented process improvement resulted in a significant reduction of SSI, but a specific correction to a flawed process that was necessary to achieve the end was not identified. Although this report demonstrates the utility of focused efforts, the durability of the rate reduction is uncertain. There will be other process improvements that must be addressed by these teams and the attention to the unmeasured detail(s) will be lost, with the risk for a gradual rise in SSI rates.

T. Pruett, MD

Impact of Vancomycin Surgical Antibiotic Prophylaxis on the Development of Methicillin-Sensitive *Staphylococcus aureus* Surgical Site Infections: Report From Australian Surveillance Data (VICNISS)

Bull AL, Worth LJ, Richards MJ (Victorian Healthcare Associated Surveillance System (VICNISS) Coordinating Centre, North Melbourne, Australia)
Ann Surg 256:1089-1092, 2012

Objective.—To compare risks for developing surgical site infection (SSI) due to *Staphylococcus aureus* when vancomycin is used for antibiotic prophylaxis with risks when a β-lactam antibiotic is administered for prophylaxis.

Background.—Vancomycin is often used as surgical antibiotic prophylaxis for major surgery. In nonsurgical populations, there is evidence that vancomycin is less effective for prevention and treatment of methicillin-sensitive *Staphylococcus aureus* (MSSA) infections. Since 2002, the Victorian Healthcare Associated Surveillance System (VICNISS) has used standardized methods for infection surveillance in Australia, including any prophylactic antibiotic agent administered before surgical procedures.

Methods.—Surveillance records were obtained for patients undergoing 4 clean surgical procedures during the period of November 2002 to June 2009. Logistic regression analysis was used to examine risk factors for infection, including age, procedure duration, American Society of Anesthesiologists score, and choice and timing of antibiotic prophylaxis.

Results.—The data set consisted of 22,549 procedures, including cardiac bypass and hip and knee arthroplasty procedures. Vancomycin prophylaxis was administered in 1610 cases and a β-lactam antibiotic for 20,939 cases. A total of 754 SSIs were recorded. The most frequent pathogens were MSSA, methicillin-resistant *Staphylococcus aureus*, and *Pseudomonas* species. The adjusted odds ratio (OR) for an SSI with MSSA was 2.79, where vancomycin prophylaxis was administered ($P < 0.001$). For methicillin-resistant *Staphylococcus aureus* infection, the adjusted OR for vancomycin was 0.44 ($P = 0.05$), whereas for *Pseudomonas* infection, it was 0.96 ($P = 0.95$).

Conclusions.—In a large Australian study population, prophylaxis with vancomycin was found to be associated with an increased risk of SSI due to MSSA when compared with prophylaxis with a β-lactam antibiotic. Given the potential for poorer surgical outcomes in the setting of indiscriminate prophylactic vancomycin use, measures to improve adherence to guidelines for restricted administration of prophylactic vancomycin are supported.

▶ Most quality measures assess the timing of antibiotic prophylaxis rather than the appropriateness of the agent. This Australian system reviewed outcomes after either vancomycin or β-lactam prophylaxis in selected cardiac and orthopedic procedures. Unfortunately, the reason why a specific antimicrobial agent was chosen was not recorded. However, there were significant differences in outcomes, with significantly more surgical site infection (SSI) in those individuals given vancomycin prophylaxis. Timing of drug administration was not perfect in this study, as only 23% of vancomycin recipients had timely administration of the drug. It is difficult to discern whether the change in SSI was associated with failure to get effective levels at the time of surgery or if the recording was flawed because of the necessity of slower infusion rates with vancomycin that made the patients fall out of compliance. It is also possible that there were unmeasured differences in the populations, such as a higher rate of methicillin-resistant *Staphylococcus aureus* (MRSA) carriage in the vancomycin group. However, none of the collected variables of the groups addressed in this report differed significantly. Fortunately, the drug did appear to have a beneficial effect in that the vancomycin group had significantly less SSI associated with MRSA.

Despite the uncertainties, the article is useful as a reminder that any one compliance measure does not tell the whole story relating to subsequent SSI generation or prevention.

T. Pruett, MD

Does This Patient Have an Infection of a Chronic Wound?
Reddy M, Gill SS, Wu W, et al (Hebrew Rehabilitation Ctr, Boston, MA; Queen's Univ, Kingston, Canada; Women's College Hosp, Toronto, Canada)
JAMA 307:605-611, 2012

Context.—Chronic wounds (those that have not undergone orderly healing) are commonly encountered, but determining whether wounds are infected is often difficult. The current reference standard for the diagnosis of infection of a chronic wound is a deep tissue biopsy culture, which is an invasive procedure.

Objectives.—To determine the accuracy of clinical symptoms and signs to diagnose infection in chronic wounds and to determine whether there is a preferred noninvasive method for culturing chronic wounds.

Data Sources.—We searched multiple databases from inception through November 18, 2011, to identify studies focusing on diagnosis of infection in a chronic wound.

Study Selection.—Original studies were selected if they had extractable data describing historical features, symptoms, signs, or laboratory markers or were radiologic studies compared with a reference standard for diagnosing infection in patients with chronic wounds. Of 341 studies initially retrieved, 15 form the basis of this review. These studies include 985 participants with a total of 1056 chronic wounds. The summary prevalence of wound infection was 53%.

Data Extraction.—Three authors independently assigned each study a quality grade, using previously published criteria. One author abstracted operating characteristic data.

Data Synthesis.—An increase in the level of pain (likelihood ratio range, 11-20) made infection more likely, but its absence (negative likelihood ratio range, 0.64-0.88) did not rule out infection. Other items in the history and physical examination, in isolation or in combination, appeared to have limited utility when infection was diagnosed in chronic wounds. Routine laboratory studies had uncertain value in predicting infection of a chronic wound.

Conclusions.—The presence of increasing pain may make infection of a chronic wound more likely. Further evidence is required to determine which, if any, type of quantitative swab culture is most diagnostic.

▶ Surgeons are often requested to address chronic wounds for the purpose of controlling potential acute infection. The reasons for consultation often vary by provider: There can be a change in the wound smell, quality of the exudate, or a plethora of other signs. This article gives a nice literature analysis, winnowing over 340 reviews down to 15 with enough consistent variables that one can assess infection in a chronic wound. Pain was the only variable that was associated with a high likelihood of acute infection (defined by quantitative deep wound culture); however, its absence did not preclude the presence of infection. The other clinical variables, either alone or in combination, were not predictive of wound infection. This article highlights the importance of diagnosis prior to moving on to conclusions. Accuracy in identification of a specific infectious problem is not always easy with chronic wounds.

T. Pruett, MD

2012 Infectious Diseases Society of America Clinical Practice Guideline for the Diagnosis and Treatment of Diabetic Foot Infections
Lipsky BA, Berendt AR, Cornia PB, et al (Univ of Washington, Seattle; Oxford Univ Hosps NHS Trust, UK; et al)
Clin Infect Dis 54:132-173, 2012

Foot infections are a common and serious problem in persons with diabetes. Diabetic foot infections (DFIs) typically begin in a wound, most often a neuropathic ulceration. While all wounds are colonized with microorganisms, the presence of infection is defined by ≥2 classic findings of inflammation or purulence. Infections are then classified into mild (superficial and limited in size and depth), moderate (deeper or more extensive), or severe (accompanied by systemic signs or metabolic perturbations). This classification system, along with a vascular assessment, helps determine which patients should be hospitalized, which may require special imaging procedures or surgical interventions, and which will require amputation. Most DFIs are polymicrobial, with aerobic gram-positive cocci (GPC), and especially staphylococci, the most common causative organisms. Aerobic gram-negative bacilli are frequently copathogens in infections that are chronic or follow antibiotic treatment, and obligate anaerobes may be copathogens in ischemic or necrotic wounds.

Wounds without evidence of soft tissue or bone infection do not require antibiotic therapy. For infected wounds, obtain a post-debridement specimen (preferably of tissue) for aerobic and anaerobic culture. Empiric antibiotic therapy can be narrowly targeted at GPC in many acutely infected patients, but those at risk for infection with antibiotic-resistant organisms or with chronic, previously treated, or severe infections usually require broader spectrum regimens. Imaging is helpful in most DFIs; plain radiographs may be sufficient, but magnetic resonance imaging is far more sensitive and specific. Osteomyelitis occurs in many diabetic patients with a foot wound and can be difficult to diagnose (optimally defined by bone culture and histology) and treat (often requiring surgical debridement or resection, and/or prolonged antibiotic therapy). Most DFIs require some surgical intervention, ranging from minor (debridement) to major (resection, amputation). Wounds must also be properly dressed and off-loaded of pressure, and patients need regular follow-up. An ischemic foot may require revascularization, and some nonresponding patients may benefit from selected adjunctive measures. Employing multidisciplinary foot teams improves outcomes. Clinicians and healthcare organizations should attempt to monitor, and thereby improve, their outcomes and processes in caring for DFIs.

▶ The article Does This Patient Have an Infection of a Chronic Wound? by M. Reddy et al is important as it sets the stage for the surgical management of the diabetic foot. Surgical goals in the management of this disorder have significant consequences for the patient. The guidelines of the Infectious Diseases Society of America make the strong recommendation (with low evidence) that an experienced surgeon aid with debridement and management of the potentially infected diabetic foot. Pain in the neuropathic extremity is often an imprecise symptom; however, the other coding mechanisms for infection can be equally vague. The importance of gaining appropriate culture, performing adequate debridement while preserving options for a functional extremity, and the wisdom to perform appropriate amputation with possibility of quicker rehabilitation is stressed within the guidelines. Often, recommendations relating to surgical management are strong but with low reliability because the literature to support them is weak. This only reinforces the importance for the surgeon to clearly understand the goals of making a clean diagnosis, performing minimal, but adequate, debridement, with the goal of good long-term function of the individual with the diabetic foot.

T. Pruett, MD

Epidemiology of *Staphylococcus aureus* Blood and Skin and Soft Tissue Infections in the US Military Health System, 2005-2010

Landrum ML, Neumann C, Cook C, et al (San Antonio Military Med Ctr, Fort Sam Houston, TX; Navy and Marine Corps Public Health Ctr, Portsmouth, VA; et al)

JAMA 308:50-59, 2012

Context.—Rates of hospital-onset methicillin-resistant *Staphylococcus aureus* (MRSA) infections are reported as decreasing, but recent rates of community-onset *S aureus* infections are less known.

Objectives.—To characterize the overall and annual incidence rates of community-onset and hospital-onset *S aureus* bacteremia and skin and soft tissue infections (SSTIs) in a national health care system and to evaluate trends in the incidence rates of *S aureus* bacteremia and SSTIs and the proportion due to MRSA.

Design, Setting, and Participants.—Observational study of all Department of Defense TRICARE beneficiaries from January 2005 through December 2010. Medical record databases were used to identify and classify all annual first-positive *S aureus* blood and wound or abscess cultures as methicillin-susceptible *S aureus* or MRSA, and as community-onset or hospital-onset infections (isolates collected >3 days after hospital admission).

Main Outcome Measures.—Unadjusted incidence rates per 100 000 person-years of observation, the proportion of infections that was due to MRSA, and annual trends for 2005 through 2010 (examined using the Spearman rank correlation test or the Mantel- Haenszel χ^2 test for linear trend).

Results.—During 56 million person-years (nonactive duty: 47 million person-years; active duty: 9 million person-years), there were 2643 blood and 80 281 wound or abscess annual first-positive Saureus cultures. Annual incidence rates varied from 3.6 to 6.0 per 100 000 person-years for *S aureus* bacteremia and 122.7 to 168.9 per 100 000 person-years for *S aureus* SSTIs. The annual incidence rates for community-onset MRSA bacteremia decreased from 1.7 per 100 000 person-years (95% CI, 1.5-2.0 per 100 000 person-years) in 2005 to 1.2 per 100 000 person-years (95% CI, 0.9-1.4 per 100 000 person-years) in 2010 ($P = .005$ for trend). The annual incidence rates for hospital-onset MRSA bacteremia also decreased from 0.7 per 100 000 person-years (95% CI, 0.6-0.9 per 100 000 person-years) in 2005 to 0.4 per 100 000 person-years (95% CI, 0.3-0.5 per 100 000 person-years) in 2010 ($P = .005$ for trend). Concurrently, the proportion of community-onset SSTI due to MRSA peaked at 62% in 2006 before decreasing annually to 52% in 2010 ($P < .001$ for trend).

Conclusion.—In the Department of Defense population consisting of men and women of all ages from across the United States, the rates of both community-onset and hospital-onset MRSA bacteremia decreased in parallel, while the proportion of community-onset SSTIs due to MRSA has more recently declined.

▶ Staying with the theme of soft tissue infections, this article was written from the perspective of the military and their concern about an increasing prevalence of methicillin-resistant *Staphylococcus aureus* (MRSA) in the community. This organism has been in the news as a dreaded, antibiotic-resistant scourge, and there has been concern that resistance to β-lactamase—resistant drugs would become as common as penicillin resistance. In a review of 5 years of medical records from the Department of Defense TRICARE beneficiaries, blood or wound cultures for first positive *S. aureus* were investigated. MRSA still represents a significant percentage of *S. aureus* infections, irrespective of whether community- or hospital-acquired (25%-45%). However, rather than replacing methicillin-sensitive *S. aureus* as the dominant clinical strain, the rate of MRSA wound infection and bacteremia has decreased over the 5-year period. This is probably a harbinger that both forms of *S. aureus* are likely to be found within the clinical arena for the foreseeable future, and it emphasizes the necessity for vigilance by providers.

T. Pruett, MD

Endoscopic Transgastric vs Surgical Necrosectomy for Infected Necrotizing Pancreatitis: A Randomized Trial
Bakker OJ, for the Dutch Pancreatitis Study Group (Univ Med Ctr Utrecht, the Netherlands; et al)
JAMA 307:1053-1061, 2012

Context.—Most patients with infected necrotizing pancreatitis require necrosectomy. Surgical necrosectomy induces a proinflammatory response and is associated with a high complication rate. Endoscopic transgastric necrosectomy, a form of natural orifice transluminal endoscopic surgery, may reduce the proinflammatory response and reduce complications.

Objective.—To compare the proinflammatory response and clinical outcome of endoscopic transgastric and surgical necrosectomy.

Design, Setting, and Patients.—Randomized controlled assessor-blinded clinical trial in 3 academic hospitals and 1 regional teaching hospital in the Netherlands between August 20, 2008, and March 3, 2010. Patients had signs of infected necrotizing pancreatitis and an indication for intervention.

Interventions.—Random allocation to endoscopic transgastric or surgical necrosectomy. Endoscopic necrosectomy consisted of transgastric puncture, balloon dilatation, retroperitoneal drainage, and necrosectomy. Surgical necrosectomy consisted of video-assisted retroperitoneal debridement or, if not feasible, laparotomy.

Main Outcome Measures.—The primary end point was the postprocedural proinflammatory response as measured by serum interleukin 6 (IL-6) levels. Secondary clinical end points included a predefined composite end point of major complications (new-onset multiple organ failure, intra-abdominal bleeding, enterocutaneous fistula, or pancreatic fistula) or death.

Results.—We randomized 22 patients, 2 of whom did not undergo necrosectomy following percutaneous catheter drainage and could not be analyzed for the primary end point. Endoscopic transgastric necrosectomy reduced the postprocedural IL-6 levels compared with surgical necrosectomy (*P* =.004). The composite clinical end point occurred less often after endoscopic necrosectomy (20% vs 80%; risk difference [RD], 0.60; 95% CI, 0.16-0.80; *P* =.03). Endoscopic necrosectomy did not cause new-onset multiple organ failure (0% vs 50%, RD, 0.50; 95% CI, 0.12-0.76; *P* =.03) and reduced the number of pancreatic fistulas (10% vs 70%; RD, 0.60; 95% CI, 0.17-0.81; *P* =.02).

Conclusion.—In patients with infected necrotizing pancreatitis, endoscopic necrosectomy reduced the proinflammatory response as well as the composite clinical end point compared with surgical necrosectomy.

Trial Registration.—isrctn.org Identifier: ISRCTN07091918.

▶ This article was chosen as a reminder that although the surgical goal of source control remains consistent, the means of achieving that end has changed dramatically. In the initial literature of surgical control of necrotizing pancreatitis, the open, transperitoneal abdomen was championed by most. Others approached necrosectomy through an extraserous approach. This article compares peroral necrosectomy of the pancreas to that of the surgical video-assisted or open approach. The primary endpoint was the generation of proinflammatory cytokines and secondary endpoints were clinical outcomes (eg, death, fistula, organ failure, bleeding). This study represents a very select group of patients. The time from the start of symptoms to necrosectomy initiation was almost 2 months. In patients that survived to this point with necrotic pancreas, the peroral debridement was associated with significantly less proinflammatory cytokine response and other clinical morbidities. However, one must wonder whether patients that did not survive to randomization would have potentially been salvaged with earlier intervention? This study is nicely done with 2 options of therapy; however, it remains to be seen whether the benefits would still be true in the event of earlier application of interventions—whether surgical or peroral debridement.

T. Pruett, MD

8 Endocrine

Adrenalectomy may improve cardiovascular and metabolic impairment and ameliorate quality of life in patients with adrenal incidentalomas and subclinical Cushing's syndrome
Iacobone M, Citton M, Viel G, et al (Univ of Padua, Italy)
Surgery 152:991-997, 2012

Background.—Adrenalectomy represents the definitive treatment in clinically evident Cushing's syndrome; however, the most appropriate treatment for patients with subclinical Cushing's syndrome (SCS) with an adrenal incidentaloma remains controversial. This study was aimed to assess whether adrenalectomy may improve cardiovascular and metabolic impairment and quality of life compared with conservative management.

Methods.—Twenty patients with adrenal incidentaloma underwent laparoscopic adrenalectomy for SCS, whereas 15 were managed conservatively. Hormonal laboratory parameters of corticosteroid secretion, arterial blood pressure (BP), glycometabolic profile, and quality of life (by the SF-36 questionnaire) were compared at baseline and the end of follow-up.

Results.—The 2 groups were equivalent concerning all the examined parameters at baseline. In the operative group, laboratory corticosteroid parameters normalized in all patients but not in the conservative-management group (P < .001). In operated patients, a decrease in BP occurred in 53% of patients, glycometabolic control improved in 50%, and body mass index decreased; in contrast, no improvement or some worsening occurred in the conservative-management group (P < .01). SF-36 evaluation improved in the operative group (P < .05).

Conclusion.—Adrenalectomy can be more beneficial than conservative management in SCS and may achieve remission of laboratory hormonal abnormalities and improve BP, glycemic control, body mass index, and quality of life.

► Subclinical Cushing's syndrome (SCS) is defined by the absence of overt clinical features of Cushing's syndrome and the presence of mild abnormalities in the pituitary-adrenal axis suggestive of adrenocorticotropic hormone (ACTH)-independent hypercortisolism as follows: (1) AM cortisol greater than 5 μg/dL after a low-dose (1 mg) overnight dexamethasone suppression test; (2) morning ACTH level less than 10; (3) urinary-free cortisol greater than 76 μg/d. The authors here compared patients who had SCS and a concomitant unilateral adrenal incidentaloma and underwent surgery with those who did not. The results are striking in their support for surgery in these patients. Table 1 in the original article from the paper documents some of the changes seen. Notable improvement was seen in blood pressure, serum glucose, and hemoglobin A1c in the patients who had surgery, whereas the control group did not see any positive changes and blood pressure worsened over the study period.

The results are impressive but must be viewed as preliminary because the patients were not randomly divided in any way—the control patient population (those who did not have surgery) was self-selected—they were the patients who refused surgery over this period. Nevertheless, the results certainly warrant a good prospective study to confirm that surgery is beneficial in patients with SCS and an adrenal adenoma.

T. J. Fahey, MD

A Clinical Prediction Score to Diagnose Unilateral Primary Aldosteronism
Küpers EM, Amar L, Raynaud A, et al (Assistance Publique-Hôpitaux de Paris, France; Georges Pompidou European Hosp, Paris, France; et al)
J Clin Endocrinol Metab 97:3530-3537, 2012

Context.—Adrenal venous sampling is recommended to assess whether aldosterone hypersecretion is lateralized in patients with primary aldosteronism. However, this procedure is invasive, poorly standardized, and not widely available.

Objective.—Our goal was to identify patients' characteristics that can predict unilateral aldosterone hypersecretion in some patients who could hence bypass adrenal venous sampling before surgery.

Design and Setting.—A cross-sectional diagnostic study was performed from February 2009 to July 2010 at a single center specialized in hypertension care.

Patients.—A total of 101 consecutive patients with primary aldosteronism who underwent adrenal venous sampling participated in the study. The autonomy of aldosterone hypersecretion was assessed with the saline infusion test.

Intervention.—Adrenal venous sampling was performed without ACTH infusion but with simultaneous bilateral sampling.

Main Outcome Measures.—Variables independently associated with a lateralized adrenal venous sampling in multivariate logistic regression were used to derive a clinical prediction rule.

Results.—Adrenal venous sampling was successful in 87 patients and lateralized in 49. All 26 patients with a typical Conn's adenoma plus serum potassium of less than 3.5 mmol/liter or estimated glomerular filtration rate of at least 100 ml/min/1.73 m^2 (or both) had unilateral primary aldosteronism; this rule had 100% specificity (95% confidence interval, 91−100) and 53% sensitivity (95% confidence interval, 38−68).

Conclusions.—If our results are validated on an independent sample, adrenal venous sampling could be omitted before surgery in patients

TABLE 2.—Concordance of AVS and Imaging Results in Patients Age 40 or Younger and Those Older Than 40 yr with PA

| | AVS Results | | |
	Unilateral Right	Unilateral Left	Bilateral
Patients ≤ 40 yr old			
Right adrenal adenoma	2	0	0
Left adrenal adenoma	0	7	0
No typical adenoma	5	1	10
Patients > 40 yr old			
Right adrenal adenoma	9	1	4
Left adrenal adenoma	0	8	1
No typical adenoma	8	8	23

with a typical Conn's adenoma if they meet at least one of two supplementary biochemical characteristics (serum potassium < 3.5 mmol/liter or estimated glomerular filtration rate ≥ 100 ml/min/1.73 m^2) (Table 2).

▶ This is an interesting proposal—to provide a rationale for avoiding adrenal vein sampling (AVS) to confirm lateralization of an adrenal adenoma as the cause of Conn's adenoma. With the recently documented possibility that there is a significantly higher incidence of primary hyperaldosteronism as an underlying cause of hypertension, it is possible that the utilization of AVS will increase substantially. The problem is that it is not a great test: AVS is invasive (with associated risk of complications), not widely available, has a significant incidence of being unsuccessful (up to 50% in some series), and is not always informative, even when thought to be successful. The authors here have identified 3 criteria that they indicate can obviate the need for AVS with 100% specificity: a typical adenoma on cross-sectional imaging + either a serum potassium < 3.5 or an estimated glomerular filtration rate of > 100 mL/min/1.73 m^2. Although this would be a wonderful addition to the management algorithm of patients with primary hyperaldosteronism, at this point it is a little early to adopt these criteria. First, the authors note that the criteria are dependent on the identification of an adenoma and a completely normal contralateral gland. This is an important point as a truly normal contralateral gland on imaging may be nearly sufficient to avoid AVS by itself in my experience. Second, the data in Table 2 show that nearly 30% of the patients in the study were 40 years old or less and really do not need another criterion for lateralization. So, the sample size is really quite small and although additional criteria to avoid referring patients for AVS are desirable, these criteria clearly need to be validated prior to widespread adoption.

T. J. Fahey, MD

What is the Best Criterion for the Interpretation of Adrenal Vein Sample Results in Patients with Primary Hyperaldosteronism?

Webb R, Mathur A, Chang R, et al (Natl Cancer Inst, Bethesda, MD; Warren F Magnuson Clinical Ctr, Bethesda, MD; et al)
Ann Surg Oncol 19:1881-1886, 2012

Background.—In patients with primary hyperaldosteronism, adrenal vein sampling (AVS) has emerged as a gold standard for distinguishing between unilateral and bilateral disease, but multiple criteria have been used and no consensus exists as to the most accurate criterion. The objective of this study was to determine which AVS criteria most accurately identify patients with unilateral surgical disease and are associated with significant clinical improvement after adrenalectomy.

Methods.—This is a retrospective analysis of AVS results in 108 patients with primary hyperaldosteronism treated at a single institution. Literature review of AVS criteria was used to distinguish between unilateral and bilateral disease.

Results.—Of the 10 AVS criteria identified in the literature, one criterion (ACTH stimulation, positioning: cortisol [adrenal]/cortisol [periphery] [Ca/Cp] >5.0 and lateralization: aldosterone/cortisol [A/C] [dominant {D}]: A/C [nondominant {ND}] >4:1) was the most accurate in identifying and correctly predicting lateralization of disease (*P* value range: <0.001— 0.0369). For this criterion, the true positive rate was 88%. The second most accurate criterion was no ACTH stimulation, positioning Ca/Cp >1.1 and lateralization: A/C (D): A/C (ND) >2:1. For this criterion, the overall true positive was 85%. However, we found no significant difference in clinical outcome based on individual criteria fulfillment.

Conclusions.—Of the multiple criteria used for AVS evaluation, one criterion has the best accuracy. With the increasing use of AVS, there should be a consensus by which these results are evaluated and surgeons recommend adrenalectomy.

▶ This study from the National Cancer Institute (NCI) provides a thoughtful comparison of current criteria that are utilized to determine lateralization for primary hyperaldosteronism. The authors applied 10 different criteria to 108 patients who were seen at the NCI and underwent adrenal vein sampling. Eighty-nine of these patients ultimately had surgery for primary hyperaldosteronism at the NCI and had records available for analysis. Of the 10 criteria, the one that was ultimately considered the most accurate combined the use of adrenocorticotropic hormone (ACTH) stimulation and then the ratio of the stimulated aldosterone to cortisol from one side to the other. For those not familiar with this technique, ACTH stimulation is performed to maximize the cortisol output at the time of adrenal vein catheterization. A ratio of adrenal vein to peripheral cortisol levels of greater than 5x is considered best to document true positioning of the catheter tip in the adrenal veins. Lateralization is then determined by a ratio of aldosterone to cortisol of greater than 4:1 from one side to the other. Although the authors do note that there was no statistical difference between the various criteria regarding success of the operation, in this series this was the best overall criteria. In this editor's experience, these are the criteria used at our institution and, really, these are the criteria that make the most sense. I agree with the authors' conclusions that a single set of criteria should be adopted for uniform reporting of adrenal vein sampling and that the criteria with the best accuracy should be used.

T. J. Fahey, MD

Resection of adrenocortical carcinoma is less complete and local recurrence occurs sooner and more often after laparoscopic adrenalectomy than after open adrenalectomy
Miller BS, Gauger PG, Hammer GD, et al (Univ of Michigan Health System, Ann Arbor; et al)
Surgery 152:1150-1157, 2012

Background.—Controversy surrounds the use of laparoscopy for resection of adrenocortical carcinoma. We evaluated the hypothesis that outcome is equivalent in patients undergoing laparoscopic adrenalectomy versus open adrenalectomy.

Methods.—This is a retrospective review of 217 patients (156 patients with stage I—III cancer) with adrenocortical carcinoma referred to a single institution between 2005 and 2011. Outcome and operative data were assessed for the subset undergoing resection with curative intent. Student *t* and Fisher exact tests and the Kaplan—Meier method were used to compare data ($P \le .05$ was considered statistically significant).

Results.—One hundred fifty-six patients (64% female; median age, 47 years [range, 18—80]; median follow-up, 26.5 months [range, 1—188]) were identified. Forty-six patients underwent laparoscopic adrenalectomy, and 110 underwent open adrenalectomy. Twenty-seven percent of laparoscopic adrenalectomy patients had stage III cancer. After laparoscopic adrenalectomy, 30% had positive margins or intraoperative tumor spill compared to 16% of the open adrenalectomy patients ($P = .04$). Overall survival for patients with stage II cancer was longer in those undergoing open adrenalectomy ($P = .002$). Time to visible tumor bed recurrence or peritoneal recurrence in stage II patients was shorter in laparoscopic adrenalectomy patients ($P = .002$).

Conclusion.—Open adrenalectomy is superior to laparoscopic adrenalectomy for adrenocortical carcinoma based on completeness of resection, site and timing of initial tumor recurrence, and survival in stage II patients. Intraoperative evaluation is insensitive for the detection of stage III tumors.

▶ The debate as to whether all operations for suspected adrenocortical carcinoma (ACC) should be done with an open or a laparoscopic approach continues. Two articles at the 2012 meeting of the American Association of Endocrine Surgeons addressed this topic—this one from the group at Michigan and the other a multicenter study from Italy (see below).

The major problem with this report—as with the MD Anderson group's report previously[1] —is that these cases are accrued from hospitals and surgeons from all over and very likely with a highly variable experience in managing suspicious adrenal masses. This point is not addressed in the report, but it would be interesting to learn what percentage of cases were referred from community hospitals as opposed to major medical centers and from experienced adrenal surgeons compared with surgeons with limited experience. It is likely that the experience level of the initial operating surgeon with adrenal masses and adrenocortical carcinoma could even be ascertained retrospectively, and this information could help sort out this controversy. Nevertheless, the group's experience as a referral center cannot be discounted. My approach is to discuss with every patient undergoing adrenalectomy for a possible malignancy the pros and cons of the laparoscopic vs open approaches.

T. J. Fahey, MD

Reference

1. Gonzalez RJ, Shapiro S, Sarlis N, et al. Laparoscopic resection of adrenal cortical carcinoma: a cautionary note. *Surgery.* 2005;138:1078-1085.

Open versus endoscopic adrenalectomy in the treatment of localized (stage I/II) adrenocortical carcinoma: Results of a multiinstitutional Italian survey
Lombardi CP, Raffaelli M, De Crea C, et al (Università Cattolica del Sacro Cuore, Rome, Italy; et al)
Surgery 152:1158-1164, 2012

Background.—We compared the oncologic effectiveness of open adrenalectomy and endoscopic adrenalectomy in the treatment of patients with localized adrenocortical carcinoma.

Methods.—One hundred fifty-six patients with localized adrenocortical carcinoma (stage I/II) who underwent R0 resection were included in an Italian multiinstitutional surgical survey. They were divided into 2 groups based on the operative approach (either conventional or endoscopic).

Results.—One hundred twenty-six patients underwent open adrenalectomy and 30 patients underwent endoscopic adrenalectomy. The 2 groups were well matched for age, sex, lesion size, and stage ($P = NS$). The mean follow-up time was similar for the 2 groups ($P = NS$). The local recurrence rate was 19% for open adrenalectomy and 21% for endoscopic adrenalectomy, whereas distant metastases were recorded in 31% of patients in the conventional adrenalectomy group and 17% in the endoscopic adrenalectomy group ($P = NS$). The mean time to recurrence was 27 ± 27 months in the conventional open adrenalectomy group and 29 ± 33 months in the endoscopic adrenalectomy group ($P = NS$). No significant differences were found between the 2 groups in terms of 5-year disease-free survival (38.3% vs 58.2%) and 5-year overall survival rates (48% vs 67%; $P = NS$).

Conclusion.—The operative approach does not affect the oncologic outcome of patients with localized adrenocortical carcinoma, if the principles of surgical oncology are respected.

► This study on adrenal cortical carcinoma (ACC) is a retrospective study from 10 centers across Italy. The patients appear to be well matched, and there were no differences in either recurrence or survival between the 2 groups. Importantly, and perhaps of some concern, there were no patients who had peritoneal carcinomatosis in either the laparoscopic or open groups. This differs from the experience seen by the Michigan group as well as the similar experience reported by the MD Anderson group.[1] Although it is possible that there is some difference in the natural behavior of the disease, it is more likely that this is an aberration of reporting or detection.

Obviously, a randomized, prospective study is needed to answer the question of whether a laparoscopic approach is equivalent to an open approach in the management of adrenocortical carcinoma. However, although everyone accepts that ACC is a highly malignant tumor, is there any reason to believe that ACC should behave differently than other cancers for which a laparoscopic approach was initially decried because of peritoneal or wound seeding? Ultimately, a careful laparoscopic approach by good surgeons proved to be equivalent (or even better) than an open approach in colorectal tumors. There is little reason to believe that ACC should be different and, ultimately, I believe that really it is the technical skill of the surgeon, not the overall approach. The bottom line— adrenal masses being removed for suspicion of malignancy should not be approached by surgeons who are not experts in the management of adrenocortical carcinoma, either laparoscopically or open. Period.

T. J. Fahey, MD

Reference

1. Gonzalez RJ, Shapiro S, Sarlis N, et al. Laparoscopic resection of adrenal cortical carcinoma: a cautionary note. *Surgery.* 2005;138:1078-1086.

Small, nonfunctioning, asymptomatic pancreatic neuroendocrine tumors (PNETs): Role for nonoperative management
Lee LC, Grant CS, Salomao DR, et al (Mayo Clinic, Rochester, MN)
Surgery 152:965-974, 2012

Background.—Controversy exists regarding the optimal management of incidentally discovered, small pancreatic neuroendocrine tumors (PNETs). Our aim was to review the outcomes of patients who underwent nonoperative and operative management.

Methods.—We retrospectively reviewed patients with nonfunctioning PNETs at our institution from January 1, 2000 to June 30, 2011. Patients were included if the tumor was sporadic and <4 cm without radiographic evidence of local invasion or metastases.

Results.—Nonoperative patients ($n = 77$, median age, 67 years; range, 31—94) had a median tumor size of 1.0 cm (range, 0.3—3.2). Mean follow-up (F/U) was 45 months (max. 153 months). Median tumor size did not change throughout F/U; there was no disease progression or disease specific mortality. In the operative group ($n = 56$, median age, 60 years; range, 27—82), median neoplasm size was 1.8 cm (range, 0.5—3.6). Mean F/U was 52 months (max. 138 months). A total of 46% of the operative patients had some type of complication, more than half due to a clinically significant pancreatic leak. No recurrence or disease specific mortality was seen in the operative group, including 5 patients with positive lymph nodes.

Conclusion.—Small nonfunctioning PNETs usually exhibit minimal or no growth over many years. Nonoperative management may be advocated when serial imaging demonstrates minimal or no growth without suspicious features.

▶ Pancreatic endocrine incidentalomas are increasingly being recognized on cross-sectional imaging. These are usually nonfunctioning, and the management of these tumors has been largely to resect, even when small. A recent experience from the Massachusetts General Hospital reinforced the need to resect these small pancreatic endocrine tumors, because the study found that 8% of tumors less than 2 cm were found to develop metastasis despite resection.[1] Here the authors argue that these small pancreatic neuroendocrine tumors can be safely followed with serial imaging and be referred for excision only if there is growth or development of suspicious features. One of the major limitations of this study is that only 29% of the 77 patients actually had cytologic confirmation that these were, in fact, pancreatic endocrine tumors. Although this editor agrees that nonoperative management is appropriate for most of these small pancreatic endocrine incidentalomas, I would consider biopsy confirmation a very important part of the algorithm. Furthermore, biopsy would permit a Ki-67 (or other, better, yet-to-be-described molecular markers) to contribute to the patient and physician decision as to how to best manage these small tumors.

T. J. Fahey, MD

Reference

1. Haynes AB, Deshpande V, Ingkakul T, et al. Implications of incidentally discovered, nonfunctioning pancreatic endocrine tumors: short-term and long-term patient outcomes. *Arch Surg.* 2011;146:534-538.

Pancreatic Enucleation: Improved Outcomes Compared to Resection
Cauley CE, Pitt HA, Ziegler KM, et al (Indiana Univ School of Medicine, Indianapolis)
J Gastrointest Surg 16:1347-1353, 2012

Introduction.—Pancreatic enucleation is associated with a low operative mortality and preserved pancreatic parenchyma. However, enucleation is an uncommon operation, and good comparative data with resection are

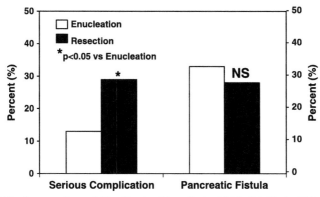

FIGURE 2.—Postoperative morbidity. (Reprinted from Cauley CE, Pitt HA, Ziegler KM, et al. Pancreatic enucleation: improved outcomes compared to resection. *J Gastrointest Surg.* 2012;16:1347-1353, with permission from The Society for Surgery of the Alimentary Tract.)

lacking. Therefore, the aim of this analysis was to compare the outcomes of pancreatic enucleation and resection.

Material and Methods.—From 1998 through 2010, 45 consecutive patients with small (mean, 2.3 cm) pancreatic lesions underwent enucleation. These patients were matched with 90 patients undergoing pancreatoduodenectomy ($n = 38$) or distal pancreatectomy ($n = 52$). Serious morbidity was defined in accordance with the American College of Surgeons—National Surgical Quality Improvement Program. Outcomes were compared with standard statistical analyses.

Results.—Operative time was shorter (183 vs. 271 min, $p < 0.01$), and operative blood loss was significantly lower (160 vs. 691 ml, $p < 0.01$) with enucleation. Fewer patients undergoing enucleation required monitoring in an intensive care unit (20% vs. 41%, $p < 0.02$). Serious morbidity was less common among patients who underwent enucleation compared to those who had a resection (13% vs. 29%, $p = 0.05$). Pancreatic endocrine (4% vs. 17%, $p = 0.05$) and exocrine (2% vs. 17%, $p < 0.05$) insufficiency were less common with enucleation. Ten-year survival was no different between enucleation and resection.

Conclusion.—Compared to resection, pancreatic enucleation is associated with improved operative as well as short- and long-term postoperative outcomes. For small benign and premalignant pancreatic lesions, enucleation should be considered the procedure of choice when technically appropriate (Fig 2).

▶ While the debate over whether to observe or resect small pancreatic endocrine incidentalomas is settled over the next few years (decades), this article details nicely the role for limited resection; that is, enucleation for small endocrine pancreatic tumors. The analysis was not restricted to pancreatic neuroendocrine tumors (PNETs), although approximately 50% of the lesions in each group were PNETs and so the conclusions certainly do apply to the management of PNETs. In virtually every category, the morbidity was lower for patients who underwent enucleation except for the development of pancreatic fistula, as shown in Fig 2 from the article. This rate of pancreatic fistula is similar to that seen in other studies of pancreatic enucleation or limited pancreatic resection and highlights the fact that even a small operation on the pancreas is associated with a substantial risk of morbidity. The long-term advantage of enucleation relates to the lower incidence of pancreatic exocrine and endocrine insufficiency. As noted in the discussion of the previous article, selection of appropriate candidates for enucleation is very important and not addressed in this report. There will be an increasing role for application of molecular markers to determine not only which lesions can be safely observed, but also which can be safely removed by enucleation or limited resection.

T. J. Fahey, MD

Calcimimetics Versus Parathyroidectomy for Treatment of Primary Hyperparathyroidism: Retrospective Chart Analysis of a Prospective Database

Keutgen XM, Buitrago D, Filicori F, et al (New York Presbyterian Hosp—Weill Cornell Med Ctr)
Ann Surg 255:981-985, 2012

Objective.—This study aims to determine the efficacy of calcimimetics in improving bone mineral density (BMD) in patients with primary hyperparathyroidism (pHPT) and compare those results to patients undergoing parathyroidectomy.

Background.—Parathyroidectomy has been shown to improve BMD in pHPT, but calcimimetics have recently been advocated as a medical alternative to parathyroidectomy for pHPT.

Materials and Methods.—We identified 17 patients that were treated with calcimimetics for pHPT. Seventeen patients with pHPT who underwent parathyroidectomy served as surgical controls. Serum calcium level, parathyroid hormone (PTH) level, and femur and spine BMD T scores were compared before and 1 year after therapy.

Results.—Both groups were demographically matched. Calcium levels normalized in 70.6% of medically versus 100% of surgically treated patients $(P = 0.026)$. PTH levels normalized in 35% of patients treated with calcimimetics versus 76% of surgical patients $(P = 0.036)$. Femur BMD improved in 18.8% of medically treated patients versus 58.8% of surgical patients $(P = 0.032)$. Spine BMD improved in 70.6% of medically treated patients versus 82.4% of surgical patients $(P = 0.69)$. Further analysis demonstrated that regardless of treatment, normalization of PTH was associated with significant improvement in femur $(P = 0.03)$ and spine BMD $(P < 0.001)$. Normalization of calcium without normalization of PTH did not impact BMD.

Conclusions.—Parathyroidectomy results in greater normalization of serum calcium and PTH levels and significantly improves cortical BMD compared to calcimimetics. Regardless of treatment, normalization of

TABLE 3.—Pre- and Posttreatment Values Within the Calcimimetic and Surgery Groups, Respectively

| Parameters | Calcimimetics | | | Surgery | | |
	Pretreatment	Posttreatment	P	Pretreatment	Posttreatment	P
Calcium (mg/dL)*	10.79	10.14	0.003	10.77	9.48	<0.001
PTH (pg/mL)†	115.8	92.8	0.082	183.2	55	0.001
Femur T score‡	−2.25	−2.4	NI§	−1.82	−1.69	0.19
Spine T score‡	−1.9	−1.45	0.045	−1.94	−1.6	0.017

*Normal Calcium Level: 8.5–10.4 mg/dL.
†Normal PTH Level 10–68 pg/mL.
‡Osteopenia: −1.5 to −2.5, Osteoporosis: >−2.5.
§NI: No improvement in BMD T score.

PTH is associated with significant improvement in spine and femur BMD, suggesting that the superior effects of surgery may be mediated by better control of PTH (Table 3).

▶ Although cinacalcet has become an integral part of the treatment of patients with secondary hyperparathyroidism, its role in the medical management of patients with primary hyperparathyroidism is uncertain. Some have advocated its use and, furthermore, some endocrinologists have used it to treat patients with primary hyperparathyroidism. The article by Keutgen demonstrates nicely that parathyroidectomy is superior to calcimimetic treatment for primary hyperparathyroidism. As shown in Table 3, parathyroidectomy facilitates better control of both the serum calcium and parathyroid hormone (PTH) levels than calcimimetic treatment, and this appears to correlate with significant improvement in the bone mineral density of cortical bone. When looking at all 34 patients together, it is apparent that the most important parameter for improvement in bone density appears to be normalization of PTH. Because most patients seen in endocrine surgeons' offices with primary hyperparathyroidism are there at least in part because of an observation of decreased bone density, this is an important point. To achieve a turnaround in the bone density, it is important to be sure that the PTH has normalized. Whether better bone density improvement is correlated with lower PTH levels is an area worthy of further study.

T. J. Fahey, MD

Abandoning Unilateral Parathyroidectomy: Why We Reversed Our Position after 15,000 Parathyroid Operations
Norman J, Lopez J, Politz D (Norman Parathyroid Ctr, Tampa, FL)
J Am Coll Surg 214:260-269, 2012

Background.—Our group championed the techniques and benefits of unilateral parathyroidectomy. As our experience has matured, it seems this limited operation might be appropriate only occasionally.

Methods.—A single surgical group's experience with 15,000 parathyroidectomies examined the ongoing differences between unilateral and bilateral techniques for 10-year failure/recurrence, multigland removal, operative times, and length of stay.

Results.—With limited experience, 100% of operations were bilateral, decreasing to 32% by the 500th operation ($p < 0.001$), and long-term failure rates increased to 6%. Failures were 11 times more likely for unilateral explorations ($p < 0.001$ vs bilateral), causing gradual increases in bilateral explorations to 97% at the 14,000[th] operation ($p < 0.001$). Ten-year cure rates are unchanged for bilateral operations, and unilateral operations show continued slow recurrence rates of 5% ($p < 0.001$). Removal of more than one gland occurred 16 times more frequently when 4 glands were analyzed ($p < 0.001$), increasing cure rates to the current 99.4% ($p < 0.001$). Of 1,060 reoperations performed for failure at another institution, intraoperative parathyroid hormone levels fell >50% in 22% of patients, yet a second adenoma was subsequently found. Operative times decreased with experience; bilateral operations taking only 5.9 minutes longer on average (22.3 vs 16.4 minutes; $p < 0.001$), which is 25 minutes less than unilateral at the 500th operation ($p < 0.001$). By the 1,000[th] operation, incision size (2.5 ± 0.2 cm), anesthesia, and hospital stay (1.6 hours) were identical for unilateral and bilateral procedures.

Conclusions.—Regardless of surgical adjuncts (scanning, intraoperative parathyroid hormone), unilateral parathyroidectomy will carry a 1-year failure rate of 3% to 5% and a 10-year recurrence rate of 4% to 6%. Allowing rapid analysis of all 4 glands through the same 1-inch incision has caused us to all but abandon unilateral parathyroidectomy.

► Dr Norman's group has been at the forefront in advancing parathyroid surgery over the years. Thus, this article, which reverses much of what Norman espoused during earlier years, came as quite a surprise to some. The concept that a unilateral or focused approach may leave behind glands that can ultimately become hyperproducing parathyroid glands in the future is understandable. However, the recurrence rates seen in the literature—and even acknowledged by Norman in this series—do not approach the 25% recurrence rate that should be expected if all of the glands identified at surgery are hyperproducing by gamma counter. Furthermore, the idea that just exposing parathyroid glands to the air and a bit of surgical steel somehow prevents them from becoming hyperplastic or abnormal in the future is, frankly, bewildering. Although Norman has made tremendous contributions—and I strongly believe that the role for unilateral parathyroid explorations is less than we previously have thought (as he has written)—it must be said that his group does not always acknowledge recurrent disease even when it is present. I have seen 2 patients with recurrent hyperparathyroidism operated on at the Norman clinic who were sent e-mails telling them that they do not have recurrent disease simply because he had seen their parathyroids—despite clear biochemical evidence of a recurrence. One presumes that these patients are registered as cures after 4-gland exploration in this report. As with all things, the truth lies somewhere in between. Unilateral exploration is still a good operation—especially if the surgery is done under local anesthesia, where it is more comfortable than a bilateral exploration if it is feasible. It seems likely that the long-term recurrence rates may be lower with bilateral exploration, if additional enlarged glands are excised. But not all patients require a bilateral exploration.

Finally, in the response to a letter written about his article,[1] Norman notes that one of the benefits of bilateral exploration is the identification of 75% more incidentally found thyroid cancers. This is, frankly, preposterous and one of the greatest flaws in Norman's thinking. It is well known that concomitant thyroid disease requiring at least fine-needle aspiration is present in 25% of patients undergoing parathyroid surgery. There is really no excuse for not getting a preoperative ultrasound in every patient undergoing parathyroidectomy and dealing with this appropriately prior to a neck exploration. Except, of course, if it was going to inhibit patient movement to the Norman parathyroid center.

T. J. Fahey, MD

Reference

1. Norman J, Lopez J, Politz D, et al. Abandoning unilateral parathyroidectomy: why we reversed our position after 15,000 parathyroid operations. *J Am Coll Surg*. 2012;215:297-300.

Is minimally invasive parathyroidectomy associated with greater recurrence compared to bilateral exploration? Analysis of more than 1,000 cases
Schneider DF, Mazeh H, Sippel RS, et al (Univ of Wisconsin, Madison)
Surgery 152:1008-1015, 2012

Background.—The durability of minimally invasive parathyroidectomy (MIP) has been questioned, and some advocate for routine open parathyroidectomy (OP). This study compared outcomes between patients treated with MIP compared with OP for primary hyperparathyroidism (PHPT).

Methods.—A retrospective review was performed to identify cases of PHPT with single adenomas (SA) between 2001 and 2011. Operations were classified as OP when both sides were explored. Kaplan-Meier estimates were plotted and compared by the log-rank test.

Results.—We analyzed 1,083 patients with PHPT with SA; 928 (85.7%) were MIP and 155 (14.3%) were OP. There was no difference in the rates of persistence (0.2% MIP vs 0% OP, $P = .61$) or recurrence (2.5% MIP vs 1.9% OP, $P = .68$) between the 2 groups. The Kaplan-Meier estimates did, however, began to separate beyond 8 years' follow-up. The OP group did experience a greater incidence of transient hypocalcemia postoperatively (1.9% vs 0.1%, $P = .01$).

Conclusion.—MIP appears equivalent to OP in single-gland disease. Although patients undergoing OP experienced more transient hypocalcemia, patients undergoing MIP appear to have a greater long-term

TABLE 3.—Outcomes

Variable	MIP ($n = 928$)	OPEN ($n = 155$)	P Value
Total failures	25 (2.7)	3 (1.9)	.58
Persistent	2 (0.2)	0	.61
Recurrent	23 (2.5)	3 (1.9)	.68
Complications	16 (1.7)	5 (3.2)	.21
Transient hoarseness	2 (0.2)	8 (5.2)	.61
Permanent hoarseness	0	2 (1.3)	.56
Transient hypocalcemia	1 (0.1)	3 (1.9)	.01
Permanent hypocalcemia	0	0	—
Bleeding/hematoma	0	1 (0.7)	.68
Other	4 (0.43)	0	.41

Data are represented as the number of patients in each category with the percentage in parentheses.

recurrence rate. Therefore, proper patient selection and counseling of these risks is necessary for either approach (Table 3).

▶ This article from Herb Chen's group at the University of Wisconsin is timely. The question as to whether a focused approach to parathyroidectomy is the best approach has been elevated to the forefront of discussion regarding parathyroid surgery, at least in part because of the publication last year by Norman's group.[1] This study attempts to avoid the controversy surrounding missed glands by including only patients who were found to have single adenomas. Table 3 from the article sums up the data. Notable findings are that only 2 patients had persistent disease in the minimally invasive parathyroidectomy (unilateral) group, which is a remarkably low number. As indicated in Table 3, there were long-term recurrences in both groups, although these appear to have stopped in the patients who underwent 4-gland exploration (open group) after 8 years. As noted in the comments on Norman's article, scientifically this does not seem to make a lot of sense. Why should performing a bilateral exploration (where only 1 gland was excised; the authors make that very clear) be associated with a reduction in long-term recurrence? In this study, the answer may lie in the number of patients that had a bilateral exploration and more than 1 gland excised. Unfortunately, that number is not divulged in this article. Is it likely that those with subclinical multigland disease were excluded by the inclusion criteria? Nevertheless, the recurrence rate for a focused exploration is far less than expected if the Norman data regarding the incidence of multigland disease are accepted. And finally, as also indicated in the article, the use of the open (bilateral exploration) approach was associated with apparently statistically nonsignificant, but clearly clinically significant, higher incidence of complications—transient and permanent hoarseness and hematoma (Table 3).

T. J. Fahey, MD

Reference

1. Norman J, Lopez J, Politz D. Abandoning unilateral parathyroidectomy: why we reversed our position after 15,000 parathyroid operations. *J Am Coll Surg*. 2012; 214:260-269.

Changes in bone mineral density after surgical intervention for primary hyperparathyroidism
Dy BM, Grant CS, Wermers RA, et al (Mayo Clinic, Rochester, MN)
Surgery 152:1051-1058, 2012

Background.—Patients with primary hyperparathyroidism often lack classic symptoms but can have reductions in bone mineral density and increased fracture risk. We sought to determine bone mineral density improvement after successful surgery and associated factors.

Methods.—A review of patients with osteopenia or osteoporosis with curative parathyroidectomy and both pre- and postoperative dual-energy X-ray absorptiometry bone mineral density scans was conducted. We compared patients with declining (<0%), moderate improvement (0.1−5%), and significant improvement (>5%) on dual-energy X-ray absorptiometry bone mineral density scans.

Results.—We identified 420 patients who underwent a dual-energy X-ray absorptiometry bone mineral density scan preoperatively and within 36 months postoperatively. At the most affected site, 38% had significant improvement, 31% moderate improvement, and 31% declining bone mineral density. Patients who significantly improved were younger ($P=.01$), had lesser preoperative dual-energy X-ray absorptiometry ($P=.001$), and had greater preoperative levels of parathyroid hormone ($P=.04$), serum calcium ($P=.03$), and preoperative urinary calcium. There was no difference in outcomes between sex and with preoperative bisphosphonate use. Average hip and spine bone mineral density had similar responses to surgery.

Conclusion.—Bone mineral density improves in up to 75% of patients after curative parathyroidectomy for primary hyperparathyroidism. The hip and lumbar spine responded similarly. Younger patients and those with severe primary hyperparathyroidism may derive the most skeletal benefits from parathyroidectomy, but the uniform positive response supports parathyroidectomy in patients with osteoporosis and possibly osteopenia.

▶ This report from the American Association of Endocrine Surgeons' annual meeting last year is the largest analysis of changes in bone mineral density after parathyroidectomy to date. The authors show very nicely that 75% of their patients had improvements in bone density after parathyroidectomy. What is not discussed is why 25% did not show improvement. The missing piece of the puzzle here is the postoperative parathyroid hormone levels (and to a lesser extent, vitamin D levels). The definition of a successful operation for parathyroidectomy used by the authors is normalization of serum calcium, which is the accepted norm. As recently shown in the report by Keutgen et al,[1] it is likely that normalization of parathyroid hormone levels is also important in the resolution of bone loss secondary to hyperparathyroidism. If additional data can be accrued to show that normalization of parathyroid hormone (PTH) is at least as important, it may be prudent to change the definition of a successful parathyroidectomy going forward and to identify the causes of persistent PTH elevations in patients who otherwise appear to have a successful parathyroidectomy.

T. J. Fahey, MD

Reference

1. Keutgen XM, Buitrago D, Filicori F, et al. Calcimimetics versus parathyroidectomy for treatment of primary hyperparathyroidism: retrospective chart analysis of a prospective database. *Ann Surg.* 2012;255:981-985.

Effect of Cinacalcet on Cardiovascular Disease in Patients Undergoing Dialysis

The EVOLVE Trial Investigators (Stanford Univ School of Medicine, Palo Alto, CA; Denver Nephrology, CO; Instituto Nacional de Ciencias Médicas y Nutrición Salvador Zubirán, Mexico City; et al)
N Engl J Med 367:2482-2494, 2012

Background.—Disorders of mineral metabolism, including secondary hyperparathyroidism, are thought to contribute to extraskeletal (including vascular) calcification among patients with chronic kidney disease. It has been hypothesized that treatment with the calcimimetic agent cinacalcet might reduce the risk of death or nonfatal cardiovascular events in such patients.

Methods.—In this clinical trial, we randomly assigned 3883 patients with moderate-to-severe secondary hyperparathyroidism (median level of intact parathyroid hormone, 693 pg per milliliter [10th to 90th percentile, 363 to 1694]) who were undergoing hemodialysis to receive either cinacalcet or placebo. All patients were eligible to receive conventional therapy, including phosphate binders, vitamin D sterols, or both. The patients were followed for up to 64 months. The primary composite end point was the time until death, myocardial infarction, hospitalization for unstable angina, heart failure, or a peripheral vascular event. The primary analysis was performed on the basis of the intention-to-treat principle.

Results.—The median duration of study-drug exposure was 21.2 months in the cinacalcet group, versus 17.5 months in the placebo group. The primary composite end point was reached in 938 of 1948 patients (48.2%) in the cinacalcet group and 952 of 1935 patients (49.2%) in the placebo group (relative hazard in the cinacalcet group vs. the placebo group, 0.93; 95% confidence interval, 0.85 to 1.02; $P = 0.11$). Hypocalcemia and gastrointestinal adverse events were significantly more frequent in patients receiving cinacalcet.

Conclusions.—In an unadjusted intention-to-treat analysis, cinacalcet did not significantly reduce the risk of death or major cardiovascular events in patients with moderate-to-severe secondary hyperparathyroidism who were undergoing dialysis. (Funded by Amgen; EVOLVE ClinicalTrials.gov number, NCT00345839.)

► Cinacalcet has become widely prescribed in the United States to prevent the complications of secondary hyperparathyroidism in dialysis patients. Although the rates of parathyroidectomy for secondary hyperparathyroidism have plummeted for this disease, the long-term benefits of medical therapy with cinacalcet vs surgical therapy for secondary hyperparathyroidism have not been well characterized. This study is an important one that addresses this question.

One major drawback of this study—which, by the way, accrued patients from 4 different continents—is that it is unclear when patients were referred for parathyroidectomy and whether early parathyroidectomy was associated with long-term benefit. As shown in the article by Keutgen et al, at least in primary hyperparathyroidism it appears that cinacalcet may not reduce calcium and parathyroid hormone as effectively as surgical parathyroidectomy.[1] So the unanswered question at the end of the day is, would earlier referral for surgical parathyroidectomy have any beneficial effect, or is the contribution of secondary hyperparathyroidism to major cardiovascular morbidity not as significant as hypothesized? This is a complicated question that will probably require an equally large and complicated study to answer.

T. J. Fahey, MD

Reference

1. Keutgen XM, Buitrago D, Filicori F, et al. Calcimimetics versus parathyroidectomy for treatment of primary hyperparathyroidism: retrospective chart analysis of a prospective database. *Ann Surg*. 2012;255:981-985.

Cinacalcet Treatment for Stable Kidney Transplantation Patients With Hypercalcemia due to Persistent Secondary Hyperparathyroidism: A Long-term Follow-up

Paschoalin RP, Torregrosa J-V, Sánchez-Escuredo A, et al (Hosp Clinic, Barcelona, Spain)
Transplant Proc 44:2588-2589, 2012

Background.—Cinacalcet is an effective treatment for hypercalcemia due to persistent hyperparathyroidism (HPT) in patients who have undergone kidney transplantation (KT). Few data are available about their long-term follow-up.

Objective.—We aimed to evaluate the long-term efficacy of cinacalcet in functioning stable KT subjects with hypercalcemia secondary to persistent HPT.

Material and Methods.—Twenty-three patients (6 men) with a stable KT showed persistent hypercalcemia (>12 months) secondary to HPT (parathyroid hormone by radioimmunoassay [iPTH] > 150 pg/mL). The mean age was 54 ± 13 years. Time after KT to beginning cinacalcet treatment was 36.5 ± 37.9 (range 12 to 172) months. Initial cinacalcet doses were

30 mg/d. Median follow-up was 53 ± 7.4 months (range 42 to 60 months). We determined serum calcium, phosphorus, alkaline phosphatase, iPTH, creatinine, and immunosuppressant concentrations at baseline as well as 3, 6, and 12 months and after every 6 months thereafter.

Results.—Initial serum calcium was 11 ± 0.65 mg/dL and mean calcium during treatment, 10.25 ± 0.81 mg/dL ($P < .001$). Initial serum phosphorus was 2.8 ± 0.58 mg/dL and mean value serum phosphorus during the treatment period, 3.13 ± 0.6 mg/dL ($P = 0.015$). Initial iPTH was 260 ± 132 pg/mL and during the treatment period; 237 ± 131 pg/mL ($P = ns$). There was no change in renal function nor in immunosuppressant blood levels. Doses of cinacalcet at the end of the follow-up were 40.4 ± 18.9 mg/d.

Conclusion.—Cinacalcet was effective for long-term control of hypercalcemia related to persistent HPT for patients with stable KT.

▶ The authors of this report look at the role of cinacalcet in patients with tertiary hyperparathyroidism after kidney transplant. The data document that there is a statistically significant decline in the serum calcium level (as well as an increase in the serum phosphorus) in patients treated with cinacalcet, and this persists for up to 5 years (the length of the study). Although the authors view this in a positive light, the decline in the serum calcium level is really not very substantial (barely into the normal range), and there is no significant decline in serum parathyroid hormone levels. While they document that there is no decline in serum creatinine over the course of the study, given the results of the study by Keutgen et al,[1] it would seem that the effects achieved by cinacalcet treatment are not adequate to prevent other complications of hyperparathyroidism. Although the authors conclude that cinacalcet should be utilized to "avoid (kidney) allograft calcifications and maintain bone health," they present no data regarding bone health in this cohort of patients. Until there are more data supporting the use of medical therapy in tertiary hyperparathyroidism, I would strongly recommend that patients with tertiary hyperparathyroidism be treated surgically.

T. J. Fahey, MD

Reference

1. Keutgen XM, Buitrago D, Filicori F, et al. Calcimimetics versus parathyroidectomy for treatment of primary hyperparathyroidism: retrospective chart analysis of a prospective database. *Ann Surg.* 2012;255:981-985.

Preoperative Diagnosis of Benign Thyroid Nodules with Indeterminate Cytology

Alexander EK, Kennedy GC, Baloch ZW, et al (Brigham and Women's Hosp and Harvard Med School, Boston, MA; Veracyte, Inc, South San Francisco, CA; Univ of Pennsylvania, Philadelphia; et al)
N Engl J Med 367:705-715, 2012

Background.—Approximately 15 to 30% of thyroid nodules evaluated by means of fine-needle aspiration are not clearly benign or malignant. Patients with cytologically indeterminate nodules are often referred for diagnostic surgery, though most of these nodules prove to be benign. A novel diagnostic test that measures the expression of 167 genes has shown promise in improving preoperative risk assessment.

Methods.—We performed a 19-month, prospective, multicenter validation study involving 49 clinical sites, 3789 patients, and 4812 fine-needle aspirates from thyroid nodules 1 cm or larger that required evaluation. We obtained 577 cytologically indeterminate aspirates, 413 of which had corresponding histopathological specimens from excised lesions. Results of a central, blinded histopathological review served as the reference standard. After inclusion criteria were met, a gene-expression classifier was used to test 265 indeterminate nodules in this analysis, and its performance was assessed.

Results.—Of the 265 indeterminate nodules, 85 were malignant. The gene-expression classifier correctly identified 78 of the 85 nodules as suspicious (92% sensitivity; 95% confidence interval [CI], 84 to 97), with a specificity of 52% (95% CI, 44 to 59). The negative predictive values for "atypia (or follicular lesion) of undetermined clinical significance," "follicular neoplasm or lesion suspicious for follicular neoplasm," or "suspicious cytologic findings" were 95%, 94%, and 85%, respectively. Analysis of 7 aspirates with false negative results revealed that 6 had a paucity of thyroid follicular cells, suggesting insufficient sampling of the nodule.

Conclusions.—These data suggest consideration of a more conservative approach for most patients with thyroid nodules that are cytologically indeterminate on fine-needle aspiration and benign according to gene-expression classifier results. (Funded by Veracyte.)

▶ This report is a follow-up study of Veracyte's initial report on the Afirma gene expression classifier.[1] It is an important report, as it confirms that molecular classification of indeterminate thyroid nodules by gene expression analysis is quite accurate, although not perfect. How this information will be utilized by clinicians going forward has yet to be determined. First, the study was fully funded by Veracyte; thus, independent validation must occur. While I strongly believe that the results will be validated (because we were the first to show that gene expression using the Affy chips could differentiate benign and malignant thyroid nodules), this still needs to happen. Second, application of the data obtained to specific patients needs to be determined. The most important use of the technology is to identify patients who have malignancy and are better off with a total thyroidectomy at the initial operation. It is my hope that molecular testing should be able to nearly completely eliminate completion thyroidectomy in the future. Whether patients with lesions classified as benign on molecular analysis will be able to forego surgery going forward is certainly unclear at this time. There are unanswered questions, such as how often should the fine-needle aspiration and gene expression classifier be repeated? Should a hemithyroidectomy be performed for a benign but potentially premalignant lesion (Bethesda IV or V lesions)? Much work remains to be done to identify the appropriate place for gene expression analysis and other molecular tests in the management of thyroid nodules.

T. J. Fahey, MD

Reference

1. Barden CB, Shister KW, Zhu B, et al. Classification of follicular thyroid tumors by molecular signature: results of gene profiling. *Clin Cancer Res*. 2003;9:1792-1800.

A Panel of Four miRNAs Accurately Differentiates Malignant from Benign Indeterminate Thyroid Lesions on Fine Needle Aspiration
Keutgen XM, Filicori F, Crowley MJ, et al (New York Presbyterian Hosp—Weill Cornell Med Ctr; et al)
Clin Cancer Res 18:2032-2038, 2012

Purpose.—Indeterminate thyroid lesions on fine needle aspiration (FNA) harbor malignancy in about 25% of cases. Hemi- or total thyroidectomy has, therefore, been routinely advocated for definitive diagnosis. In this study, we analyzed miRNA expression in indeterminate FNA samples and determined its prognostic effects on final pathologic diagnosis.

Experimental Design.—A predictive model was derived using 29 *ex vivo* indeterminate thyroid lesions on FNA to differentiate malignant from benign tumors at a tertiary referral center and validated on an independent set of 72 prospectively collected *in vivo* FNA samples. Expression levels of miR-222, miR-328, miR-197, miR-21, miR-181a, and miR-146b were determined using reverse transcriptase PCR. A statistical model was developed using the support vector machine (SVM) approach.

Results.—A SVM model with four miRNAs (miR-222, miR-328, miR-197, and miR-21) was initially estimated to have 86% predictive accuracy using cross-validation. When applied to the 72 independent *in vivo* validation samples, performance was actually better than predicted with a sensitivity of 100% and specificity of 86%, for a predictive accuracy of 90% in differentiating malignant from benign indeterminate lesions. When Hurthle cell lesions were excluded, overall accuracy improved to 97% with 100% sensitivity and 95% specificity.

Conclusions.—This study shows that the expression of miR-222, miR-328, miR-197, and miR-21 combined in a predictive model is accurate at differentiating malignant from benign indeterminate thyroid lesions on FNA. These findings suggest that FNA miRNA analysis could be a useful adjunct in the management algorithm of patients with thyroid nodules.

▶ MicroRNAs (miRNA) are small RNAs that interact with messenger (m)RNA to modify expression and translation of mRNA through sequence-specific interaction. Typically, a single miRNA will interact with multiple genes to modify gene expression. It is because of this ability to interact with and affect the expression of multiple genes that we turned to miRNA analysis as a possible tool to discriminate between benign and malignant thyroid nodules. The advantages of a miRNA test from a clinical vantage point are as follows: (1) There are fewer gene targets, which, therefore, permits a polymerase chain reaction—based approach rather than the much more costly Affymetrix-based test (the Afirma test looks at the levels of 142 genes); (2) miRNAs are much more stable than mRNA, making sample handling considerably easier (and, therefore, probably more reliable). Although clearly this test also needs independent validation, it holds promise as ultimately a better test than the Afirma test. In the end, application of this test, as with any molecular test, will require thoughtful interpretation of the results as applied to individual patients.

T. J. Fahey, MD

The *BRAF*[V600E] Mutation Is an Independent, Poor Prognostic Factor for the Outcome of Patients with Low-Risk Intrathyroid Papillary Thyroid Carcinoma: Single-Institution Results from a Large Cohort Study

Elisei R, Viola D, Torregrossa L, et al (Univ of Pisa, Italy)
J Clin Endocrinol Metab 97:4390-4398, 2012

Background.—The $BRAF^{V600E}$ mutation, the most frequent genetic alteration in papillary thyroid carcinoma (PTC), was demonstrated to be a poor prognostic factor. The aim of this study was to evaluate its prognostic significance in a large cohort of low-risk intrathyroid PTC.

Methods.—Among the 431 consecutive PTC patients, we selected 319 patients with an intrathyroid tumor and no metastases (T1-T2, N0, M0). The $BRAF^{V600E}$ mutation was analyzed by PCR-single-strand conformation polymorphism analysis and direct genomic sequencing. The correlation between the presence/absence of the mutation, the clinical-pathological features, and the outcome of the PTC patients was investigated.

Results.—The $BRAF^{V600E}$ mutation was present in 106 of 319 PTC patients (33.2%). Its prevalence was also the same in subgroups identified according to the level of risk. The $BRAF^{V600E}$ mutation correlated with multifocality, aggressive variant, absence, or infiltration of the tumoral capsule. $BRAF^{V600E}$-mutated PTC also required a higher number of radioiodine courses to obtain diseasefree status. The $BRAF^{V600E}$ mutation was the only prognostic factor predicting the persistence of the disease in these patients after 5 yr of follow-up.

Conclusions.—The $BRAF^{V600E}$ mutation was demonstrated to be a poor prognostic factor for the persistence of the disease independent from other clinical-pathological features in low-risk intrathyroid PTC patients. It could be useful to search for the $BRAF^{V600E}$ mutation in the workup of low-risk PTC patients to distinguish those who require less or more aggressive treatments. In particular, the high negative predictive value of the $BRAF^{V600E}$ mutation could be useful to identify, among low-risk PTC patients, those who could avoid 131-I treatment.

▶ The objectives of this study are laudable—to ultimately reduce unnecessary treatment of patients with small, low-risk papillary thyroid cancers. The authors propose to do this by testing for *BRAF* mutations. Although this is easy (and now a routine part of the pathology report in many centers), whether *BRAF* can be considered a poor prognostic factor is highly questionable. There are 2 major flaws in this study: (1) Nowhere do the authors state what percentage of these cases was classical papillary thyroid cancer vs follicular variant papillary thyroid carcinoma (FVPTC). Given that they mention "tumoral capsular infiltration" in multiple tables as one of the criteria analyzed as a pathologic feature, it is highly likely that there were a substantial number of FVPTCs in this cohort of patients. Additionally, the overall rate of *BRAF* positivity is rather low—another indication of a high percentage of FVPTC as opposed to classical papillary thyroid carcinoma (PTC). (2) There is no mention of lymph node status specifically for these patients, and it is highly likely that very few (or none) of these patients underwent prophylactic central neck dissections. So, without these 2 bits of information, it is possible (and even likely) that the only thing that *BRAF* mutations are associated with is classical PTC and subsequently with a higher likelihood of lymph node metastases that were not removed, leading to increased risk of residual disease. It is my strong opinion that *BRAF* mutations will soon be recognized as highly associated with classical variant PTC and that its use as an independent prognosticator with other features of classical PTC (such as lymph node metastases) will actually be very limited.

T. J. Fahey, MD

$BRAF^{V600E}$ status adds incremental value to current risk classification systems in predicting papillary thyroid carcinoma recurrence
Prescott JD, Sadow PM, Hodin RA, et al (Massachusetts General Hosp, Boston)
Surgery 152:984-990, 2012

Background.—Papillary thyroid cancer (PTC) recurrence risk is difficult to predict. No current risk classification system incorporates *BRAF* mutational status. Here, we assess the incremental value of *BRAF* mutational status in predicting PTC recurrence relative to existing recurrence risk algorithms.

Methods.—Serial data were collected for a historical cohort having undergone total thyroidectomy for papillary thyroid carcinoma (PTC) during a 5-year period. Corresponding $BRAF^{V600E}$ testing was performed

TABLE 2.—Assessment of Associations Between Individual Clinicopathologic Tumor
Variables and Time to PTC Recurrence (Events = 55)

Variable	Hazard Ratio	Confidence Interval	*P* Value
Male	2.08	1.21–3.59	.01[†]
Age at surgery (per 10 yrs)	1.02	0.85–1.23	.83
AJCC TNM, tumor stage			
T1 (<2 cm (reference))			
T2 (2–4 cm)	1.06	0.50–2.24	.88
T3 (≥4 cm or minimal extrathyroidal	2.34	1.30–4.23	.005[†]
extension)			
T4 (gross ETE)	4.30	0.58–31.9	.15
Tumor histologic subtype			
Normal risk (reference)			
Low risk*	0.00	—	—
High risk	1.20	0.29–4.94	.80
Central neck LN positivity	1.87	1.10–3.19	.02[†]
Lateral neck LN positivity	2.69	1.48–4.86	.001[†]
Lymphovascular invasion	2.89	1.45–5.73	.002[†]
Tumor multifocality	2.11	1.21–3.67	.01[†]
BRAF[V600E+]	2.62	1.17–5.88	.02[†]

AJCC TNM, American Joint Commission on Cancer Tumor-Nodes- Metastasis; ETE, extrathyroidal extension; FVPTC, follicular variant of PTC; LN, lymph node; PTC, papillary thyroid cancer.
*No patients with low risk histological subtypes recurred leading to model non-convergence.
[†]Statistically significant.

and Cox proportional hazard regression modeling, with and without *BRAF* status, was used to evaluate existing recurrence risk algorithms.

Results.—The 5-year cumulative PTC recurrence incidence within our 356 patient cohort was 15%. A total of 205 (81%) of associated archived specimens were successfully genotyped, and 110 (54%) harbored the *BRAF*[V600E] mutation. The 5-year cumulative recurrence incidence among *BRAF*[V600E] patients was 20% versus 8% among *BRAF* wild type. *BRAF*[V600E] was significantly associated with time to recurrence when added to the following algorithms: AMES (hazard ratio [HR] 2.43 [confidence interval 1.08–5.49]), MACIS category (HR 2.46 [1.09–5.54]), AJCC-TNM (HR 2.51 [1.11–5.66]), and ATA recurrence-risk category (HR 2.44 [1.08–5.50]), and model discrimination improved (incremental c-index range 0.046–0.109).

Conclusion.—The addition of *BRAF* mutational status to established risk algorithms improves the discrimination of risk recurrence in patients undergoing total thyroidectomy for PTC (Table 2).

▶ This report also looks to add *BRAF* mutation status to algorithms for recurrence of papillary thyroid carcinoma (PTC). The data show that when added to traditional classification systems (low risk vs high risk), *BRAF* status does contribute to discerning risk of recurrence. However, the authors really do not tease out whether this contribution holds up if the low-risk tumors (defined in the study as FVPTC) are removed from the analysis. Table 2 from the original article contains the heart of the data. There are 2 things to note: (1) Having gross extra-thyroidal extension (ETE) was not statistically significant in their model—this is hard to believe, as so many studies previously have found that gross ETE is associated with a higher incidence of recurrence. (2) The comparisons are all univariate. So we really do not know whether *BRAF* is an independent risk factor for recurrence or a marker for pathologic features that we already accept are risk factors for recurrence. The point is, at this time, *BRAF* status should not be used to change our current treatment algorithms for patients with PTC. There is a real danger that patients who are otherwise low risk for recurrence or dying from PTC will be treated more aggressively (given radioactive iodine and at higher doses) simply because they are *BRAF*-positive. Given that up to 80% of classical PTCs may be *BRAF*-positive, this will lead to overtreatment of many patients.

T. J. Fahey, MD

BRAFV600E Mutation Does Not Mean Distant Metastasis in Thyroid Papillary Carcinomas
Sancisi V, Nicoli D, Ragazzi M, et al (Instituto di Ricovero e Cura a Carattere Scientifico, Reggio Emilia, Italy)
J Clin Endocrinol Metab 97:E1745-E1749, 2012

Context.—The oncogenic BRAFV600E mutation has been frequently associated with aggressive behavior of papillary thyroid carcinomas. However, controversy exists on the consistency of these data, and very little is known about the relationship between this genetic alteration and the tendency of papillary thyroid carcinoma (PTC) to develop metastasis at distant sites.

Study Design.—We analyzed by direct sequencing the frequency of BRAFV600E mutation within a group of 47 highly aggressive PTC, which had developed distant metastases. As control, we analyzed the BRAFV600E mutation in a group of 75 PTC without distant metastases who were disease free for a minimum 7-yr follow-up.

Results.—The BRAFV600E mutation was present in 29.8% of the distantly metastatic PTC, whereas it was detected in about 44.0% of the control tumors.

Conclusion.—These results clearly prove that the BRAFV600E mutation is not associated with the development of distant metastases or fatal outcome in PTC and may not predict aggressive behavior in this type of tumor.

▶ In the setting of continued publication of manuscripts associating v-raf murine sarcoma viral oncogene homolog B1 (BRAF) mutation with more aggressive tumor types, these authors have analyzed tumors from patients with differentiated thyroid carcinomas—more than half of these patients died of their disease—and found that BRAF mutation is not associated with distant metastatic disease or with dying of thyroid cancer. Although I agree completely with the study conclusions, as it is likely that BRAF mutations are associated with the classical variant of papillary thyroid carcinoma and nothing more, I am not sure that this manuscript has the data to fully support the conclusions so emphatically. One of the potential problems lies in the selection of cases, which were accrued over 32 years, dating back to 1979. Additionally, the tumors were analyzed for only BRAF mutations.

Because BRAF mutations appear in some studies to be increasing over this period and Ret-PTC rearrangements decreasing, it is possible that the groups of tumors were not really comparable. Nevertheless, it is one of the first manuscripts to counter the prevailing notion that BRAF mutation is synonymous with more aggressive tumors and poorer outcomes. Further prospective studies are needed to corroborate these findings.

T. J. Fahey, MD

Undetectable Sensitive Serum Thyroglobulin (<0.1 ng/ml) in 163 Patients with Follicular Cell-Derived Thyroid Cancer: Results of rhTSH Stimulation and Neck Ultrasonography and Long-Term Biochemical and Clinical Follow-Up

Chindris AM, Diehl NN, Crook JE, et al (Mayo Clinic, Jacksonville, FL; et al)
J Clin Endocrinol Metab 97:2714-2723, 2012

Context.—Surveillance of patients with differentiated thyroid cancer (DTC) is achieved using serum thyroglobulin (Tg), neck ultrasonography (US), and recombinant human TSH (rhTSH)-stimulated Tg (Tg-stim).

Objective.—Our primary aim was to assess the utility of rhTSH Tg-stim in patients with suppressed Tg (Tg-supp) below 0.1 ng/ml using a sensitive assay. Our secondary aims were to assess the utility of US and to summarize the profile of subsequent Tg-supp measures.

Design.—This is a retrospective study conducted at two sites of an academic institution.

Patients.—A total of 163 patients status after thyroidectomy and radioactive iodine treatment who had Tg-supp below 0.1 ng/ml and rhTSH Tg-stim within 60 d of each other were included.

Results.—After rhTSH stimulation, Tg remained below 0.1 ng/ml in 94 (58%) and increased to 0.1—0.5 in 56 (34%), more than 0.5—2.0 in nine (6%), and above 2.0 ng/ml in four (2%) patients. Serial Tg-supp levels were obtained in 138 patients followed over a median of 3.6 yr. Neck US were performed on 153 patients; suspicious exams had fine-needle aspiration (FNA). All positive FNA were identified around the time of the initial rhTSH test. Six of seven recurrences were detected by US (Tg-stim > 2.0 ng/ml in one, 0.8 in one and ≤0.5 in four). One stage IV patient had undetectable Tg-stim.

Conclusion.—In patients with DTC whose T₄-suppressed serum Tg is below 0.1 ng/ml, long-term monitoring with annual Tg-supp and periodic neck US are adequate to detect recurrences. In our experience, rhTSH testing does not change management and is not needed in this group of patients.

► This article provides long-term follow-up on a moderate-sized cohort of patients with differentiated thyroid cancer who had serial thyroglobulin (Tg) measurements. The conclusions are important with regard to the treatment of these patients long term. Basically, if the serum Tg is very low, then the need to perform a Thyrogen-stimulation test evaporates. Although there were a few failures using this threshold, the results were not substantially improved by doing a Thyrogen stimulation. The implications of the data are adequate and less expensive follow-up by just obtaining serial serum Tg levels. However, it should be noted that all patients in this series did receive radioactive iodine (RAI) ablation. So, the study will raise the question as to whether all patients should receive RAI to facilitate follow-up. Additionally, the authors note that the unstimulated serum Tg was done with thyroid-stimulating hormone suppression but this is not defined in the manuscript. Did the thyroid-stimulating hormone have to be undetectable also? Or were low normal levels adequate? These are important factors in determining how to treat patients who have low-risk papillary thyroid cancer (PTC), and not all patients with low-risk PTC should get RAI just to facilitate follow-up according to these guidelines.

T. J. Fahey, MD

Lymphocytic Thyroiditis on Histology Correlates with Serum Thyroglobulin Autoantibodies in Patients with Papillary Thyroid Carcinoma: Impact on Detection of Serum Thyroglobulin

Latrofa F, Ricci D, Montanelli L, et al (Univ of Pisa, Italy)
J Clin Endocrinol Metab 97:2380-2387, 2012

Context.—Serum thyroglobulin (Tg), the marker of residual tumor in papillary thyroid carcinoma, can be underestimated in patients with Tg autoantibodies (TgAb). TgAb are due to a coexistent lymphocytic thyroiditis (LT) or the papillary thyroid carcinoma *per se*. TgAb assays are highly discordant.

Design.—We evaluated 141 patients with a clinical diagnosis of nodular thyroid disease, 32 of Hashimoto's thyroiditis, and four of Graves' disease, who underwent total thyroidectomy for an associated papillary thyroid carcinoma. Patients were classified as papillary thyroid carcinomalymphocytic thyroiditis (PTC-T) and papillary thyroid carcinoma (PTC) according to the presence or absence of LT on histology. Tg was measured before thyroid remnant ablation, when it is expectedly detectable, by an immunometric assay (IMA) and TgAb by three noncompetitive IMA and three competitive radioimmunoassays (RIA). The number of lymphocytes was compared with TgAb concentration.

Results.—Seventy-two of 177 patients (40.7%) were classified as PTC-T and 105 (59.3%) as PTC. Although the tumor stage was similar in the two groups, Tg was undetectable in more PTC-T (37 of 72) than PTC (12 of 105) ($P < 0.01$), and Tg values were lower in the former (0; 0—4.7 ng/ml) (median; 25th to 75th percentiles) than in the latter group (9.7; 2.7—24.2) ($P < 0.01$). Accordingly, the percent of positive TgAb by the six assays resulted in higher PTC-T (29.2-50.0%) than PTC (1.9—6.7%) ($P < 0.01$). Among 49 patients with undetectable Tg, TgAb were more frequently positive by IMA (57.1—63.3%) than RIA (30.6—42.9%). The number of lymphocytes correlated with TgAb concentration in all six assays (0.34 < Rho < 0.46) (all $P < 0.01$).

Conclusions.—In papillary thyroid carcinoma, LT on histology must be carefully searched for because it is frequently associated with TgAb and therefore mistakenly low or undetectable Tg. TgAb can be missed by some assays. In absence of LT, TgAb are rare.

▶ As the use of thyroglobulin (Tg) to follow patients with differentiated thyroid cancer has increased, so too has the importance of the assays used to detect Tg and Tg antibodies. This article delineates nicely the importance of the pathologist in helping to guide our trust in a negative Tg test. The presence of lymphocytic thyroiditis is associated with the presence of antibodies, and if lymphocytic thyroiditis is identified on histopathology, a negative Tg assay should be viewed with some caution. The study brings out a couple of important findings. First, in Fig 2 of the original article, the authors report the percentage of patients with positive Tg antibodies by 6 different antibody assays in patients with papillary thyroid carcinomalymphocytic (PTC) + thyroiditis, PTC without thyroiditis, and in the presence of Hashimoto's thyroiditis. As reported by Spencer last year in the *Journal of Clinical Endocrinology and Metabolism*, the sensitivity of the antibody assays can vary widely,[1] and this graph confirms that assays for Tg antibody vary in sensitivity. The immunometric assays also appear to perform better than the radioimmunoassay (RIA). Another important point that is suggested by the data displayed in Fig 2 of the original article, but brought out in the article, is that basically all the antibody assays will miss some cases where there are antibodies present. The authors looked at patients with thyroid remnants visible on the posttreatment RIA scan and found 15 patients with negative Tg but clearly visible thyroid remnants. Of these, 12 of the 15 had antibodies that were present but below the level of detection reported by the assays. The take-home message is that lymphocytic thyroiditis should be carefully documented on histopathology because it may affect the interpretation of a negative Tg postoperatively. If there is thyroiditis and a negative Tg antibody report, the reported Tg value should be viewed skeptically, especially if reported as undetectable.

T. J. Fahey, MD

Reference

1. Spencer C, Petrovic I, Fatemi S. Current thyroglobulin autoantibody (TgAb) assays often fail to detect interfering TgAb that can result in the reporting of falsely low/undetectable serum Tg IMA values for patients with differentiated thyroid cancer. *J Clin Endocrinol Metab.* 2011;96:1283-1291.

Predictors of Level II and Vb Neck Disease in Metastatic Papillary Thyroid Cancer
Merdad M, Eskander A, Kroeker T, et al (Univ of Toronto, Ontario, Canada; Mount Sinai Hosp, Ontario, Canada)
Arch Otolaryngol Head Neck Surg 138:1030-1033, 2012

Objective.—To identify predictors of levels II and Vb involvement in papillary thyroid cancer (PTC) with lateral neck metastasis.

TABLE 2.—Univariate and Multivariate Analysis of Factors Predicting Level II and Vb Metastasis in Papillary Thyroid Cancer With Lateral Neck Disease

Variable	Level II Univariate	Level Vb Univariate	Level Vb Multivariate[a]
Age of patient	0.60	0.01[b]	0.03[b]
Diameter of tumor	0.84	0.20	0.25
Sex of patient	1.00	0.51	0.85
Surgery, primary vs secondary	0.18	0.90	0.11
Pathologic features	0.47	0.11	0.22
Multifocality	0.61	1.00	0.46
Extracapsular invasion	1.00	0.12	0.47
Positive margins	0.17	0.59	0.58
Lymphovascular invasion	1.00	0.06	0.03[b]

[a]All variables were included in the logistic regression model (multivariate analysis).
[b]Reached statistical significance.

Design.—Large case series.

Setting.—High-volume tertiary care hospital.

Patients.—Consecutive sample of 185 patients who underwent 248 selective neck dissections of at least levels II to V for pathologically proven PTC.

Main Outcome Measures.—Significant independent predictors of level II and Vb metastasis, including age and pathologic variables (tumor diameter, dominant nodule cellular pathology, multifocality, extracapsular invasion, positive margins, and lymphovascular invasion).

Results.—Levels II and Vb were involved in 49.3% and 29.2% of our cohort, respectively. Age and lymphovascular invasion were independent predictors of level Vb involvement with metastasis (logistic regression: odds ratio for age = 0.92, SE = 0.03, $P = .02$; and odds ratio for lymphovascular invasion = 5.52, SE = 0.80, $P = .03$). No significant predictors were identified for level II involvement.

Conclusions.—Levels II and Vb were involved in a significant number of patients with PTC and lateral neck disease. Younger age and lymphovascular involvement were independent risk factors for level Vb involvement in patients with PTC and lateral neck metastasis. The increased risk might be of marginal clinical significance. No significant predictors were identified for level II involvement. Our findings do not favor a limited neck dissection on the basis of any of the study's clinical or pathologic variables, and we therefore recommend the routine excision of levels IIa to Vb in all patients with PTC presenting with lateral neck disease (Table 2).

▶ The authors here looked at a large series of patients with papillary thyroid cancer and lateral neck node metastases and asked whether there were any features of either the patient or the tumor that could predict whether metastatic disease could be removed by a lesser dissection. The data presented suggest that lymph node metastases to levels II and Vb are actually quite common.

Table 2 shows that only younger age and the presence of lymphovascular invasion were predictive factors of Level Vb metastases, whereas none were predictive of level II metastases. The authors conclude that all patients presenting with lateral neck metastases should undergo comprehensive neck dissection. Although I agree with the conclusions, the article does raise a red flag. It is noted in the methods that only patients who underwent comprehensive neck dissections were included in the analysis. Unfortunately, the number of patients who underwent less-than-comprehensive dissections is not divulged—although it clearly states that these patients were excluded. So, one is left wondering, when did the authors do less than a comprehensive neck dissection—and how often? And how would these numbers affect the conclusion? This is an important point, because there is definitely the potential for increased morbidity associated with more comprehensive neck dissections. Finally, although the presence of metastatic disease suggests that these levels should be removed, ultimately recurrence rates associated with comprehensive vs lesser resections need to be compared to adequately address the question as to whether a lesser dissection is just as effective as a more comprehensive dissection with perhaps lower morbidity.

T. J. Fahey, MD

9 Nutrition

Parenteral Nutrition Does not Improve Postoperative Recovery from Radical Cystectomy: Results of a Prospective Randomised Trial
Roth B, Birkhäuser FD, Zehnder P, et al (Univ of Bern, Switzerland)
Eur Urol 63:475-482, 2013

Background.—After radical cystectomy, patients are in a catabolic state because of postoperative stress response, extensive wound healing, and ileus.

Objective.—To evaluate whether recovery can be improved with total parenteral nutrition (TPN) in patients following extended pelvic lymph node dissection (ePLND), cystectomy, and urinary diversion (UD).

Design, Setting, and Participants.—We conducted a prospective, randomised, single-centre study of 157 consecutive cystectomy patients.

Intervention.—Seventy-four patients (group A) received TPN during the first 5 postoperative days, with additional oral intake ad libitum. Eighty-three patients (group B) received oral nutrition alone.

Outcome Measurements and Statistical Analysis.—The primary outcome was the occurrence of postoperative complications. Secondary outcomes were time to recovery of bowel function, biochemical nutritional (serum albumin, serum prealbumin, serum total protein) and inflammatory (C-reactive protein) parameters, length of hospital stay, and costs attributed to the TPN. The Pearson χ^2 test was used for dichotomous variables; the Wilcoxon rank sum test was used for continuous variables.

Results and Limitations.—Postoperative complications occurred in 51 patients (69%) in group A and in 41 patients (49%) in group B ($p = 0.013$), a difference resulting from group A having more infectious complications than group B (32% vs 11%; $p = 0.001$). Serum prealbumin and serum total protein were significantly lower in group B on postoperative day 7 but not on postoperative day 12. Time to gastrointestinal recovery and length of hospital stay did not differ between the two groups. The costs for TPN were €614 per patient. A potential limitation is the use of a glucose-based parenteral nutrition without lipids.

Conclusions.—Postoperative TPN is associated with a higher incidence of complications, mainly infections, and higher costs following ePLND, cystectomy, and UD versus oral nutrition alone.

▶ Previous studies have shown that use of total parenteral nutrition (TPN) can be associated with increased infectious complications in surgical and medical patients. Thus, for decades, it has been recommended that enteral nutrition accompany parenteral nutrition whenever possible. It has also been recommended that use of short-term TPN be avoided in the well-nourished patient because there is little benefit and there may be harm. This prospective, randomized trial demonstrated the harm that can occur by noting a significant increase in infectious complications when patients who were undergoing cystectomy received 5 days of total parenteral nutrition vs controls who were fed normally. In general, cystectomy patients are quite well nourished and thus would not be expected to benefit from short-term TPN. In addition, elevated blood glucose levels associated with TPN can be a major factor in increasing infectious complications. This study joins others recommending that TPN not be used routinely in postoperative surgical patients.

J. M. Daly, MD

Parenteral lipid administration to very-low-birth-weight infants—early introduction of lipids and use of new lipid emulsions: A systematic review and meta-analysis
Vlaardingerbroek H, Veldhorst MAB, Spronk S, et al (Erasmus MC—Sophia Children's Hosp, Rotterdam, Netherlands; et al)
Am J Clin Nutr 96:255-268, 2012

Background.—The use of intravenous lipid emulsions in preterm infants has been limited by concerns regarding impaired lipid tolerance. As a result, the time of initiation of parenteral lipid infusion to very-low-birth-weight (VLBW) infants varies widely among different neonatal intensive care units. However, lipids provide energy for protein synthesis and supply essential fatty acids that are necessary for central nervous system development.

Objective.—The objective was to summarize the effects of initiation of lipids within the first 2 d of life and the effects of different lipid compositions on growth and morbidities in VLBW infants.

Design.—A systematic review and meta-analysis of publications identified in a search of PubMed, EMBASE, and Cochrane databases was undertaken. Randomized controlled studies were eligible if information on growth was available.

Results.—The search yielded 14 studies. No differences were observed in growth or morbidity with early lipid initiation. We found a weak favorable association of non—purely soybean-based emulsions with the incidence of sepsis (RR: 0.75; 95% CI: 0.56, 1.00).

Conclusions.—The initiation of lipids within the first 2 d of life in VLBW infants appears to be safe and well tolerated; however, beneficial effects on growth could not be shown for this treatment nor for the type of lipid emulsion. Emulsions that are not purely soybean oil—based might be associated with a lower incidence of sepsis. Large-scale randomized controlled trials in preterm infants are warranted to determine whether early initiation of lipids and lipid emulsions that are not purely soybean oil-based results in improved long-term outcomes.

▶ The use of parenteral nutrition is critical in the low-birth-weight, preterm infant. Yet, these same children are sensitive to the amount of calories and the individual constituents (amino acids, glucose, and lipids) within the total parenteral nutrition formulation. In the study, the authors performed a meta-analysis of published reports involving early nutritional support in preterm infants.

As noted, few differences were observed across different types of lipid emulsions except for a weak association with non—purely soybean-based emulsions. However, the issue needs further resolution with larger prospective, randomized trials. These children are so delicate that greater precision is needed to determine precisely the correct amounts and composition of nutrients to be infused that will maximize growth and minimize potential complications.

J. M. Daly, MD

Randomized Controlled Trial of Early Parenteral Nutrition Cycling to Prevent Cholestasis in Very Low Birth Weight Infants

Salvador A, Janeczko M, Porat R, et al (Albert Einstein Med Ctr, Philadelphia, PA)
J Pediatr 161:229-233.e1, 2012

Objectives.—To compare the incidence of cholestasis in very low birth weight infants receiving cycled versus continuous parenteral nutrition, and to determine factors that predispose to parenteral nutrition—associated cholestasis (PNAC).

Study Design.—Preterm infants weighing ≤ 1250 g (n = 70) at birth were randomly assigned within the first 5 postnatal days to either cycle (n = 34) or continuous (n = 36) parenteral nutrition. Liver function tests were obtained at baseline, and sequentially thereafter. Cholestasis was defined as direct bilirubin > 2 mg/dL. Infants with major congenital anomalies, congenital hepatic disease, clinically apparent congenital viral infection, and those who required major abdominal surgery were excluded.

Results.—The incidence of PNAC was similar in the 2 groups (cycle 32% vs continuous 31%; $P = 1.0$). Bilirubin and transaminases were similar in both groups by repeated measures of ANOVA. Gestational age, birth weight, and Apgar scores were significantly lower, and Clinical Risk Index for Babies II scores were significantly higher in infants who developed PNAC. Using backward selection logistic regression, bronchopulmonary dysplasia, duration of parenteral nutrition, and days to full enteral nutrition emerged as factors independently associated with PNAC.

Conclusions.—Early prophylactic parenteral nutrition cycling in very low birth weight infants in this study did not reduce cholestasis. Time to full feedings is a significant predictor for PNAC in very low birth weight infants. Preterm infants with bronchopulmonary dysplasia are more likely to have PNAC as a comorbidity. The Clinical Risk Index for Babies II score may help identify those preterm infants who might benefit from future prospective prevention trials.

▶ Cholestasis results in major morbidity in preterm, very low-birth-weight infants. There are many unanswered questions related to the timing of initiation of parenteral feeding, the amounts and composition of calories, and individual nutrients that may prevent the development of cholestasis in these children. This study is very well done. Patients were stratified and then randomized properly to evaluate the method of feeding (cycled versus continuous). The rationale for this study is that cycled feeding approximates the normal circumstances, whereby feeding occurs over a 12- to 16-hour period with a rest from eating for approximately 8 hours. It is known that normal feeding is not associated with such a high incidence of cholestasis. Thus, it has been thought that a period of rest from continuous feeding may be beneficial to the liver, reduce steatosis, and improve liver function.

Despite the theoretical benefits of cycled parenteral feeding, no major differences were noted between the 2 groups. Younger age, lower birth weight, and poorer Apgar scores were associated with parenteral nutrition—associated cholestasis. It is this group of infants in which further work must be done to reduce liver dysfunction. Although early return to full enteral feeding reduced the liver abnormalities, these children often have delayed return to full enteral feeding.

J. M. Daly, MD

Influence of Shielding TPN From Photooxidation on the Number of Early Blood Transfusions in ELBW Premature Neonates

Stritzke A, Turcot V, Rouleau T, et al (Children's and Women's Health Ctr of BC, Vancouver, Canada; Res Ctr Hosp Ste-Justine, Montreal, Quebec, Canada)
J Pediatr Gastroenterol Nutr 55:398-402, 2012

Objectives.—The smallest premature neonates often receive blood transfusions early in life. Nonrestrictive transfusion policies are linked to deleterious outcomes. Exposure of total parenteral nutrition (TPN) to ambient light generates oxidation products associated with haemolysis in vitro. Shielding TPN from light limits oxidation. Our hypothesis was protecting TPN from light decreases haemolysis and therefore the need for early blood transfusions.

Methods.—Comparison of haemolysis between animals fed enterally and those receiving TPN, and exploratory case-control retrospective analysis of transfusion counts in premature infants receiving light-exposed or light-protected TPN. The statistical analysis was analysis of variance and longitudinal binomial regression model adjusting for potential covariables of transfusion counts.

Results.—In animals, TPN is associated with higher ($P < 0.05$) haemolysis compared with enteral feeds; photoprotection induces lower peroxide load with no effect on the level of haemolysis. In premature infants, light-exposed (n = 76) or light-protected (n = 57) populations exhibited similar clinical characteristics. Initial haematocrit, gestational age, and index of disease severity had a significant effect on the number of transfusions. When adjusting for these covariables, photoprotection was no longer significant.

Conclusions.—Even though peroxides are associated in vitro with haemolysis, shielding TPN from light to reduce infused peroxides does not significantly decrease the need for early transfusions in premature infants.

▶ Premature infants with low birth weight are at the greatest risk for anemia requiring blood transfusions during their growth and development while receiving total parenteral nutrition (TPN). The causes are multifactorial. The authors had an interesting hypothesis that light exposure resulted in peroxides that damaged red cells resulting in hemolysis. Enteral feeding in animals protected against the hemolysis associated with parenteral feeding, but photo protection did not reduce hemolysis associated with TPN. In a case-control study in neonates, photo protection did not reduce hemolysis when patient covariables were included in the analysis. Thus, it does not appear important at this stage to reduce the formation of peroxides by providing for photoprotection during the infusion of TPN. As newer parenteral products such as vitamins, lipids, and amino acids become available, however, this issue should be re-evaluated.

J. M. Daly, MD

Significant Reduction in Central Venous Catheter–related Bloodstream Infections in Children on HPN After Starting Treatment With Taurolidine Line Lock

Chu H-P, Brind J, Tomar R, et al (Great Ormond Street Hosp, London, UK)
J Pediatr Gastroenterol Nutr 55:403-407, 2012

Objective.—The aim of this study was to review the incidence and type of central venous catheter—related bloodstream infection in children on treatment with home parenteral nutrition (PN) before and after the introduction of taurolidine. Taurolidine is a catheter lock solution that prevents biofilm formation and has broad-spectrum bactericidal and antifungal action. Its use in pediatric patients on PN has only been reported in case studies.

Methods.—A total of 19 children were reviewed, with the diagnoses of enteropathy (8 cases), short bowel syndrome (7 cases), and gastrointestinal dysmotility (4 cases). Incidence and type of sepsis were reviewed for 8 to 12 months pre- (when heparin was used) and 2 to 33 months postintroduction of the taurolidine catheter lock.

Results.—There were 8.6 episodes of catheter-related bloodstream infections per 1000 catheter days with heparin and 1.1 episodes per 1000 catheter days with taurolidine ($P = 0.002$). A total of 14 of the 19 patients (74%) had no infections for up to 33 months after changing to taurolidine. No reports of multiresistant organisms or adverse effects with taurolidine were found.

Conclusions.—Taurolidine line lock was associated with a decreased incidence of catheter-related bloodstream infections. This finding supports its use in patients with a history of septicemia on treatment with cyclical PN.

▶ Long-term parenteral nutrition is life saving in those patients with short bowel syndrome, enteropathy, and dysmotility. However, the longer the requirement for catheter-based parenteral nutrition, the greater the risk is of bloodstream infection. Major advances have been made in enforcing absolute and strict sterile technique during insertion of the catheter as well as during dressing changes. Additionally, studies have investigated the use of antifungal agents being flushed into the catheter. This retrospective study evaluated the occurrence of catheter-based infections before and after the introduction of taurolidine as a catheter lock solution. As noted, these infections were markedly reduced with taurolidine. It will be important to replicate these results in a randomized, prospective trial, as the issue is too critical to leave to chance.

J. M. Daly, MD

Longer-Term Outcomes of Nutritional Management of Crohn's Disease in Children
Lambert B, Lemberg DA, Leach ST, et al (Univ of New South Wales, Sydney, Australia)
Dig Dis Sci 57:2171-2177, 2012

Background.—While the short-term benefits of exclusive enteral nutrition (EEN) for induction of remission in children with Crohn's disease (CD) are well documented, the longer-term outcomes are less clear.

Aim.—This retrospective study aimed to ascertain the outcomes for up to 24 months following EEN in a group of children with CD.

Methods.—Children treated with EEN as initial therapy for newly diagnosed CD over a 5-year period were identified. Details of disease activity, growth, and drug requirements over the period of follow-up were noted. Outcomes in children managed with EEN were compared to a group of children initially treated with corticosteroids.

Results.—Over this time period, 31 children were treated with EEN and 26 with corticosteroids. Twenty-six (84 %) of the 31 children treated with EEN entered remission. Children treated with EEN exhibited lower pediatric Crohn's disease activity index (PCDAI) scores at 6 months ($p = 0.02$) and received lower cumulative doses of steroids over the study period ($p < 0.0001$) than the group treated with corticosteroids. Height increments over 24 months were greater in the EEN group ($p = 0.01$). Although the median times to relapse were the same, the EEN group had a lower incidence of relapse in each time interval and survival curve analysis showed lower risk of relapse ($p = 0.008$).

Conclusions.—EEN lead to multiple benefits beyond the initial period of inducing remission for these children, with positive outcomes over 2 years from diagnosis. Of particular clinical relevance to growing children was the reduced exposure to corticosteroids.

▶ Crohn's disease (CD) in childhood can be devastating with both short- and long-term poor outcomes. Associated with the disease are nutritional debilitation and growth retardation. Thus, parenteral and enteral nutrition are often used for nutritional support and for help with disease remission. This retrospective review evaluated those patients who received early initiation of enteral nutrition support compared with those who were first placed on corticosteroids. The results showed that early enteral nutrition resulted in similar short-term remission rates as steroids while significantly improving growth in these children. In addition, over a longer period, those treated with enteral nutrition had fewer relapses and overall had lower Crohn's disease activity index scores. Thus, this long-term retrospective study has results that are bolstered by short-term prospective trial results strongly suggesting that enteral nutritional support should be initiated early after CD is diagnosed in children. This is an important study to read along with the bibliography.

J. M. Daly, MD

Continuous Parenteral and Enteral Nutrition Induces Metabolic Dysfunction in Neonatal Pigs

Stoll B, Puiman PJ, Cui L, et al (USDA/ARS Children's Nutrition Res Ctr, Houston, TX; Erasmus MC—Sophia Children's Hosp, Rotterdam, The Netherlands; et al)
JPEN J Parenter Enteral Nutr 36:538-550, 2012

Background.—We previously showed that parenteral nutrition (PN) compared with formula feeding results in hepatic insulin resistance and steatosis in neonatal pigs. The current aim was to test whether the route of feeding (intravenous [IV] vs enteral) rather than other feeding modalities (diet, pattern) had contributed to the outcome.

Methods.—Neonatal pigs were fed enterally or parenterally for 14 days with 1 of 4 feeding modalities as follows: (1) enteral polymeric formula intermittently (FORM), (2) enteral elemental diet (ED) intermittently (IEN), (3) enteral ED continuously (CEN), and (4) parenteral ED continuously (PN). Subgroups of pigs underwent IV glucose tolerance tests (IVGTT) and hyperinsulinemic-euglycemic clamps (CLAMP). Following CLAMP, pigs were euthanized and tissues collected for further analysis.

Results.—Insulin secretion during IVGTT was significantly higher and glucose infusion rates during CLAMP were lower in CEN and PN than in FORM and IEN. Endogenous glucose production rate was suppressed to zero in all groups during CLAMP. In the fed state, plasma glucose-dependent insulinotropic polypeptide (GIP), glucagon-like peptide (GLP)−1, and GLP−2 were different between feeding modalities. Insulin receptor phosphorylation in liver and muscle was decreased in IEN, CEN, and PN compared with FORM. Liver weight was highest in PN.

Steatosis and myeloperoxidase (MPO) activity tended to be highest in PN and CEN. Enterally fed groups had higher plasma GLP-2 and jejunum weight compared with PN.

Conclusions.—PN and enteral nutrition (EN) when given continuously as an elemental diet reduces insulin sensitivity and the secretion of key gut incretins. The intermittent vs continuous pattern of EN produced the optimal effect on metabolic function.

▶ Liver dysfunction with elevated enzymes and bilirubin levels and steatosis occurs commonly in patients fed with parenteral nutrition. Many theories have been used to explain such metabolic dysfunction, including underlying illnesses, using the parenteral route that bypasses the intestinal tract leading to mucosal and muscular atrophy, lymphoid attrition and transmigration of intestinal bacteria, continuous feeding vs intermittent feeding that occurs with eating, deficient nutrients in the formula, and a variety of other hypotheses. The problem of hepatic steatosis is exacerbated in the neonate. This experimental study in neonatal pigs determined that the problem was limited to continuous parenteral and enteral feeding. It did not appear to be the diet, because intermittent total enteral (elemental diet) feeding had less metabolic dysfunction than administration of the same diet continuously.

Studies such as this are important, as they can describe the metabolic milieu and the endocrine responses to such feeding, providing clues to improve management.

J. M. Daly, MD

Parenteral ω-3 Fatty Acid Lipid Emulsions for Children With Intestinal Failure and Other Conditions: A Systematic Review
Seida JC, Mager DR, Hartling L, et al (Univ of Alberta, Edmonton, Canada)
JPEN J Parenter Enteral Nutr 37:44-55, 2013

Background.—There is growing interest in the use of ω-3 fatty acid (n-3FA) lipid emulsions to prevent complications associated with parenteral nutrition. The authors systematically reviewed the evidence on the benefits and safety of n-3FA compared with standard lipid emulsions in children with intestinal disease, critical illness, trauma, or postoperative complications.

Materials and Methods.—The authors searched 4 bibliographic databases from their inception to March 2011, conference proceedings, trial registries, and reference lists. Two reviewers independently selected studies, assessed methodological quality, and rated the strength of the evidence. One reviewer extracted and a second reviewer verified data. The authors summarized findings qualitatively and conducted meta-analysis when appropriate.

Results.—Five randomized controlled trials with unclear risk of bias and 3 high-quality prospective cohort studies were included. The studies examined premature, low birth weight infants (n = 6) and children with heart disease (n = 1) or intestinal failure (n = 1). The strength of evidence was consistently low or very low across all lipid emulsion comparisons and outcomes. In young children, n-3FA emulsions resulted in improvement in some biochemical outcomes of intestinal failure—associated liver disease but no difference in mortality. Few studies examined patient-important outcomes, such as length of hospital and intensive care stay; need for transplantation, growth, and cognitive development; or the long-term effects and potential harms associated with these therapies.

Conclusions.—Currently, there is a lack of sufficient high-quality data to support the use of parenteral n-3FA lipid emulsions in children. Future trials examining long-term clinical outcomes and harms are needed.

▶ In children requiring total parenteral nutrition, it is important to use formulations that are well-tolerated and do not lead to liver dysfunction. Thus, investigators have tried a multitude of interventions, such as cyclic feeding and use of different lipid formulations. This meta-analysis evaluated the use of ω-3 fatty acids as a potential means of eliminating many of the metabolic dysfunctions that often occur with standard lipid formulations. As the authors stated, most studies had small numbers of patients and the studies were powered inadequately to draw meaningful conclusions. In addition, most studies evaluated biochemical data without measuring patient-driven data that could be much more meaningful.

Studies such as this meta-analysis are important when they bring forward negative results, prompting the reader to more critically evaluate the literature. In addition, they point out areas that are important to study in the future.

J. M. Daly, MD

Teduglutide Reduces Need for Parenteral Support Among Patients With Short Bowel Syndrome With Intestinal Failure
Jeppesen PB, Pertkiewicz M, Messing B, et al (Rigshospitalet, Copenhagen, Denmark; Dept of General Surgery and Clinical Nutrition, Warszawa, Poland; Hopital Beaujon Service de Gastroenterologie et Assistance Nutritive, Clichy, France; et al)
Gastroenterology 143:1473-1481.e3, 2012

Background & Aims.—Teduglutide, a glucagon-like peptide 2 analogue, might restore intestinal structural and functional integrity by promoting growth of the mucosa and reducing gastric emptying and secretion. These factors could increase fluid and nutrient absorption in patients with short bowel syndrome with intestinal failure (SBS-IF). We performed a prospective study to determine whether teduglutide reduces parenteral support in patients with SBS-IF.

Methods.—We performed a 24-week study of patients with SBS-IF who were given subcutaneous teduglutide (0.05 mg/kg/d; n = 43) or placebo (n = 43) once daily. Parenteral support was reduced if 48-hour urine volumes exceeded baseline values by ≥10%. The primary efficacy end point was number of responders (patients with >20% reduction in parenteral support volume from baseline at weeks 20 and 24).

Results.—There were significantly more responders in the teduglutide group (27/43 [63%]) than the placebo group (13/43 [30%]; $P = .002$). At week 24, the mean reduction in parenteral support volume in the teduglutide group was 4.4 ± 3.8 L/wk (baseline 12.9 ± 7.8 L/wk) compared with 2.3 ± 2.7 L/wk (baseline 13.2 ± 7.4 L/wk) in the placebo group ($P < .001$). The percentage of patients with a 1-day or more reduction in the weekly need for parenteral support was greater in the teduglutide group (21/39 [54%]) than in the placebo group (9/39 [23%]; $P = .005$). Teduglutide increased plasma concentrations of citrulline, a biomarker of mucosal mass. The distribution of treatment-emergent adverse events that led to study discontinuation was similar between patients given teduglutide (n = 2) and placebo (n = 3).

Conclusions.—Twenty-four weeks of teduglutide treatment was generally well tolerated in patients with SBS-IF. Treatment with teduglutide reduced volumes and numbers of days of parenteral support for patients with SBS-IF; ClinicalTrials.gov Number, NCT00798967.

▶ The treatment of patients with short bowel syndrome with intestinal failure is extremely difficult. The ultimate goal is to restore intestinal integrity and function to the point at which minimal parenteral support (nutrition plus intravenous fluids) are required for homeostasis. Therapies have included use of glutamine and growth hormone, intestinal lengthening or reversal procedures, and even intestinal transplantation. A glucagon-like peptide 2 analogue (teduglutide) has been shown to increase intestinal mucosal mass as well as function. This prospective, randomized, multinational, blinded trial was carried out to answer the question as to whether teduglutide can improve intestinal function in those with short bowel syndrome with intestinal failure.

The study was well designed, having a lead-in period when urine outputs were stabilized. Once this was done, parenteral nutrition support and intravenous fluids were decreased, measuring urine outputs to help determine intestinal absorption capabilities. Teduglutide significantly improved intestinal function with adverse events similar to those in the control group.

This study offers a major step forward for these patients who have significant impairment in their intestinal absorptive capacities. It is a must-read.

J. M. Daly, MD

The Role of ω-3 Fatty Acid Supplemented Parenteral Nutrition in Critical Illness in Adults: A Systematic Review and Meta-Analysis
Palmer AJ, Ho CKM, Ajibola O, et al (Univ of Aberdeen, UK; Univ of Malaya Med Centre, Kuala Lumpur, Malaysia)
Crit Care Med 41:307-316, 2013

Objective.—To determine whether the supplementation of parenteral nutrition with ω-3 fatty acids confers treatment benefits to critically ill adult patients.

Data Source.—We performed computerized searches for relevant articles from 1996 to June 2011 on MEDLINE, EMBASE, and the Cochrane register of controlled trials and abstracts of scientific meetings from 2005 to 2011.

Study Selection.—Randomized controlled trials of ω-3 fatty acid supplemented parenteral nutrition in critically ill adult patients admitted to the intensive therapy unit, given in addition to their routine care, compared with parenteral nutrition without ω-3 fatty acid supplementation.

Data Synthesis.—Five fully published trials and three trials published in abstract form with 391 participants have been included. Overall trial quality was poor. Mortality data were pooled from eight studies with 391 participants. No differences were found with a risk ratio for death of 0.83 (95% confidence interval 0.57, 1.20; $p = 0.32$). Data for infectious complications were available from five studies with 337 participants. No differences were found, with a risk ratio for infection of 0.78 (95% confidence interval 0.43, 1.41; $p = 0.41$). Data for intensive therapy unit and hospital length of stay were available from six and three studies with 305 and 117 participants, respectively. With respect to intensive therapy unit length of stay, no differences were observed with a mean difference of 0.57 days in favor of the ω-3 fatty acid group (95% confidence interval $-5.05, 3.90; p = 0.80$). A significant reduction in hospital length of stay of 9.49 days (95% confidence interval-16.51, -2.47; $p = 0.008$) was observed for those receiving ω-3 fatty acid supplemented parenteral nutrition, but results were strongly influenced by one small study.

Conclusions.—On the basis of this systematic review, it can be concluded that ω-3 fatty acid supplementation of parenteral nutrition does not improve mortality, infectious complications, and intensive therapy unit length of stay in comparison with standard parenteral nutrition. Although ω-3 fatty acids appear to reduce hospital length of stay, the poor methodology of the included studies and the absence of other outcome improvements mean they cannot be presently recommended.

▶ Multiple studies have evaluated the efficacy of various nutrients being infused into critically ill patients in the intensive care unit (ICU). However, many of these studies involve small numbers of patients. This meta-analysis sought to understand the potential efficacy of ω-3 fatty acid supplementation as part of parenteral nutrition in critically ill patients. Nearly 400 patients were included in the analysis of adult patients from 5 published reports and 3 abstracts. Few clinical outcome differences were observed. Thus, currently, it can be concluded that the use of ω-3 fatty acid supplementation in critically ill patients in the ICU does not reduce mortality, infectious complications, or length of stay. This therapy should not be considered the standard of care for patients in intensive care.

J. M. Daly, MD

Who should we feed? A Western Trauma Association multi-institutional
study of enteral nutrition in the open abdomen after injury
Burlew CC, the WTA Study Group (Univ of Colorado, Denver; et al)
J Trauma Acute Care Surg 73:1380-1388, 2012

Background.—The open abdomen is a requisite component of a damage
control operation and treatment of abdominal compartment syndrome.
Enteral nutrition (EN) has proven beneficial for patients with critical injury,
but its application in those with an open abdomen has not been defined. The
purpose of this study was to analyze the use of EN for patients with an open
abdomen after trauma and the effect of EN on fascial closure rates and noso-
comial infections.

Methods.—We reviewed patients with an open abdomen after injury
from January 2002 to January 2009 from 11 trauma centers.

Results.—During the 7-year study period, 597 patients required an open
abdomen after trauma. Most were men (77%) sustaining blunt trauma
(72%), with a mean (SD) age of 38 (0.7) years, an Injury Severity Score of
31 (0.6), an abdominal injury score of 3.8 (0.1), and an Abdominal Trauma
Index score of 26.8 (0.6). Of the patients, 548 (92%) had an open abdomen
after a damage control operation, whereas the remainder experienced
an abdominal compartment syndrome. Of the 597 patients, 230 (39%)
received EN initiated before the closure of the abdomen at mean (SD) day
3.6 (1.2) after injury. EN was started with an open abdomen in one quarter
of the 290 patients with bowel injuries. For the 307 patients without a bowel
injury, logistic regression indicated that EN is associated with higher fascial
closure rates (odds ratio [OR], 5.3; $p < 0.01$), decreased complication rates
(OR, 0.46; $p = 0.02$), and decreased mortality (OR, 0.30; $p = 0.01$). For the
290 patients who experienced a bowel injury, regression analysis showed no
significant association between EN and fascial closure rate (OR, 0.6;
$p = 0.2$), complication rate (OR, 1.7; $p = 0.19$), or mortality (OR, 0.79;
$p = 0.69$).

Conclusion.—EN in the open abdomen after injury is feasible. For
patients without a bowel injury, EN in the open abdomen is associated
with increased fascial closure rates, decreased complication rates, and
decreased mortality. EN should be initiated in these patients once resuscitation is completed. Although EN for patients with bowel injuries did not
seem to affect the outcome in this study, prospective randomized controlled
trials would further clarify the role of EN in this subgroup.

▶ This study is a retrospective review of nearly 600 patients who required an open
abdomen for damage control after surgery or to obviate an abdominal compartment syndrome after major injury, most of which was due to blunt trauma. As
expected, most patients were male, with nearly one-third suffering from intestinal
injury. Previous studies have shown that initiation of early enteral nutrition leads
to improved outcomes in critically ill patients, but little information is available
regarding enteral feeding of the patient with an open abdomen. Nearly one-
quarter of the patients received supplemental total parenteral nutrition. Enteral

feeding was well-tolerated with few complications. Interestingly, patients without bowel injury seemed to have improved outcomes with early enteral nutrition with better fascial healing and decreased mortality. This may be due to a selection bias in that those patients who tolerated enteral feeding were in a better category. No differences were seen in those with intestinal injury, whether fed or not. However, despite these associations, the major message is that patients with an open abdomen can have early enteral feeding started with few potential complications. This multi-institutional study bears reading.

J. M. Daly, MD

Markers of Inflammation and Coagulation May Be Modulated by Enteral Feeding Strategy
Bastarache JA, Ware LB, Girard TD, et al (Vanderbilt Univ School of Medicine, Nashville, TN)
JPEN J Parenter Enteral Nutr 36:732-740, 2012

Background.—Although enteral nutrition (EN) is provided to most mechanically ventilated patients, the effect of specific feeding strategies on circulating markers of coagulation and inflammation is unknown.

Methods.—Markers of inflammation (tumor necrosis factor [TNF]-α, interleukin [IL]-1β, interferon [IFN]-γ, IL-6, IL-8, IL-10, IL-12) and coagulation (tissue factor [TF], plasminogen activator inhibitor-1) were measured at baseline (n = 185) and 6 days (n = 103) in mechanically ventilated intensive care unit patients enrolled in a randomized controlled study of trophic vs full-energy feeds to test the hypothesis that trophic enteral feeds would be associated with decreases in markers of inflammation and coagulation compared to full-energy feeds.

Results.—There were no differences in any of the biomarkers measured at day 6 between patients who were randomized to receive trophic feeds compared to full-energy feeds. However, TF levels decreased modestly in patients from baseline to day 6 in the trophic feeding group (343.3 vs 247.8 pg/mL, $P = .061$) but increased slightly in the full-calorie group (314.3 vs 331.8 pg/mL). Lower levels of TF at day 6 were associated with a lower mortality, and patients who died had increasing TF levels between days 0 and 6 (median increase of 39.7) compared to decreasing TF levels in patients who lived (median decrease of 95.0, $P = .033$).

Conclusions.—EN strategy in critically ill patients with acute respiratory failure does not significantly modify inflammation and coagulation by day 6, but trophic feeds may have some modest effects in attenuating inflammation and coagulation.

▶ It has been well-demonstrated that enteral nutrition is the preferred method of feeding for critically ill patients in intensive care units. The major question that needs a conclusion is what type of nutrition is best for intensive care unit (ICU) patients at varying stages of stress. One method of determining the degree of stress is the measurement of circulating cytokines and various coagulation factors. It has been suggested that immunonutrition provides benefit to ICU patients by reducing the incidence of infection. In this randomized, controlled study, patients were assigned to receive either trophic or standard enteral nutrition support. Few differences were observed. However, as shown previously, lower levels of circulating tumor necrosis factor were associated with improved patient outcomes. These results were a byproduct of the randomized trial evaluating the efficacy of trophic feeding in this population. It should be noted that circulating cytokines move in various directions and may not be the best markers to use in determining the efficacy of enteral feeding.

J. M. Daly, MD

Effect of Not Monitoring Residual Gastric Volume on Risk of Ventilator-Associated Pneumonia in Adults Receiving Mechanical Ventilation and Early Enteral Feeding: A Randomized Controlled Trial

Reignier J, for the Clinical Research in Intensive Care and Sepsis (CRICS) Group (District Hosp Ctr, La Roche-sur-Yon, France; et al)
JAMA 309:249-256, 2013

Importance.—Monitoring of residual gastric volume is recommended to prevent ventilator-associated pneumonia (VAP) in patients receiving early enteral nutrition. However, studies have challenged the reliability and effectiveness of this measure.

Objective.—To test the hypothesis that the risk of VAP is not increased when residual gastric volume is not monitored compared with routine residual gastric volume monitoring in patients receiving invasive mechanical ventilation and early enteral nutrition.

Design, Setting, and Patients.—Randomized, noninferiority, open-label, multicenter trial conducted from May 2010 through March 2011 in adults requiring invasive mechanical ventilation for more than 2 days and given enteral nutrition within 36 hours after intubation at 9 French intensive care units (ICUs); 452 patients were randomized and 449 included in the intention-to-treat analysis (3 withdrew initial consent).

Intervention.—Absence of residual gastric volume monitoring. Intolerance to enteral nutrition was based only on regurgitation and vomiting in the intervention group and based on residual gastric volume greater than 250 mL at any of the 6 hourly measurements and regurgitation or vomiting in the control group.

Main Outcome Measures.—Proportion of patients with at least 1 VAP episode within 90 days after randomization, as assessed by an adjudication committee blinded to patient group. The prestated noninferiority margin was 10%.

Results.—In the intention-to-treat population, VAP occurred in 38 of 227 patients (16.7%) in the intervention group and in 35 of 222 patients (15.8%) in the control group (difference, 0.9%; 90% CI, −4.8% to 6.7%). There were no significant between-group differences in other ICU-acquired infections, mechanical ventilation duration, ICU stay length, or mortality rates. The proportion of patients receiving 100% of their calorie goal was higher in the intervention group (odds ratio, 1.77; 90% CI, 1.25-2.51; $P = .008$). Similar results were obtained in the per-protocol population.

Conclusion and Relevance.—Among adults requiring mechanical ventilation and receiving early enteral nutrition, the absence of gastric volume monitoring was not inferior to routine residual gastric volume monitoring in terms of development of VAP.

Trial Registration.—clinicaltrials.gov Identifier: NCT0113748.

▶ It has been thought for some time that enteral nutrition given via nasointestinal tube can be made safer by monitoring gastric residual volumes because high gastric volumes have been associated with reflux aspiration and pneumonia. This article is an excellent example of scientifically evaluating a past premise to determine future management principles. This multicenter trial basically found that monitoring residual gastric volumes did not prevent ventilator-associated pneumonia compared with the nonmonitored control group. It did result in a greater amount of nutrients being infused, as more attention to detail occurred in the monitored group, allowing for increases in the rate of enteral nutrient infusion when residual gastric volumes were low. The results of this trial should not be interpreted as giving rise to a laissez-faire attitude toward monitoring patients. Standard techniques, such as keeping the head of the bed elevated, making sure that feedings are only incrementally increased, and measuring abdominal girth and intestinal function, should continue. Complications of aspiration are catastrophic. Nevertheless, this trial is recommended reading because of its design and conclusions.

J. M. Daly, MD

Characteristics and Current Practice of Parenteral Nutrition in Hospitalized Patients
Wischmeyer PE, Weitzel L, Mercaldi K, et al (Univ of Colorado School of Medicine, Denver; United BioSource Corporation, Lexington, MA; et al)
JPEN J Parenter Enteral Nutr 37:56-67, 2013

Background.—For 40 years, parenteral nutrition (PN) has provided therapeutic benefits to patients unable to receive oral/enteral nutrition. Very limited published evidence exists to describe modern PN practices or characteristics of patients receiving PN. The aim of this article was to describe the characteristics of hospitalized patients receiving PN in 196 U.S. hospitals to define patient groups at risk for PN-related complications. This will provide researchers a baseline understanding about who is receiving hospital-based PN to maximize generalizability and validity of future research.

Methods.—Claims data from the Premier Perspective database, the largest inpatient clinical database in the United States, were used to evaluate hospital-based PN practices. Data gathered between January 2005 and December 2007 included a total of 106,374 patients receiving PN. A total of 68,984 adults (age ≥18 years), 34,307 infants (age <1 year), and 3083 pediatric patients (age 1—17 years) were evaluated. Key variables such as admitting diagnosis, infection rates, in-hospital mortality, and costs were extracted.

Results.—Hospitalized patients requiring PN in the United States are older and more often white than the overall hospitalized population. Hospitalized PN patients are more likely to be admitted emergently and have a higher severity of illness. Bloodstream infection rates in adult PN patients (25.5%) were considerably higher than in pediatric (14.7%) or neonatal patients (1.7%) receiving PN.

Conclusions.—These findings are the first large-scale description of "real-world" hospital-based PN practices in the United States, helping set a baseline for future PN research.

▶ This article is quite interesting because it describes relatively recent (2005–2007) data across the Premier hospital database of more than 11 million inpatients, of which approximately 1% received parenteral nutrition for an average of 8 to 10 days. Most of the parenteral nutrition was delivered outside the intensive care unit. More than 68 000 adults were included in the database review. It is interesting that much of the data come from hospitals in the South, that the parenteral nutrition group was older on average, and a higher percentage of these patients were white compared with the nonparenteral nutrition group of patients. In addition, these patients were sicker with a common diagnosis of intestinal failure. In keeping with the acute illnesses and the sicker population, infectious complications were more common in these patients compared with the nonparenteral nutrition inpatients. The higher illness severity led to longer lengths of stay on average for these patients. The study provides a glimpse as to the use of parenteral nutrition in the United States within the past 7 years and can provide guidance as to its use in expected populations and perhaps gives insight as to how complications may be lessened.

J. M. Daly, MD

Human Leukocyte Death After a Preoperative Infusion of Medium/Long-Chain Triglyceride and Fish Oil Parenteral Emulsions: A Randomized Study in Gastrointestinal Cancer Patients

Cury-Boaventura MF, Torrinhas RSMdM, de Godoy ABP, et al (Cruzeiro do Sul University, São Paulo, Brazil; Univ of São Paulo (LIM 35), Brazil; Univ of São Paulo, Brazil)
JPEN J Parenter Enteral Nutr 36:677-684, 2012

Background.—Parenteral lipid emulsions (LEs) can influence leukocyte functions. The authors investigated the effect of 2 LEs on leukocyte death in surgical patients with gastrointestinal cancer.

Material and Methods.—Twenty-five patients from a randomized, double-blind clinical trial (ID: NCT01218841) were randomly included to evaluate leukocyte death after 3 days of preoperative infusion (0.2 g fat/kg/d) of an LE composed equally of medium/long-chain triglycerides and soybean oil (MCTs/LCTs) or pure fish oil (FO). Blood samples were collected before (t0) and after LE infusion (t1) and on the third postoperative day (t2).

Results.—After LE infusion (t1 vs t0), MCTs/LCTs did not influence cell death; FO slightly increased the proportion of necrotic lymphocytes (5%). At the postoperative period (t2 vs t0), MCTs/LCTs tripled the proportion of apoptotic lymphocytes; FO maintained the slightly increased proportion of necrotic lymphocytes (7%) and reduced the percentage of apoptotic lymphocytes by 74%. In the postoperative period, MCT/LCT emulsion increased the proportion of apoptotic neutrophils, and FO emulsion did not change any parameter of apoptosis in the neutrophil population. There were no differences in lymphocyte or neutrophil death when MCT/LCT and FO treatments were compared during either preoperative or postoperative periods. MCT/LCTs altered the expression of 12 of 108 genes related to cell death, with both pro- and antiapoptotic effects; FO modulated the expression of 7 genes, demonstrating an antiapoptotic effect.

Conclusion.—In patients with gastrointestinal cancer, preoperative MCT/LCT infusion was associated with postoperative lymphocyte and neutrophil apoptosis. FO has a protective effect on postoperative lymphocyte apoptosis.

▶ For more than 40 years, it has been known that lipid emulsions can alter the cellular response to inflammation. In some instances, lipid emulsions have been infused as a means of binding circulating endotoxin and thereby diminishing the deleterious response to sepsis. In this study, the authors evaluated blood samples from 25 patients that had been entered into a randomized, prospective trial studying pure fish oil vs medium- to long-chain triglycerides and soybean oil. The lipid emulsions altered the expression of less than 10% of genes related to lymphocyte/neutrophil cell death, but it did appear that the fish oil emulsion was protective. In addition to these effects, it will be important to determine if altered cell function occurs related to cellular responses to infection and, ultimately, patient outcomes.

J. M. Daly, MD

Effects of ω-3 Fish Oil Lipid Emulsion Combined With Parenteral Nutrition on Patients Undergoing Liver Transplantation
Zhu X, Wu Y, Qiu Y, et al (Med School of Nanjing Univ, China)
JPEN J Parenter Enteral Nutr 37:68-74, 2013

Background.—The effect of parenteral nutrition (PN) support supplemented with ω-3 fatty acids was investigated in a randomized, controlled clinical trial at the Affiliated Drum Tower Hospital, Medical School of Nanjing University.

Materials and Methods.—Ninety-eight patients with the diagnosis of end-stage liver disease or hepatic cellular carcinoma were admitted for orthotopic liver transplantation at the Affiliated Drum Tower Hospital. The patients were randomly divided into 3 groups: diet group (n = 32), PN group (n = 33), and polyunsaturated fatty acid (PUFA) group (n = 33). Patients in the PN and PUFA groups received isocaloric and isonitrogenous PN for 7 days after surgery. Venous heparin blood samples were obtained for assay on days 2 and 9 after surgery. A pathological test was performed after reperfusion of the donor liver and on day 9.

Results.—Alanine aminotransferase levels were improved significantly by PUFA treatment compared with traditional PN support ($P < .05$). Compared with the results on day 9 in the PN group, a significant difference was seen in the extent of increase of the prognostic nutrition index and prealbumin in the PUFA group. The pathological results also showed that ω-3 fatty acid supplementation reduced hepatic cell injury. PUFA therapy also decreased the incidence of infectious morbidities and shortened the posttransplant hospital stay significantly.

Conclusion.—Posttransplant PN support can greatly improve metabolism of protein and nutrition states of patients. ω-3 fatty acid—supplemented PN significantly reduces injury of the transplanted liver, decreases the incidence of infectious morbidities, and shortens posttransplant hospital stay.

▶ This is a remarkable prospective, randomized trial in which patients undergoing liver transplantation were randomly assigned to receive routine intravenous fluids plus diet when able, parenteral nutrition, or parenteral nutrition supplemented with ω-3 fatty acids (polyunsaturated fatty acid [PUFA]). Importantly, improvements in nutritional indices and prealbumin were only seen in the PUFA group. In addition, patient outcomes, such as infectious complications and hospital length of stay, were significantly less in the PUFA group compared with the other 2 groups. This interesting study utilized nutrition supplements (PUFA) in patients who become malnourished because of their liver dysfunction. In general, these patients return to normal nutrition status after transplantation, but it appears that use of PUFA accelerates this process. It also appears that the use of immunonutrition with PUFA did not adversely affect the transplantation immunologic outcomes. If this work is corroborated by others, it will make major changes in our approaches to patients undergoing liver transplantation.

J. M. Daly, MD

Parenteral nutrition suppresses the bactericidal response of the small intestine
Omata J, Pierre JF, Heneghan AF, et al (Univ of Wisconsin-Madison School of Medicine and Public Health; et al)
Surgery 153:17-24, 2013

Background.—Parenteral nutrition (PN) increases infectious risk in critically ill patients compared with enteral feeding. Previously, we demonstrated that PN feeding suppresses the concentration of the Paneth cell antimicrobial protein secretory phospholipase A2 (sPLA$_2$) in the gut lumen. sPLA$_2$ and other Paneth cell proteins are released in response to bacterial components, such as lipopolysaccharide (LPS), and they modulate the intestinal microbiome. Because the Paneth cell protein sPLA$_2$ was suppressed with PN feeding, we hypothesized PN would diminish the responsiveness of the small bowel to LPS through reduced secretions and as a result exhibit less bactericidal activity.

Methods.—The distal ileum was harvested from Institute of Cancer Research mice, washed, and randomized for incubation with LPS (0, 1, or 10 μg/mL). Culture supernatant was collected and sPLA$_2$ activity was measured. Bactericidal activity of the ileum segment secretions was assessed against *Pseudomonas aeruginosa* with and without an sPLA$_2$ inhibitor at 2 concentrations, 100 nmol/L and 1 μmol/L. Institute of Cancer Research mice were randomized to chow or PN for 5 days. Tissue was collected for immunohistochemistry (IHC) and ileal segments were incubated with LPS (0 or 10 μg/mL). sPLA$_2$ activity and bactericidal activity were measured in secretions from ileal segments.

Results.—Ileal segments responded to 10 μg/mL LPS with significantly greater sPLA$_2$ activity and bactericidal activity. The bactericidal activity of secretions from LPS stimulated tissue was suppressed 50% and 70%, respectively, with the addition of the sPLA$_2$-inhibitor. Chow displayed greater sPLA$_2$ in the Paneth cell granules and secreted higher levels of sPLA$_2$ than PN before and after LPS. Accordingly, media collected from chow was more bactericidal than PN. IHC confirmed a reduction in Paneth cell granules after PN.

Conclusion.—This work demonstrates that ileal segments secrete bactericidal secretions after LPS exposure and the inhibition of the Paneth cell antimicrobial protein sPLA$_2$ significantly diminishes this. PN feeding resulted in suppressed secretion of the sPLA$_2$ and resulted in increased bacterial survival. This demonstrates that PN significantly impairs the innate immune response by suppressing Paneth cell function.

▶ Multiple studies have found an association between infectious complications and the use of parenteral nutrition in intensive care unit patients. Numerous etiologies have been described, including intestinal bacterial translocation caused by atrophy and overgrowth of Gram-negative bacteria as well as altered host intestinal immune responses. To determine the etiology of such intestinal changes to nutrition, animal studies provide the opportunity for control of feeding method and tissue examination.

In this study, the authors sought to evaluate the response of the small intestine to lipopolysaccharide (LPS), as they hypothesized that parenteral nutrition-induced intestinal atrophy and reduced Paneth cell antimicrobial protein secretory phospholipase would also reduce the intestinal response to LPS in vitro and in vivo.

Results of this study showed reduced responses to LPS in vitro when sPLA-2 was suppressed. In vivo, parenteral nutrition also suppressed sPLA-2 activity, and bactericidal activity from cultured media was significantly less. Combined, these studies showed proof of principle.

Unfortunately, animal studies of intestinal bacterial translocation and bactericidal activity do not seem to translate to the human situation in the critically ill patient. Thus, further work is required in patients to determine if these parenteral nutrition results are similar to those in animal studies.

J. M. Daly, MD

Influence of Parenteral Nutrition Delivery System on the Development of Bloodstream Infections in Critically Ill Patients: An International, Multicenter, Prospective, Open-Label, Controlled Study—EPICOS Study
Pontes-Arruda A, for the EPICOS Study Group (Fernandes Távora Hosp, Fortaleza, Brazil; et al)
JPEN J Parenter Enteral Nutr 36:574-586, 2012

Background.—Parenteral nutrition (PN) is associated with an increased risk of developing bloodstream infections (BSIs) but the impact of the PN delivery system upon BSI rates remains unclear. This was an international, multicenter, prospective, randomized, open-label, controlled trial that investigated the differences of BSIs associated with 2 different PN systems.

Methods.—Patients were randomly allocated in a 2:1:1 ratio to receive either PN delivered by a multichamber bag (MCB group), or by compounded PN made with olive oil (COM1 group) or with MCT/LCT (COM2 group). Blood cultures were performed to evaluate the incidence of BSIs, and catheter use data was collected to calculate CLAB and central venous catheter device use ratio (CVC-DUR). Secondary outcomes included the development of severe sepsis/septic shock, number of intensive care unit (ICU) and hospital days, and all-cause mortality at Day 28.

Results.—406 patients were included: 202 in the MCB group, 103 in the COM1 group, and 101 in the COM2 group. Baseline characteristics were well balanced between the 3 groups, BSIs were significantly higher in patients receiving compounded PN (46 BSIs for COM1+COM2 vs 34 BSIs for MCB; $p = 0.03$). CLAB was higher in patients receiving compounded PN (13.2 for COM1+COM2 vs 10.3 for MCB; $p < 0.0001$). No differences were observed for the secondary outcomes.

Conclusion.—Compounded PN was associated with a higher incidence of BSIs and CLABs, suggesting that the use of MCB PN may play a role in reducing the incidence of BSIs in patients who receive PN. Trial registration number: NCT00798681.

▶ The use of parenteral nutrition has long been associated with an increased risk of catheter-related infections. There are many assumed reasons, such as high glucose levels, parenteral lipid use, long-term in-dwelling catheters, use of blood and other products in the same intravenous line, and poor sterile technique when either inserting or changing the central venous site. Less commonly cited is the pharmaceutical method of creating the solution. More recently, multichambered bags have been developed that obviate the use of compounding the solution in the hospital pharmacy. This prospective, randomized study suggests that compounding significantly increased the incidence of bloodstream infections compared with the use of a multichambered bag. If replicated, this study is important for the use of long-term parenteral nutrition. It also emphasizes the critical nature of central venous catheterization in the hospitalized patient in the prevention of bloodborne infections. It also speaks to the benefits or lack thereof of using various lipid emulsions in these critically ill patients.

J. M. Daly, MD

Intestinal Adaptation Is Stimulated by Partial Enteral Nutrition Supplemented With the Prebiotic Short-Chain Fructooligosaccharide in a Neonatal Intestinal Failure Piglet Model
Barnes JL, Hartmann B, Holst JJ, et al (Univ of Illinois, Urbana-Champaign; Univ of Copenhagen, Denmark)
JPEN J Parenter Enteral Nutr 36:524-537, 2012

Background.—Butyrate has been shown to stimulate intestinal adaptation when added to parenteral nutrition (PN) following small bowel resection but is not available in current PN formulations. The authors hypothesized that pre- and probiotic administration may be a clinically feasible method to administer butyrate and stimulate intestinal adaptation.

Methods and Materials.—Neonatal piglets (48 hours old, n = 87) underwent placement of a jugular catheter and an 80% jejunoileal resection and were randomized to one of the following treatment groups: control (20% standard enteral nutrition/80% standard PN), control plus prebiotic (10 g/L short-chain fructooligosaccharides [scFOS]), control plus probiotic (1×10^9 CFU *Lactobacillus rhamnosus* GG [LGG]), or control plus synbiotic (scFOS + LGG). Animals received infusions for 24 hours, 3 days, or 7 days, and markers of intestinal adaptation were assessed.

Results.—Prebiotic treatment increased ileal mucosa weight compared with all other treatments ($P = .017$) and ileal protein compared with control ($P = .049$), regardless of day. Ileal villus length increased in the prebiotic and synbiotic group ($P = .011$), regardless of day, specifically due to an increase in epithelial proliferation ($P = .003$). In the 7-day prebiotic group, peptide transport was upregulated in the jejunum ($P = .026$), whereas glutamine transport was increased in both the jejunum and colon ($P = .001$ and .003, respectively).

Conclusions.—Prebiotic and/or synbiotic supplementation resulted in enhanced structure and function throughout the residual intestine. Identification of a synergistic prebiotic and probiotic combination may enhance the promising results obtained with prebiotic treatment alone.

▶ After major small bowel resection, intestinal adaptation is critical to the short- and long-term outcome of the patient. Enteral feeding remains the mainstay of adaptation along with pharmacological management with a variety of agents, parenteral support, and perhaps use of reverse intestinal segments. Nevertheless, it is important to maximize intestinal adaptation and absorption using whatever means possible. Butyrate stimulates colonic adaptation, which helps tremendously for salt and water absorption.

In this animal study, prebiotic (10 g/L short-chain fructooligosaccharides) supplementation had the most marked effect on intestinal villus length and protein content as well as transport of peptides and glutamine. Longer term studies would be important to determine if such supplements result in full intestinal adaptation and long-term growth and development. As the authors pointed out, the results of this study provide the foundation for a variety of products (prebiotic and probiotic) to be studied to determine the right mix of products and the correct duration of infusion to produce the maximum positive results.

J. M. Daly, MD

Ethanol Lock Therapy in Reducing Catheter-Related Bloodstream Infections in Adult Home Parenteral Nutrition Patients: Results of a Retrospective Study

John BK, Khan MA, Speerhas R, et al (Cleveland Clinic, OH)
JPEN J Parenter Enteral Nutr 36:603-610, 2012

Background.—Equivocal data demonstrate the efficacy of ethanol lock therapy (ELT) in preventing catheter-related bloodstream infections (CRBSIs) in home parenteral nutrition (HPN) patients, but it is not currently a standard of practice. The objective of this study is to investigate the efficacy of ELT in reducing the incidence of CRBSIs in HPN patients.

Methods.—Medical records from the Cleveland Clinic database of adult HPN patients with CRBSIs placed on prophylactic ELT were retrospectively studied from January 2006 to August 2009 (n = 31). Outcomes were compared pre- and post-ELT with the patients serving as their own controls. Medical-grade (70%) ethanol was instilled daily into each lumen of the central venous catheter (CVC) between PN infusion cycles. Comparative analysis was performed using McNemar's test and Wilcoxon ranked tests.

Results.—Thirty-one patients had 273 CRBSI-related admissions prior to ELT in comparison to 47 CRBSI-related admissions post-ELT. Adjusted data for only tunneled CVC pre- and post-ELT showed a similar reduction of CRBSI-related admissions from 10.1 to 2.9 per 1000 catheter days

(*P* < .001). There was also a statistically significant reduction in culture-positive CRBSIs and number of catheters changed pre- and post-ELT. There were no reported side effects or complications in any patient undergoing ELT.

Conclusions.—This study supports the efficacy and safety of ELT in reducing CRBSI-related admissions in HPN patients and potentially helps reduce the burden of CRBSI-related healthcare costs. This novel technique shows great promise as a standard prophylaxis for CRBSI in HPN patients and must be incorporated in routine practice.

▶ Catheter-based infections are a major cause of morbidity in the hospitalized patient. Numerous studies have shown that rigorous attention to detail during catheter insertion can markedly lessen the risk of catheter-based infections. Currently, most hospitals adhere to protocols for insertion that dictate specific steps to be taken during insertion to reduce contamination. However, catheters placed for long-term nutrition support have a risk associated with dressing changes, and the longer that catheter is in place, the greater the risk.

In the current retrospective study, the catheters were flushed with 70%, medical-grade alcohol daily; this treatment was associated with reduced infections and culture-positive catheters. Clearly, this study would need to be replicated in a prospective, randomized fashion. However, if this method is proven to lessen infections, it would be a major breakthrough in our care of patients on long-term parenteral nutrition.

J. M. Daly, MD

The Impact of Refeeding on Blood Fatty Acids and Amino Acid Profiles in Elderly Patients: A Metabolomic Analysis
Dror Y, Almashanu S, Lubart E, et al (The Hebrew Univ of Jerusalem, Rehovot, Tel-Hashomer, Israel; Israeli Ministry of Health, Tel-Hashomer, Israel; Geriatric Med Ctr, Shmuel Harofeh, Beer Yaakov, Israel; et al)
JPEN J Parenter Enteral Nutr 37:109-116, 2013

Background.—Refeeding of elderly frail patients after food deprivation is commonly associated with a high mortality rate.

Objective.—To evaluate the effect of refeeding on metabolite fluctuation of blood carnitine fatty acids (15 compounds) and free amino acids (14 compounds).

Methods.—Metabolite fluctuation was followed up in an exploratory, cohort, and noninterventional study in elderly and frail patients (84.5 ± 5 years) after a long period of food deprivation. Patients in the study group were refed by enteral nutrition (EN) and were followed up during 7 days for blood metabolites (n = 27). Patients in the control group (n = 26) had been fed by EN for more than 3 months. Refeeding was initiated with 10 kcal/kg/d and gradual increases of 200 kcal/d for 3 days afterwards. Blood metabolites were assayed in a sample of 25 μL.

Results.—On food deprivation, the concentrations of all even monocarboxylic carnitine fatty acids were much higher in the study group than in the EN control group (*P* < .01). Upon refeeding, a remarkable decrease in all carnitine fatty acids was observed. In addition, significant daily fluctuations were observed for most metabolites in the study group of the refed patients as compared with the EN control group (*P* < .01). The highest fluctuations were observed following refeeding in the 7 patients who later died.

Conclusion.—A significant metabolic instability is observed on refeeding even with a slow refeeding schedule of 10 kcal/kg/d. Measurement of metabolomics parameters may be used for the evaluation of malnutrition, refeeding status, and optimization of the enteral formula.

▶ Refeeding of malnourished patients is fraught with danger, and homeostasis within the body is upset during this process. Elderly, frail patients are most at risk during refeeding. This study sought to evaluate the effects of refeeding on blood carnitine fatty acids and free amino acid levels. Refeeding was accomplished in a very slow fashion starting at 10 kcal/kg/day with gradual increases of 200 kcal/day for 3 days afterward. Interestingly, a decrease in all carnitine fatty acids occurred during refeeding compared with the control group. Significant fluctuations for many metabolites, especially in the patients who then died, suggest complex metabolic mechanisms in play in these patients. It will be important to further understand this metabolic instability in order to alter feeding nutrients and caloric infusions to reduce these marked fluctuations.

J. M. Daly, MD

Effects of a diabetes-specific enteral nutrition on nutritional and immune status of diabetic, obese, and endotoxemic rats: Interest of a graded arginine supply
Breuillard C, Darquy S, Curis E, et al (Université Paris Descartes, France; et al)
Crit Care Med 40:2423-2430, 2012

Objective.—Obese and type 2 diabetic patients present metabolic disturbance–related alterations in nonspecific immunity, to which the decrease in their plasma arginine contributes. Although diabetes-specific formulas have been developed, they have never been tested in the context of an acute infectious situation as can be seen in intensive care unit patients. Our aim was to investigate the effects of a diabetes-specific diet enriched or not with arginine in a model of infectious stress in a diabetes and obesity situation. As a large intake of arginine may be deleterious, this amino acid was given in graded fashion.

Design.—Randomized, controlled experimental study.

Setting.—University research laboratory.

Subjects.—Zucker diabetic fatty rats.

Interventions.—Gastrostomized Zucker diabetic fatty rats were submitted to intraperitoneal lipopolysaccharide administration and fed for 7 days with either a diabetes-specific enteral nutrition without (G group, n = 7) or with graded arginine supply (1–5 g/kg/day) (GA group, n = 7) or a standard enteral nutrition (HP group, n = 10).

Measurements and Main Results.—Survival rate was better in G and GA groups than in the HP group. On day 7, plasma insulin to glucose ratio tended to be lower in the same G and GA groups. Macrophage tumor necrosis factor-α (G: 5.0 ± 1.1 ng/2 × 10^6 cells·hr^{-1}; GA: 3.7 ± 0.8 ng/2 × 10^6 cells·hr^{-1}; and HP: 1.7 ± 0.6 ng/2 × 10^6 cells·hr^{-1}; $p < .05$ G vs. HP) and nitric oxide (G: 4.5 ± 1.1 ng/2 × 10^6 cells·hr^{-1}; GA: 5.1 ± 1.0 ng/2 × 10^6 cells·hr^{-1}; and HP: 1.0 ± 0.5 nmol/2 × 10^6 cells·hr^{-1}; $p < .05$ G and GA vs. HP) productions were higher in the G and GA groups compared to the HP group. Macrophages from the G and GA groups exhibited increased arginine consumption.

Conclusions.—In diabetic obese and endotoxemic rats, a diabetes-specific formula leads to a lower mortality, a decreased insulin resistance, and an improvement in peritoneal macrophage function. Arginine supplementation has no additional effect. These data support the use of such disease-specific diets in critically ill diabetic and obese patients.

▶ Tight glycemic control has been shown to improve the response to major operation, wounding, stress, and infection. This is usually obtained in the surgical patient using exogenous insulin. Patients requiring feeding in the hospital are often given standard enteral diets high in sugars requiring large and often varied doses of insulin to manage their blood sugar levels. Arginine, a nonessential amino acid, has been found to stimulate insulin production and to directly enhance the immune response and wound healing. It has also been found that lower plasma levels occur in diabetic subjects during septic episodes. Thus, this study evaluated the use of a diabetic-specific enteral formula in animals given lipopolysaccharide (LPS) and then started on enteral feeding. One cannot argue with the mortality results, but it is unclear as to the mechanisms whereby 6 of 10 normal formula (HP group) animals died within 24 hours after LPS just as the enteral diet was starting. It is understandable as to the cellular differences across groups at 7 days after LPS endotoxin was administered and enteral feeding was given. Thus, tight glycemic control using a disease-specific formula appeared to be beneficial after endotoxin administration; supplemental arginine offered no increased benefit.

J. M. Daly, MD

10 Gastrointestinal

Long-Term Outcomes of an Endoscopic Myotomy for Achalasia: The POEM Procedure

Swanstrom LL, Kurian A, Dunst CM, et al (The Oregon Clinic, Portland)
Ann Surg 256:659-667, 2012

Background.—Esophageal achalasia is most commonly treated with laparoscopic myotomy or endoscopic dilation. Per-oral endoscopic myotomy (POEM), an incisionless selective myotomy, has been described as a less invasive surgical treatment. This study presents 6-month physiological and symptomatic outcomes after POEM for achalasia.

Methods.—Data on single-institution POEMs were collected prospectively. Pre- and postoperative symptoms were quantified with Eckardt scores. Objective testing (manometry, endoscopy, timed-barium swallow) was performed preoperatively and 6 months postoperatively. At 6 months, gastroesophageal reflux was evaluated by 24-hour pH testing. Pre-/postmyotomy data were compared using paired nonparametric statistics.

Results.—Eighteen achalasia patients underwent POEMs between October 2010 and October 2011. The mean age was 59 ± 20 years and mean body mass index was 26 ± 5 kg/m^2. Six patients had prior dilations or Botox injections. Myotomy length was 9 cm (7–12 cm), and the median operating time was 135 minutes (90–260). There were 3 intraoperative complications: 2 gastric mucosotomies and 1 full-thickness esophagotomy, all repaired endoscopically with no sequelae. The median hospital stay was 1 day and median return to normal activity was 3 days (3–9 days). All patients had relief of dysphagia [dysphagia score ≤ 1 ("rare")]. Only 2 patients had Eckardt scores greater than 1, due to persistent noncardiac chest pain. At a mean follow-up of 11.4 months, dysphagia relief persisted for all patients. Postoperative manometry and timed barium swallows showed significant improvements in lower esophageal relaxation characteristics and esophageal emptying, respectively. Objective evidence of gastroesophageal reflux was seen in 46% patients postoperatively.

Conclusions.—POEM is safe and effective. All patients had dysphagia relief, 83% having relief of noncardiac chest pain. There is significant though mild gastroesophageal reflux postoperatively in 46% of patients in 6-month pH studies. The lower esophageal sphincter shows normalized pressures and relaxation.

► Just when we think we have developed a superb operation, another procedure or treatment is introduced and gives us pause about the effectiveness of the current procedure and begs the question of whether the newly introduced treatment is as effective as hailed. Such is the case with the surgical approach to achalasia! Laparoscopic Heller myotomy has been a major advance in the treatment of achalasia, and over a period of 20 years it has become the primary treatment. In many centers, gastroenterologists primarily refer patients to surgeons for a laparoscopic myotomy without performing an endoscopic procedure initially. In this report, Swanstrom et al report the results of 18 patients who underwent peroral, endoscopic myotomy (POEM procedure). The early results at 6 months are certainly not long term, but they are mostly impressive. The relief of symptoms, no pain, and early (3 days) return to full activity make this an attractive procedure. However, almost half of the patients had gastroesophageal reflux following the procedure. Although reflux can be adequately treated with medication, the long-term consequences of reflux following this procedure are not fully understood. Because reflux is present in such a substantial portion of the patients, this procedure should be carefully monitored before widespread adoption. I highly recommend reading the complete manuscript, including the discussants' comments at the end of the article, for a historical perspective of the treatment of achalasia but also review of insightful questions by the discussants. Although the authors correctly advise practitioners to perform this procedure only under an institutional review protocol, my question is why were these patients not enrolled in a randomized, controlled trial since laparoscopic Heller myotomy has proven effective?

K. E. Behrns, MD

Adenocarcinomas of the Esophagogastric Junction Are More Likely to Respond to Preoperative Chemotherapy than Distal Gastric Cancer
Reim D, Gertler R, Novotny A, et al (Technische Universität München, Munich, Germany; et al)
Ann Surg Oncol 19:2108-2118, 2012

Background.—Preoperative chemotherapy has been shown to improve outcome of patients with adenocarcinoma of the esophagogastric junction (AEG) and gastric cancer (GC), and histopathologic response has been identified as an independent prognostic parameter in these patients. A recent meta-analysis has identified patients with AEG as benefiting more from preoperative chemotherapy than patients with GC. The aim of this retrospective analysis was to prove these findings in an experienced single-center large patient cohort because there are currently no recruiting prospective clinical trials.

Methods.—In a single center, 551 patients underwent preoperative platin-based chemotherapy followed by oncologic surgery for locally advanced AEG and GC. Pretherapeutic clinical parameters were correlated with histopathologic response to preoperative chemotherapy.

Results.—Histopathologic response (< 10% of residual tumor) was found in 130 patients (24%) and was significantly correlated with overall survival ($P < 0.0001$). Tumor localization at the esophagogastric junction

(GE junction), lower baseline cT stage, and baseline cN0 stage were significantly associated with histopathologic response ($P = 0.034$, $P = 0.015$, and $P = 0.002$, respectively). In subgroup analyses, the latter two predictive parameters were confirmed only for AEG ($n = 378$) but not for other GC ($n = 173$). AEG patients who were pretherapeutically staged as having cT3/4, cN0 disease ($n = 73$) were identified as the subgroup with the highest rate of histopathologic response (48%).

Conclusions.—AEG is more likely to respond to preoperative chemotherapy than GC, a finding that might help identify patients who would benefit from preoperative chemotherapy.

▶ The past 2 decades have seen a marked increase in the incidence of adenocarcinomas of the esophagogastric junction (EGJ), and this finding has led to substantial new knowledge not only about EGJ cancers but also gastric cancers. Previously, EGJ cancers were often approached as a subset of adenocarcinomas of the stomach, but new findings related to oncogenesis, epidemiology, pathology, and treatment response clearly show that not all gastric cancers are alike. This article shows, in a large retrospective study, that the response rate to neoadjuvant therapy is clearly different between EGJ cancer and cancer of the stomach. As the authors astutely point out, the major finding of the study is not that EGJ cancer can be downstaged more readily than gastric cancer, but that neoadjuvant therapy may be a predictor of tumor biology. This finding may be of paramount importance because it could dramatically alter the management of responding versus nonresponding tumors. For example, perhaps treatment strategies that aim to rapidly identify nonresponding cancers should be used so that precious treatment time is not devoted to a nonresponding tumor. These findings may markedly alter the treatment approaches to multiple cancers. It may be that short-course neoadjuvant therapy with the rapid assessment of response with novel biomarkers may be the initial approach to cancer therapy. This study nicely shows the possibilities of using the response rate to chemotherapy as a marker of tumor biology and the need for novel treatment strategies and sequencing in multiple cancers.

K. E. Behrns, MD

Disseminated Tumor Cells in Bone Marrow and the Natural Course of Resected Esophageal Cancer
Vashist YK, Effenberger KE, Vettorazzi E, et al (Univ Med Ctr Hamburg-Eppendorf, Germany)
Ann Surg 255:1105-1112, 2012

Objective.—To assess the impact of disseminated tumor cells (DTC) in bone marrow on recurrence and survival in complete resected esophageal cancer (EC).

Background.—Current modalities to predict tumor recurrence and survival in EC are insufficient. Here, we evaluated in a prospective study the prognostic relevance of DTC in bone marrow for the natural postoperative course of EC.

Methods.—We enrolled 370 consecutive EC patients (1995–2009). All tumors, 189 squamous cell carcinomas and 181 adenocarcinomas, were completely surgically resected (R0), and patients received neither neoadjuvant nor adjuvant therapy. Disseminated tumor cells were detected by an immunocytochemical cytokeratin assay in preoperatively taken bone marrow aspirates. The results were correlated with clinic-pathological parameters and clinical outcome.

Results.—Overall 120 (32.4%) patients harbored DTC in their bone marrow. Presence of DTC significantly correlated with aggressive tumor biology as indicated by increased tumor size ($P = 0.026$), regional ($P = 0.002$) and distant ($P = 0.012$) lymph node metastases, and higher relapse rate ($P < 0.001$, χ^2 test). A gradual decrease in disease-free ($P < 0.001$) and overall ($P < 0.001$, log-rank test) survival was observed between DTC-negative and DTC-positive patients and was evident in subgroup analysis stratified for nodal status, lymph node yield, lymph node ratio, and tumor subtypes. Disseminated tumor cells were identified as a strong independent prognosticator of tumor recurrence (hazard ratio [HR] 4.0, 95% confidence interval [CI]: 2.96–5.45, $P < 0.001$) and overall survival (HR 3.1, 95% CI: 2.37–4.09, $P < 0.001$, Cox regression analysis).

Conclusions.—The presence of DTC in bone marrow is a strong and independent prognostic factor in patients with resectable EC.

▶ The diagnosis, staging, and treatment of gastrointestinal (GI) cancers are rapidly evolving. For example, the role of micro RNAs (miRNAs) in the diagnosis of gastrointestinal cancers may provide new insights into diagnosis and treatment, but we still have to acquire substantial data to practically use the information on systemic miRNAs and GI cancer treatment. However, as Vashist et al show in this article, disseminated tumor cells (DTC) in the bone marrow may be used now to predict outcome and modify treatment. In this well-conducted and thought-provoking study, the findings suggest that DTC are common and present in about one-third of all esophageal cancer patients regardless of tumor subtype (squamous cell or adenocarcinoma). Furthermore, even lymph node–negative patients harbor DTC in 24% of patients, and 30% of patients with negative non-regional lymph nodes had DTC. The presence of DTC correlated with tumor size and lymph node status. Impressively, DTC predicted tumor recurrence and overall survival. This study has significant implications for the treatment of esophageal cancer patients. For example, should DTC status be included in the staging of patients? Should all patients with DTC receive neoadjuvant therapy? Would treatment with neoadjuvant therapy be beneficial? As with all good clinical studies, this provocative study provides more questions than answers. This work, however, may serve as a landmark work in the changing landscape of esophageal cancer treatment.

K. E. Behrns, MD

Gastrointestinal Adenocarcinomas of the Esophagus, Stomach, and Colon Exhibit Distinct Patterns of Genome Instability and Oncogenesis
Dulak AM, Schumacher SE, van Lieshout J, et al (Dana-Farber Cancer Inst, Boston, MA; et al)
Cancer Res 72:4383-4393, 2012

A more detailed understanding of the somatic genetic events that drive gastrointestinal adenocarcinomas is necessary to improve diagnosis and therapy. Using data from high-density genomic profiling arrays, we conducted an analysis of somatic copy-number aberrations in 486 gastrointestinal adenocarcinomas including 296 esophageal and gastric cancers. Focal amplifications were substantially more prevalent in gastric/esophageal adenocarcinomas than colorectal tumors. We identified 64 regions of significant recurrent amplification and deletion, some shared and others unique to the adenocarcinoma types examined. Amplified genes were noted in 37% of gastric/esophageal tumors, including in therapeutically targetable kinases such as ERBB2, FGFR1, FGFR2, EGFR, and MET, suggesting the potential use of genomic amplifications as biomarkers to guide therapy of gastric and esophageal cancers where targeted therapeutics have been less developed compared with colorectal cancers. Amplified loci implicated genes with known involvement in carcinogenesis but also pointed to regions harboring potentially novel cancer genes, including a recurrent deletion found in 15% of esophageal tumors where the Runt transcription factor subunit RUNX1 was implicated, including by functional experiments in tissue culture. Together, our results defined genomic features that were common and distinct to various gut-derived adenocarcinomas, potentially informing novel opportunities for targeted therapeutic interventions.

► The milestone of human genome sequencing has precipitated genomic analysis of many diseases, especially cancers. Scientists and clinicians have rapidly gathered substantial information related to the genomics of multiple cancers. The bulk of our genomic information is associated with individual cancers. However, Dulak et al performed genomic analysis across the gastrointestinal tract by examining genomic expression from nearly 500 cancers of the esophagus, stomach, colon, and rectum. In theory, these cancers may exhibit similar patterns of gene expression because they originate from changes in intestinal mucosa. Although similarities were noted across the cancers in this study, it is obvious that each cancer has unique genomic expression patterns (Fig 1 in the original article). The information acquired in this work is vital to appropriately organize the vast amount of genomic information available. Recognition of gene expression patterns at particular times in the oncogenic process may permit specific therapies that could be applied to multiple cancers. Although we frequently see studies of alterations in gene expression for certain cancers and opine that we can apply personalized medicine to these findings, we clearly need a better understanding of how groups of genes across many cancers behave in the process of oncogenesis. This work takes a major step in that direction.

K. E. Behrns, MD

Long-Term Follow-Up of Malignancy Biomarkers in Patients With Barrett's Esophagus Undergoing Medical or Surgical Treatment

de Haro LFM, Ortiz A, Parrilla P, et al (IMIM-Hosp del Mar, Barcelona, Spain; et al)
Ann Surg 255:916-921, 2012

Objective.—This study aims to compare some validated biomarkers of malignancy (Ki-67, p53, and apoptosis) between 2 groups of patients with Barrett's esophagus (BE) undergoing randomly medical or surgical treatment.

Background.—The treatment of choice to prevent the malignant progression of BE remains controversial. Translational studies using biomarkers associated with the metaplasia-tumor pathway could be useful to provide some information in this regard.

Methods.—The study group consisted of 45 patients: 20 under medical treatment with 40 mg/day of proton pump inhibitors (PPIs) and 25 after Nissen fundoplication (NFP). After a median follow-up of 8 years (range, 5−10 years), the values of Ki-67, p53, and apoptosis were analyzed in all patients before treatment (n = 45) and then 1 year (n = 45), 3 years (n = 45), 5 years (n = 45), and 10 years (n = 25) afterwards in both groups

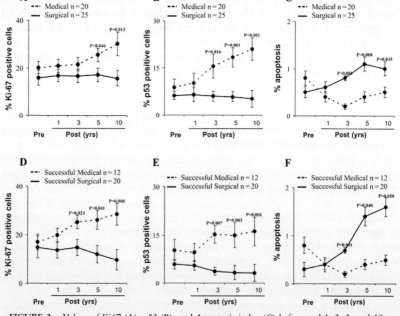

FIGURE 2.—Values of Ki67 (A), p53 (B), and Apoptosis index (C) before and 1, 3, 5, and 10 years after both types of treatment. Values of Ki67 (D), p53 (E), and Apoptosis index (F) before and 1, 3, 5, and 10 years after successful treatment in both groups. All data are expressed as mean (SE). (Reprinted from de Haro LFM, Ortiz A, Parrilla P, et al. Long-term follow-up of malignancy biomarkers in patients with Barrett's esophagus undergoing medical or surgical treatment. *Ann Surg.* 2012;255:916-921. © Southeastern Surgical Congress.)

of treatment. These values were also analyzed in 2 subgroups of patients with successful medical and surgical treatment.

Results.—Both Ki-67 and p53 remained stable after NFP, whereas they increased progressively in patients under PPIs with statistically significant differences between the 2 groups. Conversely, the apoptotic index increased progressively after NFP and decreased in the patients under PPIs with significant differences at 3, 5, and 10 years of follow-up. On comparing the subgroups of successful treatment the same differences were found.

Conclusions.—Barrett's epithelium remains more stable after a long-term follow-up in patients with BE treated surgically than in those under PPIs even in the absence of abnormal rates of acid reflux (Fig 2).

▶ The development of Barrett esophagus in patients with gastroesophageal reflux is an ominous sign because the rate of progression to esophageal adenocarcinoma is high, with estimates of increased cancer risk at 30- to 125-fold. Strict biopsy surveillance programs have been developed to monitor the epithelium in patients with Barrett esophagus, and multiple studies have demonstrated equipoise in patients treated with medical therapy or surgical therapy to prevent adenocarcinoma. Thus, as a surgical community, we are confronted with the options of treating these high-risk patients with life-long proton pump inhibitors or antireflux surgery, and we are unable to counsel patients on the best prophylactic option. However, in this study by Martinez de Haro et al, surgical therapy was associated with improved long-term biomarker status in patients who had a fundoplication compared with proton pump inhibitor therapy. The results demonstrated that Ki-67, a marker of proliferation; p53, a marker of potential malignancy; and apoptosis, an indicator of cell death, were reflective of decreased likelihood of progression to malignancy (Fig 2). Thus, surgical therapy may be a better long-term prophylactic option. Though the reasons that surgery may decrease the risk of cancer are not enunciated, it is important to note that the barrier function of a fundoplication may result in decreased esophageal epithelium exposure to bile. Several studies have demonstrated that the combination of acid exposure with bile can lead to long-term unstable esophageal epithelium. This study poignantly demonstrates the utility of studying biomarkers in addition to standard histopathology. In addition, this carefully conducted study also shows the benefit to long-term follow-up to monitor biomarkers for malignancy.

K. E. Behrns, MD

Minimally invasive versus open oesophagectomy for patients with oesophageal cancer: a multicentre, open-label, randomised controlled trial
Biere SSAY, van Berge Henegouwen MI, Maas KW, et al (VU Univ Med Centre, Amsterdam, Netherlands; Academic Med Centre, Amsterdam, Netherlands; et al)
Lancet 379:1887-1892, 2012

Background.—Surgical resection is regarded as the only curative option for resectable oesophageal cancer, but pulmonary complications occurring in more than half of patients after open oesophagectomy are a great

TABLE 2.—Primary and Secondary Outcomes for the Intention-to-Treat Population

	OO (N=56)	MIO (N=59)	p Value
Primary outcomes			
Pulmonary infection within 2 weeks	16 (29%)	5 (9%)	0·005
Pulmonary infection in-hospital	19 (34%)	7 (12%)	0·005
Secondary outcomes			
Hospital stay (days)*	14 (1–120)	11 (7–80)	0·044
Short-term quality of life[†]			
SF 36[†]			
Physical component summary	36 (6; 34–39)	42 (8; 39–46)	0·007
Mental component summary	45 (11; 40–50)	46 (10; 41–50)	0·806
EORTC C30[†]			
Global health	51 (21; 44–58)	61 (18; 56–67)	0·020
OES 18[‡]			
Talking	37 (39; 25–49)	18 (26; 10–26)	0·008
Pain	19 (21; 13–26)	8 (11; 5–11)	0·002
Total lymph nodes retrieved*	21 (7–47)	20 (3–44)	0·852
Resection margin[§]			0·080
R0	47 (84%)	54 (92%)	··
R1	5 (9%)	1 (2%)	··
pStage¶			0·943
0	0 (0%)	1 (2%)	··
I	4 (7%)	4 (7%)	··
IIa	16 (29%)	17 (29%)	··
IIb	6 (11%)	9 (15%)	··
III	14 (25%)	11 (19%)	··
IV	5 (9%)	4 (7%)	··
No residual tumour or lymph-node metastasis	7 (13%)	9 (15%)	··
Mortality‖			0·590
30-day mortality	0 (0%)	1 (2%)	··
In-hospital mortality	1 (2%)	2 (3%)	··

Data are n (%), median (range), or mean (SD, 95% CI), unless otherwise indicated. OO=open oesophagectomy. MIO=minimally invasive oesophagectomy. SF 36=Short Form 36 Health Survey (version 2). EORTC=European Organization for Research and Treatment of Cancer Quality of Life Questionnaires.
*Skewed distribution, Mann-Whitney test applied.
[†]Measures general aspects of health; scores range from 0 to 100, with higher scores representing better well-being.
[‡]Assesses several aspects of oesophageal function; scores range from 0 to 100, with lower scores indicating better function. Only statistically significant domains presented.
[§]Defined as >1 mm from a resection margin.
¶Staging based on the American Joint Committee on Cancer, 6th edn; four patients in each group did not undergo resection due to metastasis or irresectability of the tumour.
‖Death from any cause.

concern. We assessed whether minimally invasive oesophagectomy reduces morbidity compared with open oesophagectomy.

Methods.—We did a multicentre, open-label, randomised controlled trial at five study centres in three countries between June 1, 2009, and March 31, 2011. Patients aged 18–75 years with resectable cancer of the oesophagus or gastro-oesophageal junction were randomly assigned via a computer-generated randomisation sequence to receive either open transthoracic or minimally invasive transthoracic oesophagectomy. Randomisation was stratified by centre. Patients, and investigators undertaking interventions, assessing outcomes, and analysing data, were not masked to group assignment. The primary outcome was pulmonary infection within the first 2 weeks after surgery and during the whole stay in hospital. Analysis was by intention to treat. This trial is registered with the Netherlands Trial Register, NTR TC 2452.

Findings.—We randomly assigned 56 patients to the open oesophagectomy group and 59 to the minimally invasive oesophagectomy group. 16 (29%) patients in the open oesophagectomy group had pulmonary infection in the first 2 weeks compared with five (9%) in the minimally invasive group (relative risk [RR] $0 \cdot 30$, 95% CI $0 \cdot 12-0 \cdot 76$; $p = 0 \cdot 005$). 19 (34%) patients in the open oesophagectomy group had pulmonary infection in-hospital compared with seven (12%) in the minimally invasive group ($0 \cdot 35$, $0 \cdot 16-0 \cdot 78$; $p = 0 \cdot 005$). For in-hospital mortality, one patient in the open oesophagectomy group died from anastomotic leakage and two in the minimally invasive group from aspiration and mediastinitis after anastomotic leakage.

Interpretation.—These findings provide evidence for the short-term benefits of minimally invasive oesophagectomy for patients with resectable oesophageal cancer (Table 2).

▶ Thoracoscopic resection of the esophagus was reported by Cuschieri in 1994[1] and was popularized in the United States by Luketich et al in 2003[2] when they reported 222 minimally invasive esophagectomies. Surprisingly, the operation was never validated by a randomized controlled trial. However, these authors have now conducted that trial and established the pulmonary benefits of minimally invasive esophagectomy. The results showed that the occurrence of pulmonary infection in the first 2 weeks postoperatively was 29% in the open esophagectomy group versus 9% in the esophagectomy group. Furthermore, these data held true for the in-hospital infection rates (Table 2). The mortality did not differ between groups and the oncologic assessment was similar. The patients, however, did seem to experience less discomfort with the minimally invasive approach. This study confirms important findings that markedly improve the care of the patient with esophageal cancer. The minimally invasive approach should be considered the standard of care, and surgeons who perform esophageal surgery should have this procedure in their armamentarium. The benefits to the patients are quite clear, and the minimally invasive procedure should be the default. However, it is a bit curious that it took us 18 years to clearly establish the benefits of this operation.

K. E. Behrns, MD

References

1. Cuschieri A. Thoracoscopic subtotal oespphagectomy. *Endosc Surg Allied Techno.* 1994;2:21-25.
2. Luketich JD, Alvelo-Rivera M, Bunaventura PO, et al. Minimally invasive esophagectomy: outcomes in 222 patients. *Ann Surg.* 2003;238:486-494.

Preoperative Chemoradiotherapy for Esophageal or Junctional Cancer

van Hagen P, for the CROSS Group (Erasmus Univ Med Ctr, Rotterdam, The Netherlands; et al)

N Engl J Med 366:2074-2084, 2012

Background.—The role of neoadjuvant chemoradiotherapy in the treatment of patients with esophageal or esophagogastric-junction cancer is not well established. We compared chemoradiotherapy followed by surgery with surgery alone in this patient population.

Methods.—We randomly assigned patients with resectable tumors to receive surgery alone or weekly administration of carboplatin (doses titrated to achieve an area under the curve of 2 mg per milliliter per minute) and paclitaxel (50 mg per square meter of body-surface area) for 5 weeks and concurrent radiotherapy (41.4 Gy in 23 fractions, 5 days per week), followed by surgery.

Results.—From March 2004 through December 2008, we enrolled 368 patients, 366 of whom were included in the analysis: 275 (75%) had adenocarcinoma, 84 (23%) had squamous- cell carcinoma, and 7 (2%) had large-cell undifferentiated carcinoma. Of the 366 patients, 178 were randomly assigned to chemoradiotherapy followed by surgery, and 188 to surgery alone. The most common major hematologic toxic effects in the chemoradiotherapy–surgery group were leukopenia (6%) and neutropenia (2%); the most common major nonhematologic toxic effects were anorexia (5%) and fatigue (3%). Complete resection with no tumor within 1 mm of the resection margins (R0) was achieved in 92% of patients in the chemoradiotherapy–surgery group versus 69% in the surgery group ($P < 0.001$). A pathological complete response was achieved in 47 of 161 patients (29%) who underwent resection after chemoradiotherapy. Postoperative complications were similar in the two treatment groups, and in-hospital mortality was 4% in both. Median overall survival was 49.4 months in the chemoradiotherapy–surgery group versus 24.0 months in the surgery group. Overall survival was significantly better in the chemoradiotherapy–surgery group (hazard ratio, 0.657; 95% confidence interval, 0.495 to 0.871; $P = 0.003$).

Conclusions.—Preoperative chemoradiotherapy improved survival among patients with potentially curable esophageal or esophagogastric-junction cancer. The regimen was associated with acceptable adverse-event rates. (Funded by the Dutch Cancer Foundation [KWF Kankerbestrijding]; Netherlands Trial Register number, NTR487.)

▶ The use of neoadjuvant therapy for esophageal or esophagogastric junction cancer has been studied in randomized trials, but the results of these studies have been conflicting for several reasons. However, Hagen et al conducted a multicenter, randomized trial that compared neoadjuvant chemoradiotherapy plus surgery (n = 171) versus surgery alone (n = 186) in patients with well-defined tumors of the esophagus and gastroesophageal junction. Patients with both adenocarcinoma and squamous cell cancers were included. Patients in the neoadjuvant therapy arm received 5 cycles of carboplatin and paclitaxel and 5 weeks of concurrent external beam radiotherapy (41.4 Gy). The results demonstrated hematologic toxicity of 6% or less, although 1 patient died as a result of neoadjuvant therapy. The margin-negative resection rate was significantly higher in the neoadjuvant group (92%) compared with the surgery group alone (69%). Survival was significantly better in the neoadjuvant group compared with the surgery-alone group regardless of tumor type (Fig 2 in the original article). So why do the results of this study confer benefit to neoadjuvant therapy when other studies failed to demonstrate this benefit? The answer lies in strict selection criteria that did not include proximal gastric tumors or tumors that were not carefully stratified by size and length, depth of invasion, and nodal status. This study demonstrates a remarkable improvement in survival for patients with esophageal or junctional cancers and therefore sets the standard for patients that meet the study criteria and should be treated with neoadjuvant therapy. Of note, the study does not specifically address the nutritional status of these patients, but personal experience suggests that many of these patients require laparoscopic placement of jejunal feeding tubes before initiation of neoadjuvant chemoradiotherapy.

K. E. Behrns, MD

Predicting Risk for Venous Thromboembolism With Bariatric Surgery: Results From the Michigan Bariatric Surgery Collaborative

Finks JF, for the Michigan Bariatric Surgery Collaborative and from the Center for Healthcare Outcomes and Policy (Univ of Michigan, Ann Arbor; et al)

Ann Surg 255:1100-1104, 2012

Objective.—We sought to identify risk factors for venous thromboembolism (VTE) among patients undergoing bariatric surgery in Michigan.

Background.—VTE remains a major source of morbidity and mortality after bariatric surgery. It is unclear which factors should be used to identify patients at high risk for VTE.

Methods.—The Michigan Bariatric Surgery Collaborative maintains a prospective clinical registry of bariatric surgery patients. For this study, we identified all patients undergoing primary bariatric surgery between June 2006 and April 2011 and determined rates of VTE. Potential risk factors for VTE were analyzed using a hierarchical logistic regression model, accounting for clustering of patients within hospitals. Significant risk factors were used to develop a risk calculator for development of VTE after bariatric surgery.

Results.—Among 27,818 patients who underwent bariatric surgery during the study period, 93 patients (0.33%) experienced a VTE complication, including 51 patents with pulmonary embolism. There were 8 associated deaths. Significant risk factors included previous history of VTE (OR 4.15, CI 2.42−7.08); male gender (OR 2.08, CI 1.36−3.19); operative time more than 3 hours (OR 1.86, CI 1.07−3.24); BMI category (per 10 units) (OR 1.37, CI 1.06−1.75); age category (per 10 years) (OR 1.25, CI

1.03—1.51); and procedure type (reference adjustable gastric band): duodenal switch (OR 9.45, CI 2.50—35.97); open gastric bypass (OR 6.48, CI 2.17—19.41); laparoscopic gastric bypass (OR 3.97, CI 1.77—8.91); and sleeve gastrectomy (OR 3.50, CI 1.30—9.34). Nearly 97% of patients had a predicted VTE risk less than 1%.

Conclusions.—In this population-based study, overall VTE rates were low among patients undergoing bariatric surgery. The use of an empirically based risk calculator will allow for the development of a risk-stratified approach to VTE prophylaxis.

▶ The development of registries and large data sets has given surgeons new tools to assess perioperative care. With thousands of patients in these disease-specific registries, we can determine preoperative patient characteristics that are associated with the likelihood of a complication. In many cases, these studies have resulted in the generation of a risk calculator that allows the surgeon to enter the individual patient characteristics so that risk can be assessed and risk-modifying patient care initiated prior to an operation. Finks et al used the Michigan Bariatric Surgery Collaborative in assessment of the risk of venous thromboembolism (VTE) in patients undergoing bariatric surgery. Nearly 28 000 patients were included in the study, and only 93 patients developed a VTE (0.33%). Eight patients in the study died, and factors associated with the development of a VTE included a previous VTE, male gender, operating time greater than 3 hours, increasing body mass index, and procedure type. In descending order of frequency, the procedure types associated with the greatest likelihood of VTE were duodenal switch, open gastric bypass, laparoscopic gastric bypass, sleeve gastrectomy, and laparoscopic adjustable band. Assessment using a risk calculator established that 97% of patients had a risk of VTE less than 1%. This work confirms the power of large data sets to not only assess risk but to change perioperative treatment in high-risk patients. Surgeons should use this information on a regular basis to assess risk and modify perioperative care in the appropriate patient populations.

K. E. Behrns, MD

Metabolic Surgery for Non-Obese Type 2 Diabetes: Incretins, Adipocytokines, and Insulin Secretion/Resistance Changes in a 1-Year Interventional Clinical Controlled Study
Geloneze B, Geloneze SR, Chaim E, et al (Univ of Campinas, Brazil)
Ann Surg 256:72-78, 2012

Objective.—To compare duodenal-jejunal bypass (DJB) with standard medical care in nonobese patients with type 2 diabetes and evaluate surgically induced endocrine and metabolic changes.

Methods.—Eighteen patients submitted to a DJB procedure met the following criteria: overweight, diabetes diagnosis less than 15 years, current insulin treatment, residual β-cell function, and absence of autoimmunity. Patients who refused surgical treatment received standard medical care (control group). At baseline, 3, 6, and 12 months after surgery, insulin sensitivity and production of glucagon-like peptide-1 and glucose-insulinotropic polypeptide were assessed during a meal tolerance test. Fasting adipocytokines and dipeptidyl-peptidase-4 concentrations were measured.

Results.—The mean age of the patients was 50 (5) years, time of diagnosis: 9 (2) years, time of insulin usage: 6 (5) months, fasting glucose: 9.9 (2.5) mmol/dL, and HbA$_{1c}$ (glycosylated hemoglobin) level: 8.9% (1.2%). Duodenal-jejunal bypass group showed greater reductions in fasting glucose (22% vs 6% in control group, $P < 0.05$) and daily insulin requirement (93% vs 15%, $P < 0.01$). Twelve patients from DJB group stopped using insulin and showed improvements in insulin sensitivity and β-cell function ($P < 0.01$), and reductions in glucose-insulinotropic polypeptide levels ($P < 0.001$), glucagon during the first 30 minutes after meal ($P < 0.05$), and leptin levels ($P < 0.05$). Dipeptidyl-peptidase-4 levels increased after surgery ($P < 0.01$), but glucagon-like peptide-1 levels did not change.

Conclusions.—Duodenal-jejunal bypass improved insulin sensitivity and β-cell function and reduced glucose-insulinotropic polypeptide, leptin, and glucagon production. Hence, DJB resulted in better glycemic control and reduction in insulin requirement but DJB did not result in remission of diabetes.

▶ Multiple studies have recently found that Roux-en-Y gastric bypass decreases insulin requirements and improves diabetic control in obese patients. This effect is noticeable prior to significant weight loss in many patients. However, whether bypass of the foregut would result in improved blood sugar control in nonobese patients has not been demonstrated. Geloneze et al show in a modest sample (N = 18) of nonobese, insulin-requiring patients, that bypass of the proximal gut is associated with greater decreases in serum glucose concentrations and daily insulin requirement than patients treated with a medical regimen. Of note, two-thirds of the patients treated with duodenojejunal bypass were insulin free and showed increased β-cell function. It is important to recognize, however, that duodenojejunal bypass did not result in remission of diabetes. The study was carefully designed to measure multiple hormonal and incretin changes during the study period. Leptin concentrations were decreased, and this may lead to less insulin resistance and improved glucose regulation. Although this study is relatively small and other trials are necessary, this study takes the important step of demonstrating an effect of foregut bypass in nonobese patients. This study also sheds light on basic pathophysiology that is fundamental to improving our understanding of the relationship between foregut function and glucose metabolism.

K. E. Behrns, MD

Health Care Use During 20 Years Following Bariatric Surgery

Neovius M, Narbro K, Keating C, et al (Univ of Gothenburg, Sweden; Region Västra Götaland, Gothenburg, Sweden; Deakin Univ, Melbourne, Australia; et al)
JAMA 308:1132-1141, 2012

Context.—Bariatric surgery results in sustained weight loss; reduced incidence of diabetes, cardiovascular events, and cancer; and improved survival. The long-term effect on health care use is unknown.

Objective.—To assess health care use over 20 years by obese patients treated conventionally or with bariatric surgery.

Design, Setting, and Participants.—The Swedish Obese Subjects study is an ongoing, prospective, nonrandomized, controlled intervention study conducted in the Swedish health care system that included 2010 adults who underwent bariatric surgery and 2037 contemporaneously matched controls recruited between 1987 and 2001. Inclusion criteria were age 37 years to 60 years and body mass index of 34 or higher in men and 38 or higher in women. Exclusion criteria were identical in both groups.

Interventions.—Of the surgery patients, 13% underwent gastric bypass, 19% gastric banding, and 68% vertical-banded gastroplasty. Controls received conventional obesity treatment.

Main Outcome Measures.—Annual hospital days (follow-up years 1 to 20; data capture 1987-2009; median follow-up 15 years) and nonprimary care outpatient visits (years 2-20; data capture 2001-2009; median follow-up 9 years) were retrieved from the National Patient Register, and drug costs from the Prescribed Drug Register (years 7-20; data capture 2005-2011; median follow-up 6 years). Registry linkage was complete for more than 99% of patients (4044 of 4047). Mean differences were adjusted for baseline age, sex, smoking, diabetes status, body mass index, inclusion period, and (for the inpatient care analysis) hospital days the year before the index date.

Results.—In the 20 years following their bariatric procedure, surgery patients used a total of 54 mean cumulative hospital days compared with 40 used by those in the control group (adjusted difference, 15; 95% CI, 2-27; *P* =.03). During the years 2 through 6, surgery patients had an accumulated annual mean of 1.7 hospital days vs 1.2 days among control patients (adjusted difference, 0.5; 95% CI, 0.2 to 0.7; *P* < .001). From year 7 to 20, both groups had a mean annual 1.8 hospital days (adjusted difference, 0.0; 95% CI, −0.3 to 0.3; *P* =.95). Surgery patients had a mean annual 1.3 nonprimary care outpatient visits during the years 2 through 6 vs 1.1 among the controls (adjusted difference, 0.3; 95% CI, 0.1 to 0.4; *P* =.003), but from year 7, the 2 groups did not differ (1.8 vs 1.9 mean annual visits; adjusted difference, −0.2; 95% CI, −0.4 to 0.1; *P* =.12). From year 7 to 20, the surgery group incurred a mean annual drug cost of US $930; the control patients, $1123 (adjusted difference, −$228; 95% CI, −$335 to −$121; *P* < .001).

Conclusions.—Compared with controls, surgically treated patients used more inpatient and nonprimary outpatient care during the first 6-year period after undergoing bariatric surgery but not thereafter. Drug costs from years 7 through 20 were lower for surgery patients than for control patients. *Trial Registration.*—clinicaltrials.gov Identifier: NCT01479452.

▶ The short-term outcomes of bariatric surgery are evident with weight loss and improved blood glucose control. Most of the long-term data are measured in terms of a few years and generally show that patients regained some of the earlier lost weight. Few studies, however, have follow-up extending to 20 years. The work by Neovius et al comes from the Swedish Obese Subjects study in which surgery patients (N = 2010) were compared with 2037 matched controls. Most of the patients in the surgery arm had an outdated procedure, vertical-banded gastroplasty (68%). The study was designed to examine hospital stays, nonprimary care outpatient visits, and medication costs. The findings showed that during the first 6 years, surgical patients had increased hospital stays and nonprimary care outpatient visits. However, from years 7 to 20, no difference was apparent in these parameters. Surgical patients had lower medication costs largely because of the need for fewer medications for diabetes mellitus and cardiovascular disease. The increased hospital stays and nonprimary care outpatient visits in the 6 years following surgery are not surprising because the complete beneficial effect of bariatric surgery will not occur for some time. In addition, with successful bariatric surgery many patients have plastic surgery for removal of excess skin and subcutaneous tissue. These data are important because they demonstrate that in the long run, bariatric surgery is not associated with increased health care resources.

K. E. Behrns, MD

Bariatric Surgery versus Intensive Medical Therapy in Obese Patients With Diabetes
Schauer PR, Kashyap SR, Wolski K, et al (Cleveland Clinic, OH; et al)
N Engl J Med 366:1567-1576, 2012

Background.—Observational studies have shown improvement in patients with type 2 diabetes mellitus after bariatric surgery.

Methods.—In this randomized, nonblinded, single-center trial, we evaluated the efficacy of intensive medical therapy alone versus medical therapy plus Roux-en-Y gastric by-pass or sleeve gastrectomy in 150 obese patients with uncontrolled type 2 diabetes. The mean (± SD) age of the patients was 49 ± 8 years, and 66% were women. The average glycated hemoglobin level was 9.2 ± 1.5%. The primary end point was the proportion of patients with a glycated hemoglobin level of 6.0% or less 12 months after treatment.

Results.—Of the 150 patients, 93% completed 12 months of follow-up. The proportion of patients with the primary end point was 12% (5 of 41 patients) in the medical-therapy group versus 42% (21 of 50 patients) in the gastric-bypass group ($P = 0.002$) and 37% (18 of 49 patients) in the sleeve-gastrectomy group ($P = 0.008$). Glycemic control improved in all three groups, with a mean glycated hemoglobin level of 7.5 ± 1.8% in the

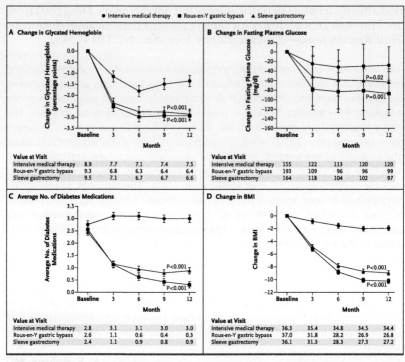

FIGURE 1.—Changes in Measures of Diabetes Control from Baseline. Values for change in glycated hemoglobin (Panel A), change in fasting plasma glucose (Panel B), the average number of diabetes medications (Panel C), and change in body-mass index (BMI) (Panel D) were plotted at 3, 6, 9, and 12 months. Least-square means and standard errors from a repeated measures model are plotted for glycated hemoglobin, average number of medications, and BMI; medians and interquartile ranges are plotted for fasting plasma glucose. P values are for the comparison between each surgical group and the medical-therapy group and were calculated from a repeated-measures model that considers data over time. (Reprinted from Schauer PR, Kashyap SR, Wolski K, et al. Bariatric surgery versus intensive medical therapy in obese patients with diabetes. *N Engl J Med.* 2012;366:1567-1576. © 2012 Massachusetts Medical Society.)

medical-therapy group, 6.4 ± 0.9% in the gastric-bypass group ($P < 0.001$), and 6.6 ± 1.0% in the sleeve-gastrectomy group ($P = 0.003$). Weight loss was greater in the gastric-bypass group and sleeve-gastrectomy group (−29.4 ± 9.0 kg and −25.1 ± 8.5 kg, respectively) than in the medical-therapy group (−5.4 ± 8.0 kg) ($P < 0.001$ for both comparisons). The use of drugs to lower glucose, lipid, and blood-pressure levels decreased significantly after both surgical procedures but increased in patients receiving medical therapy only. The index for homeostasis model assessment of insulin resistance (HOMA-IR) improved significantly after bariatric surgery. Four patients underwent reoperation. There were no deaths or life-threatening complications.

Conclusions.—In obese patients with uncontrolled type 2 diabetes, 12 months of medical therapy plus bariatric surgery achieved glycemic control in significantly more patients than medical therapy alone. Further study will be necessary to assess the durability of these results. (Funded by Ethicon Endo-Surgery and others; ClinicalTrials.gov number, NCT00432809.) (Fig 1).

▶ The merits of bariatric surgery on systemic diseases such as cardiovascular ailments and diabetes have been studied and debated extensively. More recently, the prompt improvement in blood glucose in some patients following bariatric surgery has been examined to determine the mechanisms of this response. Schauer et al contributed significantly to this body of knowledge with a randomized, single-center trial that compared intensive medical therapy alone to Roux-en-Y gastric bypass or sleeve gastrectomy in patients with uncontrolled type 2 diabetes. The primary endpoint was glycated hemoglobin of 6% or less at 12 months. The results were notable in that 42% and 37% of the gastric bypass and sleeve gastrectomy patients, respectively, attained the endpoint, whereas 12% in the medical therapy arm did so. Furthermore, blood glucose concentrations, diabetic medications, and weight loss were all more significantly improved in the surgery arms of the trial (Fig 1). This well-designed and conducted trial clearly shows the value of clinical trials in surgical patients and how a trial such as this will lead to further studies examining the physiologic and pathophysiologic responses that lead to improved glucose metabolism. Importantly, this trial also shows that persistence pays off in surgical investigation. Little more than a decade ago, bariatric surgery was not held in high esteem. However, bariatric surgeons improved the approach and results with laparoscopic techniques and now are conducting highly visible clinical trials that are providing much-needed information regarding metabolic syndrome and the effects on cardiovascular diseases and diabetes. This article highlights the persistence in bariatric surgery and the continued pursuit of physiologic research by surgeons.

K. E. Behrns, MD

Bariatric Surgery and Prevention of Type 2 Diabetes in Swedish Obese Subjects

Carlsson LMS, Peltonen M, Ahlin S, et al (Insts of Medicine, Gothenburg, Sweden; et al)

N Engl J Med 367:695-704, 2012

Background.—Weight loss protects against type 2 diabetes but is hard to maintain with behavioral modification alone. In an analysis of data from a nonrandomized, prospective, controlled study, we examined the effects of bariatric surgery on the prevention of type 2 diabetes.

Methods.—In this analysis, we included 1658 patients who underwent bariatric surgery and 1771 obese matched controls (with matching performed on a group, rather than individual, level). None of the participants had diabetes at baseline. Patients in the bariatric-surgery cohort underwent banding (19%), vertical banded gastroplasty (69%), or gastric bypass (12%); nonrandomized, matched, prospective controls received usual

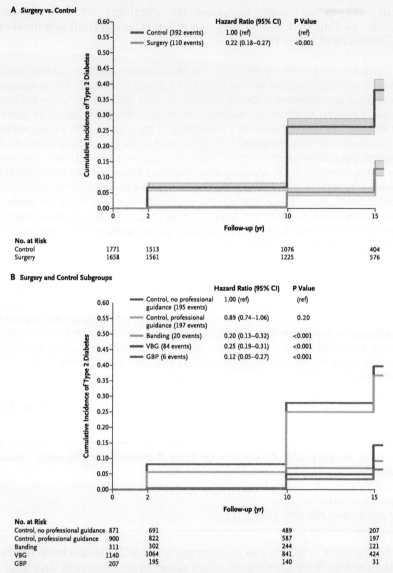

FIGURE 1.—Cumulative Incidence of Type 2 Diabetes. Panel A shows the Kaplan–Meier unadjusted estimates of the cumulative incidence of type 2 diabetes in the bariatric-surgery group and the control group. The light shading represents the 95% confidence interval. The adjusted hazard ratio with bariatric surgery was 0.17 (95% confidence interval, 0.13 to 0.21). Panel B shows the Kaplan–Meier unadjusted estimates of the incidence of type 2 diabetes in subgroups defined in the control group according to receipt or no receipt of professional guidance to lose weight and in the surgery group according to the method of bariatric surgery: gastric banding, vertical banded gastroplasty (VBG), or gastric bypass (GBP). (Reprinted from Carlsson LMS, Peltonen M, Ahlin S, et al. Bariatric surgery and prevention of type 2 diabetes in Swedish obese subjects. *N Engl J Med.* 2012;367:695-704, © 2012, Massachusetts Medical Society.)

care. Participants were 37 to 60 years of age, and the body-mass index (BMI; the weight in kilograms divided by the square of the height in meters) was 34 or more in men and 38 or more in women. This analysis focused on the rate of incident type 2 diabetes, which was a prespecified secondary end point in the main study. At the time of this analysis (January 1, 2012), participants had been followed for up to 15 years. Despite matching, some baseline characteristics differed significantly between the groups; the baseline body weight was higher and risk factors were more pronounced in the bariatric-surgery group than in the control group. At 15 years, 36.2% of the original participants had dropped out of the study, and 30.9% had not yet reached the time for their 15-year follow-up examination.

Results.—During the follow-up period, type 2 diabetes developed in 392 participants in the control group and in 110 in the bariatric-surgery group, corresponding to incidence rates of 28.4 cases per 1000 person-years and 6.8 cases per 1000 person-years, respectively (adjusted hazard ratio with bariatric surgery, 0.17; 95% confidence interval, 0.13 to 0.21; $P < 0.001$). The effect of bariatric surgery was influenced by the presence or absence of impaired fasting glucose ($P = 0.002$ for the interaction) but not by BMI ($P = 0.54$). Sensitivity analyses, including end-point imputations, did not change the overall conclusions. The postoperative mortality was 0.2%, and 2.8% of patients who underwent bariatric surgery required reoperation within 90 days owing to complications.

Conclusions.—Bariatric surgery appears to be markedly more efficient than usual care in the prevention of type 2 diabetes in obese persons. (Funded by the Swedish Research Council and others; ClinicalTrials.gov number, NCT01479452) (Fig 1).

▶ In recent years, significant evidence has indicated that bariatric surgery can markedly improve or cure type 2 diabetes. Although the mechanisms of action of improved blood glucose control with bariatric surgery remain under investigation, the body of literature suggests that bariatric surgery should be considered as a treatment for obesity-associated type 2 diabetes.

In this *New England Journal of Medicine* article, the authors demonstrated that type 2 diabetes can be prevented with bariatric surgery. In a case-matched study of approximately 1700 patients per group, the incidence of type 2 diabetes was reduced by 78% in the bariatric surgery patients compared with the incidence rate in the control population (Fig 1). Somewhat surprisingly, the type of bariatric surgery (banding vs bypass vs vertical banded gastroplasty) was not associated with a difference in the incidence of diabetes (Fig 1B). Certainly, we know that each of these operations is associated with varying amounts of weight loss, and the study did not correlate weight loss with the incidence of diabetes. It would be interesting to discern if there is a threshold of weight loss required to prevent diabetes. Likely this will be a goal of the randomized study the authors propose. This study is important because it is the first to show that bariatric surgery can prevent type 2 diabetes. Obviously, further randomized studies with standardized bariatric surgery approaches are needed to better match the group and to permit investigation of the mechanism of action, but this study provides a breakthrough message.

K. E. Behrns, MD

Single Incision Laparoscopic Cholecystectomy Is Associated With a Higher Bile Duct Injury Rate: A Review and a Word of Caution
Joseph M, Phillips MR, Farrell TM, et al (Univ of North Carolina, Chapel Hill)
Ann Surg 256:1-6, 2012

Objective.—To compare the incidence of bile duct injuries during single incision laparoscopic cholecystectomy (SILC) in relation to the accepted historic rate of 0.4% to 0.5% for standard laparoscopic cholecystectomy (SLC).

Background.—Technically, SILC is more challenging than SLC. The role and benefit of SILC in patient care has yet to be defined. Bile duct injuries have been reported in several series of SILC.

Method.—A comprehensive database search of MEDLINE, EMBASE, CINAHL, and PubMed Central was performed to generate all reported cases of SILC to present. The search was limited to reports of 20 or more patients based on current literature of existing SILC learning curves. Data were analyzed using the Student t test and χ^2 analyses where appropriate.

Results.—A total of 76 candidate studies were identified; 45 studies met inclusion criteria for an aggregate total of 2626 patients. Most SILCs were performed in the absence of acute cholecystitis (90.6%). The aggregate complication rate was 4.2%, and complications were graded according to the Dindo-Clavien Classification System. Nineteen bile duct injuries were identified for a SILC-associated bile duct injury rate of 0.72%.

Conclusions.—There seems to be an increase in the rate of bile duct injuries during SILC when compared with historic rates during SLC. Because most SILCs are performed in optimal conditions, such as lack of acute inflammation, we urge caution in applying this technique to inflamed gallbladder pathology. Controlled trials are needed before conclusions are made regarding safety of SILC.

▶ Joseph et al present a relevant and timely study of the complication rate, in particular the frequency of bile duct injury, in patients undergoing single-incision laparoscopic cholecystectomy (SILC). The authors conducted a literature review and identified studies that reported 20 or more SILC procedures with a total of 2626 patients from 45 included studies. The data demonstrate that 19 patients had bile duct injuries for an injury rate of 0.72%. Most of the injuries were Strasberg "type A," which are defined as a bile leak from a minor duct that remains in continuity with the common bile duct. Of note, more than 90% of the patients had the SILC performed for a noninflamed gallbladder; thus, the operative conditions were presumably ideal or at least appropriate for SILC. Although a bile duct injury rate of 0.72% may appear acceptable, especially when most of the injuries were minor, this rate is increased markedly compared to the commonly reported rate of 0.4% to 0.5% for standard laparoscopic cholecystectomy. Therefore, the authors correctly surmise that surgeons should proceed with caution with this technique. Bile duct injuries can lead to major morbidity with reconstructive surgery, and the personal productive time lost and social costs for the patient are substantial. Surgeons should adopt this method cautiously and be quick to convert from an SILC to a standard laparoscopic or open cholecystectomy. Given the limited benefits of SILC over standard laparoscopic cholecystectomy, we should not accept a higher rate of bile duct injuries or overall complications for this procedure. Our goal should be to decrease the current rate of bile duct injuries; any technique that cannot meet these standards should be abandoned.

K. E. Behrns, MD

Endoscopic Ultrasound-Guided Transmural and Percutaneous Transhepatic Gallbladder Drainage Are Comparable for Acute Cholecystitis
Jang JW, Lee SS, Song TJ, et al (Univ of Ulsan College of Medicine, Seoul, Korea; Inje Univ Ilsanpaik Hosp, Koyang, Korea)
Gastroenterology 142:805-811, 2012

Background & Aims.—Endoscopic ultrasound-guided transmural gallbladder drainage (EUS-GBD) is an alternative to percutaneous transhepatic gallbladder drainage (PTGBD) for patients with acute, high-risk, or advanced-stage cholecystitis who do not respond to initial medical treatment and cannot undergo emergency cholecystectomy. However, the technical feasibility, efficacy, and safety of EUS-GBD and PTGBD have not been compared.

Methods.—Fifty-nine patients with acute cholecystitis, who did not respond to initial medical treatment and were unsuitable for an emergency cholecystectomy, were chosen randomly to undergo EUS-GBD (n = 30) or PTGBD (n = 29). The technical feasibility, efficacy, and safety of EUS-GBD and PTGBD were compared.

Results.—EUS-GBD and PTGBD showed similar technical (97% [29 of 30] vs 97% [28 of 29]; 95% 1-sided confidence interval lower limit, -7%; $P = .001$ for noninferiority margin of 15%) and clinical (100% [29 of 29] vs 96% [27 of 28]; 95% 1-sided confidence interval lower limit, -2%; $P = .0001$ for noninferiority margin of 15%) success rates, and similar rates of complications (7% [2 of 30] vs 3% [1 of 29]; $P = .492$ in the Fisher exact test) and conversions to open cholecystectomy (9% [2 of 23] vs 12% [3 of 26]; $P = .999$ in the Fisher exact test). The median postprocedure pain score was significantly lower after EUS-GBD than after PTGBD (1 vs 5; $P < .001$ in the Mann—Whitney U test).

Conclusions.—EUS-GBD is comparable with PTGBD in terms of the technical feasibility and efficacy; there were no statistical differences in the safety. EUS-GBD is a good alternative for high-risk patients with acute cholecystitis who cannot undergo an emergency cholecystectomy.

▶ Most patients with acute cholecystitis are candidates for laparoscopic cholecystectomy, which is most readily performed immediately after the diagnosis is ascertained. A small, select patient population may require percutaneous transhepatic gallbladder drainage (PTGBD) for temporary or permanent relief of symptoms. Heretofore, PTGBD has been the only established method of gallbladder drainage, and it is not suitable for patients with ascites or coagulopathy. However, Jang et al performed a randomized trial of PTGBD with endoscopic ultrasound-guided gallbladder drainage (EUS-GBD) in patients who were deemed initially unfit for cholecystectomy. EUS-GBD was performed by puncturing and draining the gallbladder through the prepyloric antrum or the duodenal bulb and placing a nasobiliary tube through a dilated tract. In brief, the results of the study showed that EUS-GBD was noninferior to PTGBD in terms of technical feasibility, clinical response rate, complications, and ultimately conversion to open cholecystectomy. EUS-GBD, however, was associated with less pain than PTGBD. This single endoscopist experience nicely shows that EUS can be effectively used to gain access to and drain an acutely inflamed gallbladder. Thus, this procedure likely has a role in the treatment of acute cholecystitis. However, drainage of the gallbladder by either the percutaneous or endoscopic approaches should be relatively uncommon. Notably, in this study, 16% of patients had these procedures performed. Furthermore, medical treatment was classified as a failure after only 24 hours of antibiotics, an insufficient time to establish adequate tissue levels. Importantly, nearly 88% of patients ultimately underwent cholecystectomy within 5 to 6 days. This approach begs the question of whether a true indication existed for the drainage procedures. What changed dramatically that the patient became an operative candidate within 5 days? Could these patients really not have undergone a cholecystectomy? As emerging technology allows us to offer new treatments, we need to ensure that these approaches are indeed indicated.

K. E. Behrns, MD

Liver Transplantation for Nonalcoholic Steatohepatitis: The New Epidemic
Agopian VG, Kaldas FM, Hong JC, et al (Dumont-UCLA Transplant and Liver Cancer Ctrs, Los Angeles, CA; et al)
Ann Surg 256:624-633, 2012

Objective.—To analyze incidence, outcomes, and utilization of health care resources in liver transplantation (LT) for nonalcoholic steatohepatitis (NASH).

Summary of Background Data.—With the epidemic of obesity and metabolic syndrome in nearly 33% of the US population, NASH is projected to become the leading indication for LT in the next several years. Data on predictors of outcome and utilization of health care resources after LT in NASH is limited.

Methods.—We conducted an analysis from our prospective database of 144 adult NASH patients who underwent LT between December 1993 and August 2011. Outcomes and resource utilization were compared with other common indications for LT. Independent predictors of graft and patient survival were identified.

Results.—The average Model for End-Stage Liver Disease score was 33. The frequency of NASH as the primary indication for LT increased from 3% in 2002 to 19% in 2011 to become the second most common indication for LT at our center behind hepatitis C. NASH patients had significantly longer operative times (402 vs 322 minutes; $P < 0.001$), operative blood loss (18 vs 14 packed red blood cell units; $P = 0.001$), and posttransplant length of stay (35 vs 29 days; $P = 0.032$), but 1-, 3-, and 5-year graft (81%, 71%, 63%) and patient (84%, 75%, 70%) survival were comparable with other diagnoses. Age greater than 55 years, pretransplant intubation, dialysis, hospitalization, presence of hepatocellular carcinoma on explant, donor age greater than 55 years, and cold ischemia time greater than 550 minutes were significant independent predictors of survival for all patients, whereas body mass index greater than 35 was a predictor in NASH patients only.

Conclusions.—We report the largest single institution experience of LT for NASH. Over a 10-year period, the frequency of LT for NASH has increased 5-fold. Although outcomes are comparable with LT for other indications, health care resources are stressed significantly by this new and increasing group of transplant candidates.

▶ Nonalcoholic steatohepatitis (NASH) has become one of the most frequently diagnosed liver diseases and it is often accompanied by significant comorbidities of the metabolic syndrome including abdominal obesity, hypertension, diabetes mellitus, and dyslipidemia. Although the manifestations of NASH may be subclinical in some cases, it also may cause substantial hepatic injury that results in cirrhosis and end-stage liver disease. Agopian et al demonstrate in this work that 144 of 1294 patients undergoing liver transplant between 1993 and 2011 developed liver disease that required transplantation. The incidence of transplantation for NASH increased 5-fold in the past decade. The results demonstrated that patient and graft survival were equal to or better than the most common indicators for liver transplantation. However, the resource consumption for this group of especially ill patients was greater than that of patients who underwent transplantation for other diagnoses. Patients who were deemed high risk by multivariate analysis included those patients with a body mass index greater than 35 and those patients requiring pretransplant hemodialysis. This article is enlightening and should create consternation in the medical community because it highlights the scope of the problem of patients with advanced liver disease from NASH. Although liver transplantation may be an effective treatment for NASH, the sheer prevalence of NASH suggests that we need to treat NASH well before patients develop advanced liver disease. As the discussants point out, bariatric surgery may be an effective treatment in some patients. However, it is clear that we need a bona fide national education program to address the obesity epidemic so we can limit health care resource consumption for this devastating disease.

K. E. Behrns, MD

Long-Term Survival, Nutritional Autonomy, and Quality of Life After Intestinal and Multivisceral Transplantation
Abu-Elmagd KM, Kosmach-Park B, Costa G, et al (Univ of Pittsburgh Med Ctr, PA)
Ann Surg 256:494-508, 2012

Objective.—To assess long-term survival, graft function, and health-related quality of life (QOL) after visceral transplantation.

Background.—Despite continual improvement in early survival, the long-term therapeutic efficacy of visceral transplantation has yet to be defined.

Methods.—A prospective cross-sectional study was performed on 227 visceral allograft recipients who survived beyond the 5-year milestone. Clinical data were used to assess outcome including graft function and long-term survival predictors. The socioeconomic milestones and QOL measures were assessed by clinical evaluation, professional consultation, and validated QOL inventory.

Results.—Of 376 recipients, 227 survived beyond 5 years, with conditional survival of 75% at 10 years and 61% at 15 years. With a mean follow-up of 10 ± 4 years, 177 (92 adults, 85 children) are alive, with 118 (67%) recipients 18 years or older. Nonfunctional social support and noninclusion of the liver in the visceral allograft are the most significant survival risk factors. Nutritional autonomy was achievable in 160 (90%) survivors, with current serum albumin level of 3.7 ± 0.5 gm/dL and body mass index of 25 ± 6 kg/m^2. Despite coexistence or development of neuropsychiatric disorders, most survivors were reintegrated to society with self-sustained socioeconomic status. In parallel, most of the psychological, emotional, and social QOL measures significantly ($P < 0.05$) improved after transplantation. Current morbidities with potential impact on global health included dysmotility (59%), hypertension (37%), osteoporosis (22%), and diabetes (11%), with significantly ($P < 0.05$) higher incidence among adult recipients.

Conclusions.—With new tactics to further improve long-term survival including social support measures, visceral transplantation has achieved excellent nutritional autonomy and good QOL.

▶ Intestinal transplantation has had a checkered history, but with persistence by groups of focused transplant centers the benefits of this life-saving operation have been realized. Abu-Elmagd et al have played a primary role in advancing our knowledge in intestinal and multivisceral transplantation and have applied this information to enhance functional survival after these operations. In this comprehensive report, the authors demonstrated that 60% of patients survived more than 5 years and that 90% of these patients had a functional gastrointestinal tract with excellent weight gain. In addition, approximately 1 in 4 patients experienced neuropsychiatric disorders; however, the vast majority of patients obtained high school or college degrees despite the stresses of chronic disease and the necessary treatment. This article is a bit unique in that it goes beyond relaying the bare results of intestinal transplantation. This report tells a story! It tells how patients function after surgical treatment of a devastating disease. We now know how these patients live because the authors were diligent in assessing quality of life. As we move to patient-centered care, we need to focus on patient satisfaction and functional outcomes.

K. E. Behrns, MD

Laparoscopic Distal Pancreatectomy: Trends and Lessons Learned Through an 11-Year Experience
Kneuertz PJ, Patel SH, Chu CK, et al (Emory Univ School of Medicine, Atlanta, GA; et al)
J Am Coll Surg 215:167-176, 2012

Background.—As compared with open distal pancreatectomy, laparoscopic distal pancreatectomy (LDP) is associated with lower morbidity and shorter hospital stays. Existing reports do not elucidate trends in patient selection, technique, and outcomes over time. We aimed to determine outcomes after LDP at a specialized center, analyze trends of patient selection and operative technique, and validate a complication risk score (CRS).

Study Design.—Patients undergoing LDP between January 2000 and January 2011 were identified and divided into 2 equal groups to represent our early and recent experiences. Demographics, tumor characteristics, operative technique, and perioperative outcomes were examined and compared between groups. A CRS was calculated for the entire cohort and examined against observed outcomes.

Results.—A total of 132 LDPs were attempted, of which 8 (6.1%) were converted to open procedures. Thirty-day overall and major complication rates were 43.2% and 12.9%, respectively, with mortality <1%. Pancreatic fistulas occurred in 28 (21%) patients, of which 14 (11%) were clinically significant. Recent LDPs (n = 66) included patients with increasingly severe comorbidities (Charlson scores >2, 40.9% vs 16.7%, $p = 0.003$), more proximal tumors (74.2% vs 26.2%, $p < 0.001$), more extended resections (10.6 vs 8.3 cm, $p < 0.001$), shorter operative times (141 vs 172 minutes, $p = 0.007$), and less frequent use of a hand port (25.8% vs 66.6%, $p < 0.001$). No significant differences were found in perioperative outcomes between the groups. As compared with the hand access technique, the total laparoscopic approach was associated with shorter hospital stays (5.3 vs 6.8 days, $p = 0.032$). Increasing CRS was associated with longer operative time, significant fistulas, wound infections, blood transfusions, major complications, ICU readmissions, and rehospitalizations.

Conclusions.—This large, single-institution series demonstrates that despite a shift in patient selection to sicker patients with more proximal tumors, similar perioperative outcomes can be achieved with laparoscopic distal pancreatectomy. The CRS appears to be a reliable preoperative assessment tool for assessing other adverse perioperative outcomes in addition to predicting overall complications and fistulas as originally published.

▶ Pancreatic surgery has experienced rapid evolution in the past few decades, with markedly improved mortality rates and the introduction of minimally invasive approaches to pancreatic disease. Laparoscopic pancreatectomy has gradually evolved to include not only distal pancreatectomy, but also laparoscopic pancreatoduodenectomy performed by a select group of surgeons and institutions. Although laparoscopic distal pancreatectomy has been performed with increasing frequency, the overall rate of adoption has been slow. Kneuertz et al, however, demonstrate that laparoscopic distal pancreatectomy has evolved and should be the procedure of choice for benign and malignant pathologies of the pancreas. Their work nicely shows that patients with more complex disease have been treated by laparoscopic resection without diminution of outcomes. Furthermore, patients with complex pancreatic pathologies and significant comorbidities have good outcomes with laparoscopic pancreatic resection. Importantly, the authors have clearly evolved the technical approach as well with increasing use of the medial-to-lateral approach, which offers increased margin resection for malignant or potentially malignant tumors and allows more precise anatomic landmarks and dissection. However, this series of patients does demonstrate the continued need for evolution of the techniques because hand-assisted laparoscopic pancreatectomy has few solid indications. Almost all distal pancreatic resections can be performed by the total laparoscopic approach. Also, it appears that splenic preservation has fallen out of favor, but this operation, although technically challenging, should be offered to patients with benign disease and perhaps in cases in which the chance for malignancy is low. Nonetheless, this work demonstrates the evolution of laparoscopic pancreatic surgery for distal lesions and clearly shows that this approach should be the procedure of choice for most pathologies.

K. E. Behrns, MD

Patient Readmission and Mortality after Surgery for Hepato-Pancreato-Biliary Malignancies
Schneider EB, Hyder O, Wolfgang CL, et al (Johns Hopkins Univ School of Medicine, Baltimore, MD; Johns Hopkins Hosp, Baltimore, MD)
J Am Coll Surg 215:607-615, 2012

Background.—The incidence and associated risk factors for readmission after hepato-pancreato-biliary surgery are poorly characterized. The objective of the current study was to compare readmission after pancreatic vs hepatobiliary surgical procedures, as well as to identify potential factors associated with higher readmission within 30 days of discharge.

Study Design.—Using Surveillance, Epidemiology and End Results—Medicare linked data from 1986—2005, we identified 9,957 individuals aged 66 years and older who underwent complex hepatic, biliary, or

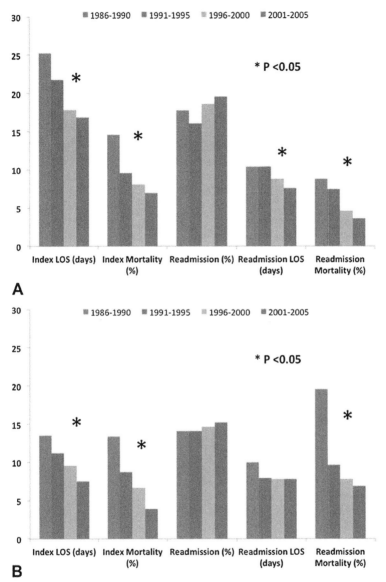

FIGURE 1.—Data on index admission length of stay (LOS), mortality, as well as incidence of readmission, readmission LOS, and readmission mortality for pancreas procedures (A) and hepatobiliary procedures (B). (Reprinted from the Journal of the American College of Surgeons. Schneider EB, Hyder O, Wolfgang CL, et al. Patient readmission and mortality after surgery for hepato-pancreato-biliary malignancies. *J Am Coll Surg.* 2012;215:607-615, Copyright 2012, with permission from the American College of Surgeons.)

pancreatic procedures for cancer treatment and were eligible for analysis. In-hospital morbidity, mortality, and 30-day readmission were examined.

Results.—Primary surgical treatment consisted of a pancreatic (46.7%), hepatic (50.0%), or biliary (3.4%) procedure. Mean patient age was

72.6 years and most patients were male (53.2%). The number of patients with multiple preoperative comorbidities increased over time (patients with Elixhauser's comorbidity score > 13: 1986–1990, 47.0% vs 2001–2005, 62.9%; $p < 0.001$). Pancreatic operations had higher inpatient mortality vs hepatobiliary procedures (9.2% vs 7.3%; $p < 0.001$). Mean length of stay after pancreatic procedures was longer compared with hepatobiliary procedures (19.7 vs 10.3 days; $p < 0.001$). The proportion of patients readmitted after a pancreatic (1986–1990, 17.7%; 1991–1995, 16.1%; 1996–2000, 18.6%; 2001–2005, 19.6%; $p = 0.15$) or hepatobiliary (1986–1990, 14.3%; 1991–1995, 14.1%; 1996–2000, 15.2%; 2001–2005, 15.5%; $p = 0.69$) procedure did not change over time. Factors associated with increased risk of readmission included preoperative Elixhauser comorbidities > 13 (odds ratio = 1.90) and prolonged index hospital stay ≥ 10 days (odds ratio = 1.54; both $p < 0.05$). During the readmission, additional morbidity and mortality were 46.5% and 8.0%, respectively.

Conclusions.—Although the incidence of readmission did not change across the time periods examined, readmission was higher among patients undergoing a pancreatic procedure vs a hepatobiliary procedure. Other factors associated with risk of readmission included number of patient comorbidities and prolonged hospital stay. Readmission was associated with additional short-term morbidity and mortality (Fig 1).

▶ Readmission rates to acute care hospitals have captured the attention of many hospital administrators and physicians because the Center for Medicare and Medicaid Services has tied readmission rates to reimbursement. Although most hospital readmissions are for chronic medical illnesses, high-risk operations in patients with significant comorbidities carry a substantial readmission rate. Schneider et al provide a retrospective look at readmission rates for hepato-pancreato-biliary surgery for malignancy using the Surveillance, Epidemiology and End Results-Medicare Database from 1986–2005. This work is illuminating for several reasons. First, and most importantly, patients who are readmitted after these surgical procedures have a shorter long-term survival. Second, contrary to popular belief, the pressure to have shorter index lengths of stay has not influenced the readmission rate. Third, although index length of stay and mortality have decreased for these procedures, the rate of readmission has not changed over several years (Fig 1). In addition, the data show that patients with more comorbidities have poorer outcomes than those patients with fewer comorbidities. Collectively, these findings suggest that surgeons need to carefully select patients for these operations and that patients with significant comorbidities may not be good candidates. Certainly, appropriateness of care (patient selection for an operation) is an important quality metric, and we need to wrap our arms around this elusive goal and begin defining appropriate-risk patients.

K. E. Behrns, MD

Lipid-Modifying Therapies and Risk of Pancreatitis: A Meta-analysis

Preiss D, Tikkanen MJ, Welsh P, et al (BHF Glasgow Cardiovascular Res Centre, UK; Helsinki Univ Hosp, Finland; et al)
JAMA 308:804-811, 2012

Context.—Statin therapy has been associated with pancreatitis in observational studies. Although lipid guidelines recommend fibrate therapy to reduce pancreatitis risk in persons with hypertriglyceridemia, fibrates may lead to the development of gallstones, a risk factor for pancreatitis.

Objective.—To investigate associations between statin or fibrate therapy and incident pancreatitis in large randomized trials.

Data Sources.—Relevant trials were identified in literature searches of MEDLINE, EMBASE, and Web of Science (January 1, 1994, for statin trials and January 1, 1972, for fibrate trials, through June 9, 2012). Published pancreatitis data were tabulated where available (6 trials). Unpublished data were obtained from investigators (22 trials).

Study Selection.—We included randomized controlled cardiovascular end-point trials investigating effects of statin therapy or fibrate therapy. Studies with more than 1000 participants followed up for more than 1 year were included.

Data Extraction.—Trial-specific data described numbers of participants developing pancreatitis and change in triglyceride levels at 1 year. Trial-specific risk ratios (RRs) were calculated and combined using random-effects model meta-analysis. Between-study heterogeneity was assessed using the I^2 statistic.

Results.—In 16 placebo- and standard care—controlled statin trials with 113 800 participants conducted over a weighted mean follow-up of 4.1 (SD, 1.5) years, 309 participants developed pancreatitis (134 assigned to statin, 175 assigned to control) (RR, 0.77 [95% CI, 0.62-0.97; P =.03; I^2 = 0%]). In 5 dose-comparison statin trials with 39 614 participants conducted over 4.8 (SD, 1.7) years, 156 participants developed pancreatitis (70 assigned to intensive dose, 86 assigned to moderate dose) (RR, 0.82 [95% CI, 0.59-1.12; P =.21; I^2 = 0%]). Combined results for all 21 statin trials provided RR 0.79 (95% CI, 0.65-0.95; P =.01; I^2 = 0%). In 7 fibrate trials with 40 162 participants conducted over 5.3 (SD, 0.5) years, 144 participants developed pancreatitis (84 assigned to fibrate therapy, 60 assigned to placebo) (RR, 1.39 [95% CI, 1.00-1.95; P =.053; I^2 = 0%]).

Conclusion.—In a pooled analysis of randomized trial data, use of statin therapy was associated with a lower risk of pancreatitis in patients with normal or mildly elevated triglyceride levels.

▶ Acute pancreatitis generally results from 2 primary etiologic sources—gallstones and alcohol use. Hypertriglyceridemia may also cause pancreatitis but at a much lower frequency than gallstones or alcohol. In addition, the therapy for hypertriglyceridemia, namely the use of statins, has been implicated as an additional cause of pancreatitis though the data to support this supposition are weak. Thus, patients with hypertriglyceridemia may be at risk for pancreatitis from both the disease itself and from the therapy. Preiss et al sought to address this question by performing a meta-analysis to determine the rate of pancreatitis following treatment with a statin or a fibrate, a class of drugs that increase the cholesterol content in bile and, hence, the possibility of gallstone-induced pancreatitis. This was a well-designed trial that included only high-quality studies with more than 1000 patients and 1-year follow-up. Furthermore, the heterogeneity to the trials was nil. The results demonstrated that statin therapy was actually associated with a decreased risk of pancreatitis. In addition, fibrate therapy was associated with a 1.39 risk ratio of pancreatitis with 935 patients needing treatment for the cause of pancreatitis in 1 patient. Thus, this analysis demonstrates that the risk of pancreatitis from these lipid-lowering agents is nonexistent or small. This work is an important contribution to medical and surgical disciplines because we on occasion ascribe a diagnosis of medication-induced pancreatitis to agents like statins when, in fact, we should be seeking other causes of pancreatitis.

K. E. Behrns, MD

Dehydration Is the Most Common Indication for Readmission After Diverting Ileostomy Creation

Messaris E, Sehgal R, Deiling S, et al (Penn State Milton S. Hershey Med Ctr, Hershey, PA)
Dis Colon Rectum 55:175-180, 2012

Background.—Early readmission after discharge from the hospital is an undesirable outcome. Ileostomies are commonly used to prevent symptomatic anastomotic complications in colorectal resections.

Objective.—The aim of this study was to identify factors predictive of readmission after colectomy/proctectomy and diverting loop ileostomy.

Design.—This study is a retrospective review.

Patients.—Patients were included who underwent colon and rectal resections with ileostomy at our institution. Sex, age, type of disease, comorbidities, elective vs urgent procedure, type of ileostomy, operative method, steroid use, ASA score, and the use of diuretics were evaluated as potential factors for readmission.

Main Outcome Measures.—The primary outcomes measured were the need for readmission and the presence of dehydration (ostomy output ≥1500 mL over 24 hours and a blood urea nitrogen/creatinine level ≥20, or physical findings of dehydration).

Results.—Six hundred three loop ileostomies were created mostly in white (95.3%), male (55.6%) patients undergoing colon or rectal resections. IBD was the most common indication at 50.9%, with rectal cancer at 16.1%, and other at 31.0%. The 60-day readmission rate was 16.9% (n = 102) with the most common cause dehydration (n = 44, 43.1%). Regression analysis demonstrated that the laparoscopic approach ($p = 0.02$), lack of epidural anesthesia ($p = 0.004$), preoperative use of steroids ($p = 0.04$), and postoperative use of diuretics ($p = 0.0001$) were highly predictive for readmission.

Furthermore, regression analysis for readmission for dehydration identified the use of postoperative diuretics as the sole risk factor ($p = 0.0001$).

Limitations.—This study is limited by the retrospective analysis of data, and it does not capture patients that were treated at home or in clinic.

Conclusion.—Readmission after colon or rectal resection with diverting loop ileostomy was high at 16.9%. Dehydration was the major cause for readmission. Patients receiving diuretics are at increased risk for readmission for dehydration. High-risk patients should be treated more cautiously as inpatients and closely monitored in the outpatient setting to help reduce dehydration and readmission.

▶ Small bowel or colonic stomas are associated with increased risks in both the immediate and long-term postoperative periods. Ileostomies are particularly troublesome for immediate issues with dehydration and electrolyte imbalance. Not infrequently, these complications result in readmission to the hospital. In this study, Messaris et al examined 603 patients, who were discharged with a diverting ileostomy, to determine the rate of readmission. Of note, 16.9% of the patients were readmitted largely for dehydration (44%). A predictive factor for readmission for dehydration was the postoperative use of diuretics. Indeed, readmission of postsurgical patients is under heavy scrutiny, and achieving the balance of timely discharge with the associated decreased length of stay versus the risk of readmission is challenging many surgical services. However, perhaps we should conceptually change our care processes and not consider the patient dismissed from our care just because they leave the hospital. Too often we look to discharge the patient to decrease the patient census and lighten the work load. Although we certainly see patients following hospital discharge, perhaps we should develop postdischarge care protocols that would decrease the readmission rate. For instance, following ileostomy creation we should discharge the patient with a care protocol that includes phone follow-up and instructions that detail fluid and food intake, ostomy output, indications for a visit with a local physician, and indicators for the immediate return to the surgical service. We need to develop the concept of a continuum of postsurgical care that extends to home care protocols that can be followed by patients and home health service providers. These protocols will be of primary importance if we are to limit postoperative readmissions.

K. E. Behrns, MD

Can the New American Joint Committee on Cancer Staging System Predict Survival in Rectal Cancer Patients Treated With Curative Surgery Following Preoperative Chemoradiotherapy?
Moon SH, Kim DY, Park JW, et al (Research Inst and Hosp, Goyang, Korea; et al)
Cancer 118:4961-4968, 2012

Background.—Although ypStage has been known as a strong prognosticator of recurrence and survival, the detailed interaction of ypT and ypN classification on a survival rate has never been evaluated.

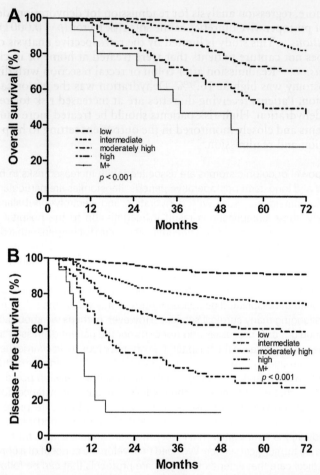

FIGURE 2.—Graphs show (A) overall survival and (B) disease-free survival according to risk group. Low: ypT0-isN0, ypT1N0, ypT2N0; intermediate: ypT0-2N1, ypT3N0; moderately high: ypT0-2N2, ypT3N1, ypT4N0; high: ypT3N2, ypT4N1-2; M+, distant metastasis (+). (Reprinted from Cancer. Moon SH, Kim DY, Park JW, et al. Can the new American Joint Committee on Cancer staging system predict survival in rectal cancer patients treated with curative surgery following preoperative chemoradiotherapy? Cancer. 2012;118:4961-4968, Copyright 2012, American Cancer Society. This material is reproduced with permission of Wiley-Liss, Inc., a subsidiary of John Wiley & Sons, Inc., _www.interscience.wiley.com.)

Methods.—Between October 2001 and December 2007, in total, 960 patients with locally advanced rectal cancer were enrolled retrospectively at 3 centers. Five-year overall survival (OS) and disease-free survival (DFS) rate were calculated for each ypTN classification.

Results.—The ypT classification interacted with ypN classification to affect survival in most categories. Patients with ypStage 0 and I cancers showed a >90% 5-year OS (ypStage 0, 96.5%; ypStage I, 92.9%; $P = .346$) and 5-year DFS (ypStage 0, 90.2%; ypStage I, 90.7%; $P = .879$). Among ypStage III subgroups, large differences in 5-year OS (ypStage

IIIA, 90.1%; ypStage IIIB, 68.3%; ypStage IIIC, 40.5%; $P < .001$) and 5-year DFS (ypStage IIIA, 74.8%; ypStage IIIB, 55.1%; ypStage IIIC, 12.3%; $P < .001$) were observed. OS and DFS in patients with ypStage IIIA disease were similar to or greater than those in patients with ypStage IIA or IIB/IIC disease. Four patient risk groups were defined: 1) low (ypT0-isN0, ypT1N0, ypT2N0), 2) intermediate (ypT0-2N1, ypT3N0), 3) moderately high (ypT0-2N2, ypT3N1, ypT4N0), and 4) high risk (ypT3N2, ypT4N1-2). Risk grouping showed a narrower range of survival rate compared with ypStage grouping.

Conclusions.—ypStage in rectal cancer, defined according to the 7th edition of the American Joint Committee on Cancer staging system, predicts survival for most ypNT classifications. However, patients with ypStage I rectal cancer have a similar prognosis to those with ypStage 0 cancer, and risk grouping reflects more precise survival outcomes than ypStage (Fig 2).

▶ The treatment of rectal cancer has been in evolution for nearly a decade since the German Rectal Cancer Study Group demonstrated the value of preoperative chemoradiotherapy. The sequencing of preoperative chemoradiotherapy prior to curative surgery has markedly altered the treatment and given rise to new questions about the role and extent of operative therapy. However, to appropriately address these questions, it is imperative that our staging systems, through which we accurately communicate and compare our results, differentiate outcomes. Moon et al retrospectively reviewed the medical records of 960 patients from 3 centers to determine if the new seventh edition of the American Joint Committee on Cancer (AJCC) staging system accurately predicted survival in patients with rectal cancer. The results demonstrated that the staging system, in most instances, accurately reflects the outcomes. However, the risk grouping developed by Gunderson et al in 2001 provides more precise staging (Fig 2). This study is important because we should continually review and compare our staging systems to ensure that they accurately predict outcomes, as clinical treatment decisions are based on accurate staging. However, 2 significant limitations of the study should be addressed: (1) a standardized approach to the delivery of chemoradiotherapy was not applied and (2) surgical therapy resulted in a lymph node harvest of 12 nodes or greater in only a little over 50% of the patients. Nonetheless, this work demonstrates the strengths and weaknesses of the AJCC staging system for rectal cancer and should be referred to frequently.

K. E. Behrns, MD

Safe and Early Discharge After Colorectal Surgery Due to C-Reactive Protein: A Diagnostic Meta-Analysis of 1832 Patients
Warschkow R, Beutner U, Steffen T, et al (Kantonsspital St Gallen, Switzerland)
Ann Surg 256:245-250, 2012

Objective.—To assess the predictive value of C-reactive protein (CRP) level for postoperative infectious complications after colorectal surgery.

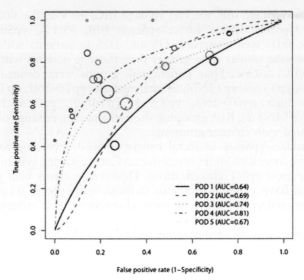

FIGURE 2.—Summary receiver operating characteristic curves postoperative infectious complications. Summary receiver operating characteristic curves were plotted for POD 1 to 5 to compare the diagnostic performance of CRP for the prediction of postoperative infectious complications. Each circle represents one study and is sized according to its weight (≅ inverse variance). AUC is the area under the curve. (Reprinted from Warschkow R, Beutner U, Steffen T, et al. Safe and early discharge after colorectal surgery due to C-reactive protein: a diagnostic meta-analysis of 1832 patients. *Ann Surg.* 2012;256:245-250. © Southeastern Surgical Congress.)

Background.—Postoperative infectious complications after colorectal surgery are frequent and associated with relevant short- and long-term sequelae. Therefore, the identification of a diagnostic tool for early recognition of postoperative infectious complications is of cardinal importance.

Methods.—A meta-analysis was performed for diagnostic studies evaluating CRP as a predictor for postoperative infectious complications on days 1 to 5 after colorectal surgery.

Results.—Six studies including a total of 1832 patients were identified. The best performance of CRP to predict postoperative infectious complications was on postoperative day 4, on which the mean CRP cutoff value was 135 mg/L (SD: 10 mg/L), the pooled sensitivity 68% (95% CI: 57%−79%), the specificity 83% (95% CI: 77%−90%) and the negative predictive value 89% (95% CI: 87%−92%). The pooled area under the receiver operating characteristic curve was 0.81 (95% CI: 0.73−0.89).

Conclusions.—This diagnostic meta-analysis of 1832 patients—the first in the literature—provides compelling evidence that C-reactive protein on postoperative day 4 has a high negative predictive value for infectious complications of 89%. Therefore, CRP measurement allows safe and early discharge of selected patients after colorectal surgery (Fig 2).

▶ The rising costs of health care have placed a premium on the duration of hospital stays for acute illnesses, and thus early discharge of patients is economically advantageous for hospitals and payers. However, early discharge of nonselect patients may lead to an increased rate of readmission, now a measure of quality and likely a parameter that will be incorporated in pay-for-performance reimbursement models. Therefore, the surgeon often faces the conundrum of discharging a patient early with a likelihood that the patient will return with a yet to-be identified complication. Warschkow et al have provided data that may help select patients for appropriate early discharge. They performed a meta-analysis of 1832 patients who underwent colorectal surgery and had a C-reactive protein (CRP) concentration determined at multiple time points postoperatively. They found that a patient with a CRP of less than 135 mg/L on postoperative day 4 had an 89% chance of not being readmitted to the hospital (Fig 2). This important finding may lead to a number of studies that will examine markers for safe and early discharge from the hospital. Although within the surgical and medical community, we bemoan regulations that may penalize us for longer lengths of stay, this work demonstrates the resolve and adaptability of identifying markers of safe early discharge. We should continue to seek biomarkers for multiple phases of caring including selection for an operation, early discharge, and candidacy for adjuvant therapy so that our care processes are more selectively applied.

K. E. Behrns, MD

Hospital Cost Analysis of a Prospective, Randomized Trial of Early vs Interval Appendectomy for Perforated Appendicitis in Children

Myers AL, Williams RF, Giles K, et al (Univ of Tennessee Health Science Ctr, Memphis; et al)

J Am Coll Surg 214:427-435, 2012

Background.—The methods of surgical care for children with perforated appendicitis are controversial. Some surgeons prefer early appendectomy; others prefer initial nonoperative management followed by interval appendectomy. Determining which of these two therapies is most cost-effective was the goal of this study.

Design.—We conducted a prospective, randomized trial in children with a preoperative diagnosis of perforated appendicitis. Patients were randomized to early or interval appendectomy. Overall hospital costs were extracted from the hospital's internal cost accounting system and the two treatment groups were compared using an intention-to-treat analysis. Nonparametric data were reported as median ± standard deviation (or range) and compared using a Wilcoxon rank sum test.

Results.—One hundred thirty-one patients were randomized to either early (n = 64) or interval (n = 67) appendectomy. Hospital charges and costs were significantly lower in patients randomized to early appendectomy. Total median hospital costs were $17,450 (range $7,020 to $55,993) for patients treated with early appendectomy vs $22,518 (range $4,722 to $135,338) for those in the interval appendectomy group. Median hospital costs more than doubled in patients who experienced an adverse event ($15,245 vs $35,391, $p < 0.0001$). Unplanned readmissions also increased costs significantly and were more frequent in patients randomized to interval appendectomy.

Conclusions.—In a prospective randomized trial, hospital charges and costs were significantly lower for early appendectomy when compared with interval appendectomy. The increased costs were related primarily to the significant increase in adverse events, including unplanned readmissions, seen in the interval appendectomy group.

▶ Determining the optimal surgical treatment for conditions that may be managed either immediately in the acute inflammatory setting or in a delayed fashion after the acute inflammation has subsided is often difficult to study because of the numerous variables involved and the diverse opinions of surgeons. Furthermore, the economic consequences of early versus delayed intervention are often not considered in randomized, clinical trials because the clinical variables, which determine patient outcomes, must be determined prior to any cost analysis. Therefore, Myers et al should be congratulated for completing this 2-study process that first determined that clinical outcomes are improved with early intervention and, subsequently, that early intervention is associated with less cost than delayed treatment. This study nicely showed that delayed intervention was more costly because the patients had a longer hospital stay, experienced more adverse events, and had a delayed return to normal activities. This study confirms previous findings that early intervention is associated with improved outcomes and decreased costs, and early intervention should thus become the default mode of treatment for children with perforated appendicitis. Whether these findings can or should be translated to other clinical conditions such as acute cholecystitis in adults is unknown. However, perhaps we should adopt early intervention as the primary approach and determine if delayed intervention is inferior. Finally, this study is important because, as the authors noted, it is an outstanding example of clinical work that determines outcome as defined by the Patient-Centered Outcomes Research Institute that was established by the Patient Protection and Affordable Care Act of 2010.

K. E. Behrns, MD

Appendectomy Timing: Waiting Until the Next Morning Increases the Risk of Surgical Site Infections
Teixeira PG, Sivrikoz E, Inaba K, et al (Los Angeles County + Univ of Southern California Med Ctr)
Ann Surg 256:538-543, 2012

Objective.—To investigate the association between time from admission to appendectomy (TTA) and the incidence of perforation and infectious complications.

Background.—Immediate appendectomy to prevent perforation has been challenged by recent studies supporting a semielective approach to acute appendicitis.

Methods.—Patients admitted with appendicitis from July 2003 to June 2011 were reviewed. Age, sex, admission white blood cell count, surgical approach (open vs laparoscopic), TTA, and pathology report were abstracted. Primary outcomes included perforation and surgical site infection (SSI). Logistic regression was performed both to identify independent predictors of perforation and to investigate the association between TTA and SSI.

Results.—Over 8 years, 4529 patients were admitted with appendicitis and 4108 (91%) patients underwent appendectomy. Perforation occurred in 23% (n = 942) of these patients. Logistic regression identified 3 independent predictors of perforation: age 55 years or older [odds ratio (95% confidence interval) OR (95% CI), 1.66 (1.21−2.29); $P = 0.002$], white blood cell count more than 16,000 [OR (95% CI), 1.38 (1.15−1.64); $P < 0.001$], and female sex [OR (95% CI), 1.20 (1.02−1.41); $P = 0.02$]. Delay to appendectomy was not associated with higher perforation rate. However, after controlling for age, leukocytosis, sex, laparoscopic approach, and perforation, TTA of more than 6 hours was independently associated with an increase in SSI [OR (95% CI), 1.54 (1.01−2.34); $P = 0.04$]. Delay of more than 6 hours resulted in a significant increase in SSI from 1.9% to 3.3% among patients with nonperforated appendicitis [OR (95% CI), 2.16 (1.03−4.52); $P = 0.03$], raising the incidence of SSI in nonperforated appendicitis to levels similar to those with perforation (3.3% vs 3.9%, $P = 0.47$).

Conclusions.—In this series, appendectomy delay did not increase the risk of perforation but was associated with a significantly increased risk of SSI in patients with nonperforated appendicitis. Prompt surgical intervention is warranted to avoid additional morbidity in this population.

▶ The past decade has witnessed the evolution of semielective operative care of the patient with acute appendicitis. Many of the patients that require appendectomy now have surgery as the first case of the day rather than undergoing an appendectomy in the middle of the night. Although convenient for the health care team, the data supporting this approach have been controversial. In this article, Teixeira et al contribute significant and compelling information about the timing of surgical treatment of patients that need an appendectomy. They found that a delay to surgical treatment of longer than 6 hours did not increase the risk of perforation, but was associated with an increased risk of surgical site infection, which was defined as a wound infection or intra-abdominal abscess. Importantly, the authors note that the complication profile of patients with a nonperforated appendicitis becomes more like that of a patient with a perforated appendix when the time to appendectomy is greater than 6 hours. This is likely a costly transformation in terms of risk to the patient and health care resource usage. Even though a formal cost analysis was not performed in this study, the risks to the patients are important and the costs at individual hospitals are likely overplayed. However, if a hospital offers acute care to patients with appendicitis, then it should be willing to offer expeditious surgical treatment. The argument should not pit the patient's well-being against the hospital margin. Hospitals and care providers must live the patient-first health care model and clearly delineate the type of health care they wish to provide. Not all hospitals need to provide a broad array of services to all patients, and in fact, regionalization of care may be a cost-effective approach.

K. E. Behrns, MD

Appendectomy by Residents Is Safe and Not Associated With a Higher Incidence of Complications: A Retrospective Cohort Study
Graat LJ, Bosma E, Roukema JA, et al (St Elisabeth Hosp, Tilburg, The Netherlands)
Ann Surg 255:715-719, 2012

Objective.—The purpose of this retrospective cohort study was to investigate whether current practice where residents perform appendectomies affects quality of care. Therefore, we investigated whether there was a difference in incidence of complications and mortality in appendectomies performed by surgeons (S), supervised residents (SR), or unsupervised residents (UR).

Background.—Appendicitis is among the most frequent conditions requiring urgent surgery. Admittance and surgery are often managed by residents. Recent studies have shown that laparoscopic appendectomy can be safely performed by residents. It is not known whether these results are applicable on appendectomies in general.

Methods.—All patients undergoing appendectomy in our hospital between January 1, 2000, and December 31, 2009, were included in the analysis. Patients undergoing appendectomy by surgeons, supervised residents,

---

TABLE 3.—Outcomes After Operation

	S, n (%)	SR, n (%)	UR, n (%)	S vs SR	S vs UR	SR vs UR
					P	
Patients, n	333	557	561			
Total hospital stay, days, median (minimum—maximum)†	4 (1—89)	4 (1—80)	4 (1—59)	0.538	0.077	0.003
Patients readmitted	30 (9)	41 (5)	35 (6)	0.375	0.143	0.478
Patients with complications	68 (20)	94 (17)	92 (16)	0.209	0.149	0.872
No. complications per patient, median (minimum—maximum)†	0 (0—5)	0 (0—7)	0 (0—6)	0.178	0.085	0.686
Patients with an intra-abdominal abscess	17 (5)	24 (4)	24 (4)	0.622	0.621	1.000
Patients with a wound-infection	10 (3)	20 (4)	24 (4)	0.705	0.371	0.645
Patients with reoperations	25 (8)	37 (7)	31 (6)	0.683	0.255	0.455
No. operations per patient, median (minimum—maximum)†	1 (1—4)	1 (1—7)	1 (1—5)	0.665	0.255	0.428
In-hospital mortality	1 (0)	1 (0)	2 (0)	1.000	1.000	1.000

S indicates surgeon; SR, supervised resident; UR, unsupervised resident.
*All *P* values calculated by the Fisher exact test, unless stated otherwise.
†Mann—Whitney *U* test.

and unsupervised residents were compared. Primary endpoints were complications and mortality.

Results.—During the study period, 1538 patients were operated. The risk of complications (S: 20% vs SR: 17% vs UR: 16%; $P = 0.209$, S vs SR; $P = 0.149$, S vs UR; and $P = 0.872$, SR vs UR) and mortality (S: 0.3% vs SR: 0.2% vs UR: 0.4%, $P = 1.000$ for all comparisons) were similar in all groups. In the multivariate model, the odds ratio for complications in the group operated by supervised residents was 0.84 (95% CI: 0.58−1.22, $P = 0.357$) versus 0.81 (95% CI: 0.55−1.18, $P = 0.265$) in the unsupervised residents group.

Conclusions.—Current practice where residents perform appendectomies either unsupervised or supervised by an experienced surgeon should not be discouraged. We found that it is safe and does not lead to more complications or negatively affect quality of care (Table 3).

▶ Graat et al performed a retrospective review of a carefully managed database to determine the impact of resident performance on patient outcome following open or laparoscopic appendectomy. Complications were determined for 3 groups of surgeons: surgeons, supervised residents, and unsupervised residents. The results showed that the patients in each group were evenly matched, and no difference in outcome was notable (Table 3). Furthermore, when adjusting for multiple factors, multivariate logistic regression failed to show any difference in complications among the surgeon groups. However, this work must be put in the context of an article[1] published just 1 month earlier that shows resident participation is an independent risk factor, by 27%, for complications. It is important to note that in the study by Graat et al in the Netherlands, resident supervision is not required, and thus, 561 patients in this study arm had an appendectomy performed by an unsupervised resident. Conversely, in the Scarborough et al study, presumably most, if not all, of the operations were supervised by a faculty member. Thus, one may anticipate that the Graat et al study would identify resident participation as a risk factor for complications. There is no readily identifiable explanation for the major difference in the findings of these studies. However, an important question to ask may be "what are our alternatives?" Certainly, we need to train the next generation of surgeons to deliver high-quality care with few complications, and perhaps in the United States we need to reexamine how we train residents or surgeons to care for patients with appendicitis such that resident involvement results in no detriment in care.

K. E. Behrns, MD

Reference

1. Scarborough JE, Bennett KM, Pappas TN. Defining the impact of resident participation on outcomes after appendectomy. *Ann Surg.* 2012;255:577-582.

Transanal endoscopic microsurgery: safe for midrectal lesions in morbidly obese patients

Kumar AS, Chhitwal N, Coralic J, et al (Washington Hosp Ctr, DC)
Am J Surg 204:402-405, 2012

Background.—Transanal endoscopic microsurgery is a safe option for proximal rectal tumors in morbidly obese patients for whom transabdominal pelvic dissection often is fraught with morbidity.

Methods.—From a database of 318 patients who underwent transanal endoscopic microsurgery, we report a retrospective case-control study of 9 patients with a body mass index range of 35 to 66 with sessile rectal lesions 6 to 15 cm from the anal verge who underwent transanal endoscopic microsurgery. Case subjects were compared with 15 controls and matched for age, tumor type, and level of tumor. The average body mass index of controls was 30 ($P < .001$). By using t test analysis, perioperative outcomes (surgical time, blood loss, and hospital length of stay) and postoperative complications were compared.

Results.—Sessile tumors were located 7 to 11 cm from the anal verge with a diameter of 1 to 4 cm. Patient and tumor factors such as age, distal tumor margin from anal verge, and tumor diameter were not significantly different between case subjects and controls. Surgical blood loss, surgical time, and hospital length of stay were not significantly different between the 2 groups. One complication occurred among the cases. No complications occurred in the control group. All patients had complete surgical resections with negative margins.

Conclusion.—Transanal endoscopic microsurgery in morbidly obese patients is a safe, feasible, and a viable alternative to low anterior resection (Table 3).

▶ The increasing number of morbidly obese patients who require surgery has presented significant technical and management challenges to surgeons. The technical difficulties may even preclude performance of the optimal operation, whereas management issues related to poor wound healing from diabetes and cardiopulmonary issues substantially increase morbidity. Therefore, alternative surgical approaches should be considered. Kumar et al addressed the issue of surgical removal of rectal tumors in morbidly obese patients by performing

TABLE 3.—Results: Intraoperative and Postoperative Variables

	Patients With BMI >35 (Group 1)		Patients With BMI ≤35 (Group 2)			
	Mean	SD	Mean	SD	P Value	
Blood loss, mL	72.5	131.5	27.3	42.6	.22	NS
Surgical time, min	104	39	145	.19	.19	NS
Hospital length of stay, d	.66	.7	.26	.45	.11	NS

NS = nonsignificant; SD = standard deviation.

transanal microsurgery. This surgical technique has become popular for T1 rectal cancers, and use of this procedure may therefore limit morbidity in obese patients. This case-matched study showed that the outcomes from this procedure did not differ between obese and nonobese patients (Table 3). Even though this study is small, it provides proof that alternative approaches to surgical removal of rectal lesions is possible in obese patients. Furthermore, this study may foreshadow the use of approaches such as natural orifice translumenal endosurgery in patients in whom a transabdominal approach may lead to increased risk and complications. As general surgeons know, a surgical site infection in a morbidly obese patient leads to substantial increases in resource utilization and ultimately results in an incisional hernia, which itself is associated with increased morbidity in morbidly obese patients. As surgeons encounter more morbidly obese patients, we need to strongly consider operative approaches that will limit morbidity, and this study highlights one such approach.

K. E. Behrns, MD

Autologous Expanded Adipose-Derived Stem Cells for the Treatment of Complex Cryptoglandular Perianal Fistulas: A Phase III Randomized Clinical Trial (FATT 1: Fistula Advanced Therapy Trial 1) and Long-term Evaluation
Herreros MD, Garcia-Arranz M, Guadalajara H, et al (La Paz Univ Hosp, Madrid, Spain)
Dis Colon Rectum 55:762-772, 2012

Background.—Autologous adipose-derived stem cells may represent a novel approach for the management of complex fistula-in-ano. After successful phase I and II clinical trials, a phase III trial was performed to investigate the safety and efficacy.

Design.—In this multicenter, randomized, single-blind, add-on clinical trial, 200 adult patients from 19 centers were randomly assigned to receive 20 million stem cells (group A, 64 patients), 20 million adipose-derived stem cells plus fibrin glue (group B, 60 patients), or fibrin glue (group C, 59 patients) after closure of the internal opening. Fistula healing was defined as reepithelization of the external opening and absence of collection >2 cm by MRI. If the fistula had not healed at 12 weeks, a second dose (40 million stem cells in groups A and B) was administered. Patients were evaluated at 24 to 26 weeks (primary end point) and at 1 year (long-term follow-up).

Results.—All results are according to the "blinded evaluator" assessment. After 24 to 26 weeks, the healing rate was 39.1%, 43.3%, 37.3% in groups A, B, and C ($p = 0.79$). At 1 year, the healing rates were 57.1%, 52.4%, and 37.3 % ($p = 0.13$). On analysis of the subpopulation treated at the technique's pioneer center, healing rates were 54.55%, 83.33%, and 18.18%, at 24 to 26 weeks ($p < 0.001$). No SAEs were reported.

Conclusions.—In treatment of complex fistula-in-ano, a dose of 20 or 60 million adipose-derived stem cells alone or in combination with fibrin glue was considered a safe treatment, achieving healing rates of approximately

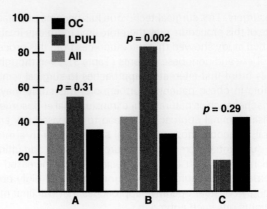

FIGURE 6.—Efficacy at 24 weeks when divided by center. *p* values correspond to the χ^2 test to measure the association between grouped center and efficacy rate at 24/26 weeks (ie, efficacy rate LPUH vs OC). LPUH = La Paz University Hospital; OC = other centers. (Reprinted from Herreros MD, Garcia-Arranz M, Guadalajara H, et al. Autologous expanded adipose-derived stem cells for the treatment of complex cryptoglandular perianal fistulas: a phase III randomized clinical trial (FATT 1: Fistula Advanced Therapy Trial 1) and long-term evaluation. *Dis Colon Rectum.* 2012;55:762-772, with permission from The ASCRS.)

40% at 6 months and of more than 50% at 1-year follow-up. It was equivalent to fibrin glue alone. No statistically significant differences were found when the 3 groups where compared. Clinical trials registration: www. clinicaltrials.gov, identifier NCT00475410; Sponsor, Cellerix SA (Fig 6).

▶ Herreros et al conducted one of the first phase III randomized trials using autologous, adipose-derived stem cells (ASC) for the treatment of complex, perianal fistulas. The study design included 3 arms: treatment with ASC alone, ASC plus fibrin glue, or fibrin glue alone. The results showed no statistically significant difference in the treatment arms, though patients treated with ASC tended to have improved outcomes. Importantly, a center difference in treatment outcomes was noted with the pioneering center demonstrating better outcomes than other centers, especially in the group of patients treated with ASC and fibrin glue (Fig 6). The reasons for these differences are not readily apparent, but suggest that experience with the treatment improves outcomes. This study is important not only because it introduces a novel approach to the treatment of perianal fistula but it provides proof of concept of the use of autologous ASC in the treatment of complex wounds. These types of studies advance our knowledge in the use of autologous stem cell therapy and will lead to markedly different treatment approaches.

K. E. Behrns, MD

Prospective, Long-Term Comparison of Quality of Life in Laparoscopic Versus Open Ventral Hernia Repair

Colavita PD, Tsirline VB, Belyansky I, et al (Carolinas Med Ctr, Charlotte, NC)
Ann Surg 256:714-723, 2012

Objectives.—To compare laparoscopic ventral hernia repair (LVHR) versus open ventral hernia repair (OVHR) for quality of life (QOL), complications, and recurrence in a large, prospective, multinational study.

Introduction.—As recurrence rates have decreased for LVHR and OVHR, QOL has become an extremely important differentiating outcomes measure.

Methods.—A prospective, international database was queried from September 2007 to July 2011 for LVHR and OVHR. Carolinas Comfort Scale (CCS) was utilized to quantify QOL (pain, movement limitation, and mesh sensation) preoperatively and at 1, 6, and 12 months postoperatively.

Results.—A total of 710 repairs included 402 OVHR and 308 LVHR. Demographics were mean age 57.1 ± 13.3 years, 49.6% male, 21.7% recurrent hernias, mean body mass index of 30.3 ± 6.6, and mean defect size of 89.4 ± 130.8. Preoperatively, 56.9% had pain, and 53.2% experienced movement limitation. At 1-month follow-up, 587 (82.7%) patients were provided CCS scores; more LVHR patients experienced pain ($P < 0.001$) and movement limitations ($P < 0.001$). At 6 and 12 months, there were no differences in QOL with 466 (65.6%) and 478 (67.3%) patients responding, respectively. After controlling for confounding variables, LVHR was independently associated with more frequent discomfort [odds ratio (OR) = 1.9, confidence interval (CI): 1.2−3.1], movement limitation (OR = 1.6, CI: 1.0−2.7), and overall symptoms (OR = 1.6, CI: 1.0−2.6) at 1 month. LVHR resulted in a shorter length of stay (LOS) ($P < 0.001$) and fewer infections ($P = 0.004$), but overall complication rates were equal. Recurrence rates were also equal ($P = 0.66$).

Conclusion.—In the largest, prospective QOL study comparing LVHR and OVHR, LVHR is associated with a decrease in QOL in the short term. LOS and infection rates are decreased in LVHR, but overall complication and recurrence rates are equal.

▶ Ventral hernia formation following surgery has been a perplexing, persistent problem for general surgeons. The recurrence rate is high and postoperative pain and discomfort frequently provide daily reminders that repair of the hernia is not a be-all and end-all. The introduction of the laparoscopic repair was greeted with enthusiasm because smaller incisions and perhaps less abdominal wall dissection would be accompanied with less postoperative pain. Colavita et al have provided important data that compare quality of life after open repair with laparoscopic repair. The authors used prospectively, patient-reported data that provided a surprising result—laparoscopic repair is associated with worse short-term quality of life outcomes! Patients who underwent laparoscopic repair had more pain and movement limitations at 1 month. At 6 months of follow-up, no differences were apparent. Importantly, the recurrence rate was not different between the groups. However, patients with laparoscopic repair had a lower infection rate and a shorter length of stay. Though the results of this study are surprising, the prospective nature of this study highlights the necessity to closely follow patients and accurately report data even though the results may not support our preconceived biases.

K. E. Behrns, MD

Randomized, Controlled, Blinded Trial of Tisseel/Tissucol for Mesh Fixation in Patients Undergoing Lichtenstein Technique for Primary Inguinal Hernia Repair: Results of the TIMELI Trial
Campanelli G, Pascual MH, Hoeferlin A, et al (Univ of Insubria-Varese, Italy; Hospital Universitario 12 de Octubre, Madrid, Spain; Hernienpraxis-Mainz, Germany; et al)
Ann Surg 255:650-657, 2012

Objective.—Test the hypothesis that fibrin sealant mesh fixation can reduce the incidence of postoperative pain/numbness/groin discomfort by up to 50% compared with sutures for repair of inguinal hernias using the Lichtenstein technique.

Background.—Inguinal hernia repair is the most common procedure in general surgery, thus improvements in surgical techniques, which reduce the burden of undesirable postoperative outcomes, are of clinical importance.

Methods.—A randomized, controlled, patient-and evaluator-blinded study (Tissucol/Tisseel for MEsh fixation in LIchtenstein hernia repair [TIMELI]; trial NCT00306839) was conducted among patients eligible for Lichtenstein repair of uncomplicated unilateral primary inguinal small—medium sized hernia. Patients were subject to mesh fixation with either fibrin sealant or sutures. Main outcome measures were visual analogue scale (VAS) assessments for "pain," "numbness," and "groin discomfort" on a scale of 0 = best and 100 = worst outcome. The primary endpoint was a composite that evaluated the prevalence of chronic disabling complications (VAS score > 30 for pain/numbness/groin discomfort) at 12 months after surgery.

Results.—In total, 319 patients were randomized between January 2006 and April 2007 (159 fibrin sealant, 160 sutures). At 12 months, the prevalence of 1 or more disabling complication was significantly lower in the fibrin sealant group than in the sutures group (8.1% vs 14.8%; $P = 0.0344$). Less pain was reported in the fibrin sealant group than in the sutures group at 1 and 6 months ($P = 0.0132$; $P = 0.0052$), as reflected by a lower proportion of patients using analgesics in the fibrin group over the study duration (65.2% vs 79.7%; $P = 0.0009$). Only 3 of 316 patients (0.9%) experienced recurrence. The incidences of wound-healing complications and other adverse events were comparable between groups.

Conclusions.—Fibrin sealant for mesh fixation in Lichtenstein repair of small—medium sized inguinal hernias is well tolerated and reduces the rate of pain/numbness/groin discomfort by 45% relative to sutures without increasing hernia recurrence (NCT00306839).

▶ Campanelli et al conducted a well-designed clinical trial to determine the postoperative complications of pain, numbness, and groin discomfort (a composite primary endpoint) in patients undergoing unilateral, small-sized, inguinal hernia Lichtenstein repairs with either fibrin sealant or suture fixation. The authors predicted that fibrin sealant would decrease the composite endpoint by 50%, although they judged that many more patients would experience these moderate-severe symptoms than actually happened. The results showed that 8.1% of the fibrin sealant group had postoperative complications that met the primary outcome, whereas 14.8% of patients in the suture group experienced these complications. Even though this difference appears small, it is important because of the large number of patients that underwent inguinal hernia repair. As the authors mention, 1 key outcome that was not studied was cost. Fibrin sealants are typically rather expensive, whereas suture is relatively cheap. However, a key point of this study and any subsequent adoption of the findings is that surgeons must embrace flexibility and change. Many experienced surgeons hold near to their heart some basic tenets and materials of surgery. For example, sutures are an integral part of surgery and any other fixation material is subpar because suture has been the mainstay for many years. Despite the importance of tradition and history and surgery, the dogmatic principles of surgery are changing and we must adapt to allow improvements in care. Importantly, we need to take the lead in embracing change and conducting novel studies that will improve care of patients.

K. E. Behrns, MD

Randomized Clinical Trial of Total Extraperitoneal Inguinal Hernioplasty vs Lichtenstein Repair: A Long-term Follow-up Study
Eker HH, Langeveld HR, Klitsie PJ, et al (Erasmus Med Ctr, Rotterdam, The Netherlands; et al)
Arch Surg 147:256-260, 2012

Hypothesis.—Mesh repair is generally preferred for surgical correction of inguinal hernia, although the merits of endoscopic techniques over open surgery are still debated. Herein, minimally invasive total extraperitoneal inguinal hernioplasty (TEP) was compared with Lichtenstein repair to determine if one is associated with less postoperative pain, hypoesthesia, and hernia recurrence.

Design.—Prospective multicenter randomized clinical trial.

Setting.—Academic research.

Patients.—Six hundred sixty patients were randomized to TEP or Lichtenstein repair.

Main Outcome Measures.—The primary outcome was postoperative pain. Secondary end points were hernia recurrence, operative complications, operating time, length of hospital stay, time to complete recovery, quality of life, chronic pain, and operative costs.

Results.—At 5 years after surgery, TEP was associated with less chronic pain (*P* =.004). Impairment of inguinal sensibility was less frequently seen after TEP vs Lichtenstein repair (1% vs 22%, *P* < .001). Operative complications were more frequent after TEP vs Lichtenstein repair (6% vs 2%, *P* < .001), while no difference was noted in length of hospital stay. After TEP, patients had faster time to return to daily activities (*P* < .002) and less absence from work (*P* =.001). Although operative costs were higher for TEP, total costs were comparable for the 2 procedures, as were overall hernia recurrences at 5 years after surgery. However, among experienced surgeons, significantly lower hernia recurrence rates were seen after TEP (*P* < .001).

Conclusions.—In the short term, TEP was associated with more operative complications, longer operating time, and higher operative costs; however, total costs were comparable for the 2 procedures. Chronic pain and impairment of inguinal sensibility were more frequent after Lichtenstein repair. Although overall hernia recurrence rates were comparable for both procedures, hernia recurrence rates among experienced surgeons were significantly lower after TEP. Patient satisfaction was also significantly higher after TEP. Therefore, TEP should be recommended in experienced hands.

Trial Registration.—clinicaltrials.gov Identifier: NCT00788554.

▶ Debate over the optimal operative approach to repair an inguinal hernia has raged since the introduction of laparoscopic methods. Numerous studies have addressed a variety of techniques, but most investigations compared multiple techniques, both open and laparoscopic, without long-term follow-up. Eker et al have now added important long-term follow-up data that focused the role of surgeon experience on patient outcomes of pain and recurrence. They nicely show that total extraperitoneal (TEP) repair is associated with decreased long-term postoperative pain and groin dysesthesias. Among experienced surgeons, the rate of recurrence was lower after TEP. Surgeon experience appears to be a critical variable in the outcome after these procedures. It is interesting to note that the least- experienced surgeons (< 10 procedures) had a recurrence rate of zero in the Lichtenstein group, whereas the recurrence rate was 25% in the TEP group. Alternatively, the most experienced surgeons (> 25 procedures) was 0.5% and 4% for the TEP and Lichenstein groups, respectively. Notably, the authors comment that the criterion for the most experienced surgeons may have been set too low. Clearly, these findings point to the fact that experience plays an important role in patient outcome, and perhaps long-term mentorship or coaching would be a valuable life-long teaching tool.

K. E. Behrns, MD

Development and Validation of a Comprehensive Curriculum to Teach an Advanced Minimally Invasive Procedure: A Randomized Controlled Trial

Palter VN, Grantcharov TP (Univ of Toronto, Ontario, Canada)

Ann Surg 256:25-32, 2012

Objective.—To develop and validate a comprehensive ex vivo training curriculum for laparoscopic colorectal surgery.

Background.—Simulators have been shown to be viable systems for teaching technical skills outside the operating room; however, integration of simulation training into comprehensive curricula remains a major challenge in modern surgical education. Currently, no curricula have been described or validated for advanced laparoscopic procedures.

Methods.—This prospective, single-blinded randomized controlled trial allocated 25 surgical residents to receive either conventional residency training or a comprehensive training curriculum for laparoscopic colorectal surgery. The curriculum consisted of proficiency-based psychomotor training on a virtual reality simulator, cognitive training, and participation in a cadaver lab. The primary outcome measure in this study was surgical performance in the operating room. All participants performed a laparoscopic right colectomy, which was video recorded and assessed using 2 previously validated assessment tools. Secondary outcome measures were knowledge relating to the execution of the procedure, assessed with a multiple-choice test, and technical performance on the simulator.

Results.—Curricular-trained residents demonstrated superior performance in the operating room compared with conventionally trained residents (global score 16.0 [14.5−18.0] versus 8.0 [6.0−14.5], $P = 0.030$; number of operative steps performed 16.0 [12.5−17.5] versus 8.0 [6.0−14.5], $P = 0.021$; procedure-specific score 71.1 [54.4−81.6] versus 51.1 [36.7−74.4], $P = 0.122$). Curricular-trained residents scored higher on the multiple-choice test (10 [9−11] versus 7.5 [5.3−7.5], $P = 0.047$), and outperformed conventionally trained residents in 7 of 8 tasks on the simulator.

Conclusions.—Participation in a comprehensive ex vivo training curriculum for laparoscopic colorectal surgery results in improved technical knowledge and improved performance in the operating room compared with conventional residency training. Reg. ID#NCT 01371136.

▶ Palter and Grantcharov conducted a randomized, single-blind, controlled trial to determine if surgical residents exposed to a comprehensive curriculum for laparoscopic colectomy resulted in enhanced operative performance. This well-conducted study compared surgical performance in a conventionally trained group of surgical residents with that in a group of residents who were trained by an integrated curriculum that included virtual reality training, cognitive training, and cadaver training. The results demonstrate convincingly that residents trained through a multimodal approach that includes a well-defined curriculum performed significantly better than conventionally trained surgical residents. This study adds credence to the use of other instructional programs, like the Fundamentals of Laparoscopic Surgery and the Fundamentals of Endoscopic Surgery, which use a comprehensive curriculum along with skills acquisition sessions to teach residents surgical procedures. While incorporating this type of training in surgical residencies is important, these data and others suggest that this training model should be the standard for all new procedures. For example, percutaneous heart valve replacement is a new procedure that requires didactic and skills training. This model of training and the accompanying assessment will become the norm for surgical training of residents and experienced surgeons alike. We should embrace these new models that will instill a culture of safety and examine the proficiency of surgeons before we enter the operating room.

K. E. Behrns, MD

Nutritional screening for risk prediction in patients scheduled for abdominal operations
Kuppinger D, Hartl WH, Bertok M, et al (Univ School of Medicine, Munich, Germany; et al)
Br J Surg 99:728-737, 2012

Background.—Increased risks related to surgery might reflect the nutritional status of some patients. Such a group might benefit from perioperative nutritional support. The purpose of this study was to identify the relative importance of nutritional risk screening along with established medical, anaesthetic and surgical predictors of postoperative morbidity and mortality.

Methods.—This prospective observational study enrolled consecutive eligible patients scheduled for elective abdominal operations. Data were collected on nutritional variables (body mass index, weight loss, food intake), age, sex, type and extent of operation, underlying disease, American Society of Anesthesiologists grade and co-morbidities. A modified composite nutritional screening tool (Nutritional Risk Screening, NRS 2002) currently recommended by European guidelines was used. Relative complication rates were calculated with multiple logistic regression and cumulative proportional odds models.

Results.—Some 653 patients were enrolled of whom 132 (20·2 per cent) sustained one or more postoperative complications. The frequency of this event increased significantly with a lower food intake before hospital admission. No other individual or composite nutritional variable provided comparable or better risk prediction (including NRS 2002). Other factors significantly associated with severe postoperative complications were ASA grade, male sex, underlying disease, extent of surgical procedure and volume of transfused red cell concentrates.

Conclusion.—In abdominal surgery, preoperative investigation of feeding habits may be sufficient to identify patients at increased risk of complications. Nutritional risk alone, however, is not sufficient to predict individual risk of complications reliably.

▶ The preoperative nutritional state of a patient has long been known to influence the postoperative outcome and risk of complications. Furthermore, the complete recovery of patients with nutritional deficits is prolonged. Therefore, careful and accurate assessment of a patient's preoperative nutritional status is important so that intervention may be instituted prior to an operation. However, the screening tools used to assess nutritional risk are often complicated and cumbersome in the clinical setting. In this article, Kuppinger et al perform a thorough and elegant analysis of preoperative nutritional and other parameters that may predict risk of postoperative complications. Although the analysis is complicated, the result is straightforward in that decreased food intake in the weeks preceding operative intervention are highly predictive of postoperative complications. Physiologically, this makes sense. Even though we measure serum markers of nutrition, albumin, prealbumin, and others, changes in these serum markers may lag behind predictors like food intake. By the time the albumin or prealbumin concentration is decreasing, the patient is significantly in the catabolic state. Thus, decreased food intake may be the first nutritional parameter that is predictive of a postoperative outcome. This work also nicely points out that sometimes we don't need an expensive test to determine the patient's risk; we can just talk to them about the changes in their daily living patterns and readily determine that they have had marked changes in physical function as a result of physiologic decline.

K. E. Behrns, MD

Wound Protectors Reduce Surgical Site Infection: A Meta-Analysis of Randomized Controlled Trials
Edwards JP, Ho AL, Tee MC, et al (Univ of Calgary, Canada; Univ of British Columbia, Canada)
Ann Surg 256:53-59, 2012

Objective.—A meta-analysis of randomized clinical trials (RCTs) was conducted to evaluate whether wound protectors reduce the risk of surgical site infection (SSI) after gastrointestinal and biliary tract surgery.

Background.—The effectiveness of impervious wound edge protectors for reduction of SSI remains unclear.

Methods.—A systematic review was conducted in Medline, EMBASE, and the Cochrane Library to identify RCTs that evaluate the risk of SSI after gastrointestinal and biliary surgeries with and without the use of an impervious wound protector. The pooled risk ratio was estimated with random-effect meta-analysis. Sensitivity analyses were performed to examine the impact of structural design of wound protector, publication year, study quality, inclusion of emergent surgeries, preoperative antibiotic administration, and bowel preparation on the pooled risk of SSI.

Results.—Of the 347 studies identified, 6 RCTs representing 1008 patients were included. The use of a wound protector was associated with a significant decrease in SSI (RR $= 0.55, 95\%$ CI $0.31-0.98, P = 0.04$). There was a nonsignificant trend toward greater protective effect in studies using a dual ring protector (RR $= 0.31, 95\%$ CI $0.14-0.67, P = 0.003$), rather than a single ring protector (RR $= 0.83, 95\%$ CI $0.38-1.83, P = 0.64$). Publication year ($P = 0.03$) and blinding of outcome assessors ($P = 0.04$) significantly modified the effect of wound protectors on SSI.

Conclusions.—Our results suggest that wound protectors reduce rates of SSI after gastrointestinal and biliary surgery.

▶ Surgical site infection (SSI) remains a troublesome complication that is associated with high financial and societal costs. Many interventions have been introduced to decrease the occurrence of SSI, and while some treatments have decreased the incidence of SSI, the rate remains high, especially in colon surgery, in which an incidence of 15% or more is not uncommon. Wound protectors have been in use for several years with varying rates of adoption, and literature reports suggest that the use of these devices is not universally associated with a decreased risk of SSI. However, the studies reported have varied in design and rigor. Edwards et al conducted a well-defined, rigorous meta-analysis that included 6 studies and 1008 patients. The results showed that wound protectors do, indeed, decrease the risk of SSI. However, not all wound protectors may be associated with the same effect. This study shows that the dual-ring wound protectors tended to be more effective than the single ring with a drape. Furthermore, more recent studies included in the meta-analysis showed that the rate of SSI was decreasing over the years with the use of these devices. This suggests that other factors are involved, and the findings could be attributed to processes like perioperative temperature and glucose control, process measures included in the surgical care improvement project. Importantly, the authors note that only 10 patients would have to be treated with a wound protector to prevent a single SSI. This is an excellent therapeutic ratio. Unfortunately, because this study is a meta-analysis, cost savings from this treatment could not be assessed. Certainly, any future randomized trials should be very large and assess the financial implications of the use of wound protectors. This well-designed study, however, indicates that not only should we use wound protectors but likely the best result is obtained with a dual ring design.

K. E. Behrns, MD

Trends for Incidence of Hospitalization and Death Due to GI Complications in the United States From 2001 to 2009
Laine L, Yang H, Chang S-C, et al (Yale Univ School of Medicine, New Haven, CT; AstraZeneca, Wilmington, DE)
Am J Gastroenterol 107:1190-1195; 2012

Objectives.—Studies from the 1990s through mid-2000s report variable decreases in upper gastrointestinal (UGI) complications and differ regarding changes in lower gastrointestinal (LGI) complications. We determined

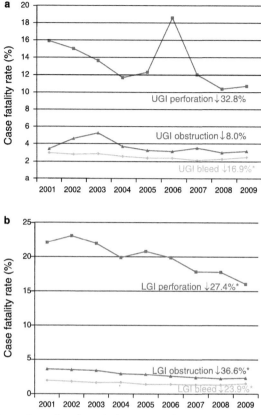

FIGURE 3.—Age- and sex-adjusted case fatality rates (%) for upper gastrointestinal (UGI) complications (a) and lower gastrointestinal (LGI) complications (b). *$P < 0.05$ for trend. (Reprinted by permission from Macmillan Publishers Ltd: American Journal of Gastroenterology, Laine L, Yang H, Chang S-C, et al. Trends for incidence of hospitalization and death due to GI complications in the United States from 2001 to 2009. *Am J Gastroenterol.* 2012;107:1190-1195. Copyright 2012.)

incidence and case fatality of hospitalizations for GI complications in the United States over the past decade.

Methods.—We used a national inpatient database to calculate yearly projections from 2001–2009 for incidence and case fatality of hospitalizations with primary discharge diagnoses of UGI and LGI complications (bleeding, perforation, and obstruction) and of undefined GI bleeding.

Results.—Age/sex-adjusted incidence of GI complications decreased nonsignificantly from 236.1 to 223.7/100,000 population from 2001–2009. Components were UGI complications (85.0 to 66.0/100,000), LGI complications (100.3 to 104.4/100,000), and undefined bleeding (50.8 to 53.3/ 100,000). Decreases were seen in UGI bleeding (78.4 to 60.6/100,000), peptic ulcer bleeding (48.7 to 32.1/100,000), LGI bleeding (41.8 to 35.7/ 100,000), and colonic diverticular bleeding (30.4 to 23.9/100,000), whereas LGI obstruction increased (55.0 to 66.0/100,000). Age/sex-adjusted case fatality decreased from 3.78 to 2.70%. 2009 case fatality rates were 2.45% for UGI bleeding, 3.00% for undefined bleeding, 1.47% for LGI bleeding, 2.30% for LGI obstruction, 10.7% for UGI perforation, and 16.0% for LGI perforation. Case fatality increased with age, but was 3.54% in patients >75 years with bleeding or obstruction.

Conclusions.—Hospitalizations for UGI complications are decreasing in the United States owing to a decrease in UGI bleeding. LGI complications are relatively stable, with a decrease in LGI bleeding and a larger increase in LGI obstruction. Case fatality owing to bleeding or obstruction is low, increasing with age but remaining < 5% even in the elderly (Fig 3).

▶ The emphasis on health care reform, with special attention to the economics of health care delivery, makes it essential that providers and leaders in the field understand the changing demographics of disease. Often practitioners are focused on the microcosm of the diseases they treat, and we fail to look outside our area of specific interest. However, this article provides excellent information about the changing demographics of gastrointestinal (GI) disease. The results of this large database study demonstrate changes in hospitalization from 2001 to 2009 and show that complications necessitating hospitalization for upper GI diseases have decreased during the study period. Furthermore, the incidence of upper GI bleeding from peptic ulcer disease also decreased markedly. Importantly, the fatality rate for upper GI diseases also decreased substantially (Fig 3). Interestingly, the incidence of hospitalization related to lower GI bleeding decreased, but complications related to lower GI (small bowel and colon) obstruction increased. The fatality from lower GI diseases also decreased significantly. This article is important because it allows us to examine resource allocation for GI diseases. Certainly, further information regarding the increasing incidence of lower GI obstruction is warranted. In addition, GI surgeons should contribute these types of demographic data related to surgical intervention in patients with GI diseases.

K. E. Behrns, MD

Thromboprophylaxis and Major Oncologic Surgery Performed With Epidural Analgesia
Shouhed D, Amersi F, Sibert T, et al (Cedars Sinai Med Ctr, Los Angeles, CA)
JAMA Surg 148:81-84, 2013

Objective.—To evaluate clinical outcomes in patients with cancer undergoing major abdominal surgery who received preoperative indwelling epidural catheters (ECs) and no postoperative thromboprophylaxis.

Design.—Retrospective analysis of a prospective database.

Setting.—Tertiary referral medical center.

Patients.—Between January 1, 2009, and July 31, 2011, 119 patients, with a mean age of 64.5 years (range, 34-95 years), underwent major abdominal oncologic surgery with an indwelling EC.

Main Outcome Measures.—Records of all patients were reviewed for age, duration of surgery, hospital length of stay, and clinical outcomes. All patients underwent lower extremity venous duplex ultrasonography prior to hospital discharge.

Results.—The average operative time was 338 minutes. Mean (SD) intensive care unit stay was 2.8 (1.4) days (range, 1-7 days). Patients ambulated by postoperative day 1 or 2. Most ECs were removed on postoperative day 4. There were no major complications from the EC. Fifty-two patients (44%) were treated with deep venous thrombosis prophylaxis on postoperative day 4 after removal of the EC. Lower extremity duplex studies showed 8 patients (6.7%) had an acute thrombus. One patient (0.8%) developed an asymptomatic proximal deep venous thrombosis and 7 patients (5.9%) developed distal superficial thrombi. No patient developed a pulmonary embolus.

Conclusions.—Thromboembolic complications following major abdominal surgery for cancer may be reduced with the use of ECs. Epidural catheters may directly prevent deep venous thrombosis through sympathetic blockade, resulting in increased blood flow to the lower extremities. This effect may also be attributable to earlier ambulation. These results suggest that patients who have an EC and do not receive concurrent postoperative thromboprophylaxis do not have an increased risk for thromboembolic events.

▶ Hopefully by now we have all incorporated thromboprophylaxis into our practices, and this should certainly include patients with cancer. In a review of 26 randomized, controlled trials evaluating 7639 patients with cancer undergoing surgery, the rate of deep venous thrombosis (DVT) without prophylaxis was found to be 35.2%, whereas 12.7% of patients receiving chemical prophylaxis had a DVT, and the combination of treatment with heparin and mechanical prophylaxis decreased the rate to 5%.[1] At the same time, the use of epidural analgesia has become more commonplace with the development of in-house acute pain services. Advantages of perioperative epidurals include reduced rates of myocardial infarction, ileus, and respiratory depression. Unfortunately, chemical thromboprophylaxis increases the risk of epidural hematoma with epidural analgesia. This study reviewed the outcome of 119 patients with various malignancies undergoing abdominal or pelvic surgery with an epidural placed preoperatively. While the epidural was in place, sequential compression devices were used without chemical prophylaxis. After the epidural was removed, 44% of patients also had chemical prophylaxis. The DVT rate was 6.7%, and all patients were successfully treated for DVT after epidural removal without any pulmonary embolism (PE). Epidural analgesia may contribute to lower DVT rates by decreasing sympathetic activity, which leads to improved lower extremity blood flow, limiting procoagulant activity, and lowering blood viscosity. We often try to minimize the risk of DVT until a fatal PE occurs with one of our patients, so diligence with DVT prophylaxis remains paramount.

J. Hines, MD

Reference

1. Weinmann EE, Salzman EW. Deep-vein thrombosis. *N Engl J Med.* 1994;331: 1630-1641.

Long-Term Outcomes of the Australasian Randomized Clinical Trial Comparing Laparoscopic and Conventional Open Surgical Treatments for Colon Cancer: The Australasian Laparoscopic Colon Cancer Study Trial

Bagshaw PF, the Australasian Laparoscopic Colon Cancer Study Group (Univ of Otago, Christchurch, New Zealand)
Ann Surg 256:915-919, 2012

Objective.—We report a multicentered randomized controlled trial across Australia and New Zealand comparing laparoscopic-assisted colon resection (LCR) with open colon resection (OCR) for colon cancer.

Background.—Colon cancer is a significant worldwide health issue. This trial investigated whether the short-term benefits associated with LCR for colon cancer could be achieved safely, without survival disadvantages, in our region.

Methods.—A total of 601 patients with potentially curable colon cancer were randomized to receive LCR or OCR. Primary endpoints were 5-year overall survival, recurrence-free survival, and freedom from recurrence rates, compared using an intention-to-treat analysis.

Results.—On April 5, 2010, 587 eligible patients were followed for a median of 5.2 years (range, 1 week-11.4 years) with 5-year confirmed follow-up data for survival and recurrence on 567 (96.6%). Significant differences between the 2 trial groups were as follows: LCR patients were older at randomization, and their pathology specimens showed smaller distal resection margins; OCR patients had some worse pathology parameters, but there were no differences in disease stages. There were no significant differences between the LCR and OCR groups in 5-year follow-up of overall survival (77.7% vs 76.0%, $P = 0.64$), recurrence-free survival (72.7% vs 71.2%, $P = 0.70$), or freedom from recurrence (86.2% vs 85.6%, $P = 0.85$).

Conclusions.—In spite of some differences in short-term surrogate onco-logical markers, LCR was not inferior to OCR in direct measures of survival and disease recurrence. These findings emphasize the importance of long-term data in formulating evidence-based practice guidelines.

▶ Laparoscopic approaches for many abdominal procedures have become commonplace and allow for reduced postoperative ileus, improved physiologic parameters, and accelerated recovery from surgery. The use of laparoscopy for cancer surgery has been a matter of debate, however. Questions include the immunologic implications of laparoscopic surgery, the adequacy and standardization of laparoscopic techniques, the risk for disease recurrence, and the impact on survival. Laparoscopic surgery for the colon was first described in the 1990s.[1]

In the initial reports of laparoscopic procedures for adenocarcinoma of the colon, a prohibitive port-site metastasis rate tempered the enthusiasm for this approach, but now these issues appear to be resolved. Laparoscopic surgery for colorectal cancer has been well studied, and the Australasian Laparoscopic Colon Cancer Study Trial reports the long-term outcomes from its randomized trial comparing laparoscopic with open resection. The group has reported previously significant improvement in the rate of return to gastrointestinal function and length of hospital stay for laparoscopic resection, but increased operative time. Those patients converted to an open operation had increased rates of pneumonia, urinary tract infections, and surgical site infections. In this report with a median follow-up of 5.2 years, no difference was identified in overall or cancer-free survival. Interestingly, only about two-thirds of patients with stage III disease received adjuvant treatment. Recurrence in the laparoscopic group tended to be found in the liver, but in the open patients these were found in the lung and peritoneum. Of the recurrences, 61.9% were identified within the first 24 months. Several reliable studies have confirmed that in experienced hands laparoscopic surgery for colon cancer has results similar to open surgery and has several short-term advantages. Surprisingly, though, most colon cancer surgery is still performed using an open technique.

J. Hines, MD

Reference

1. Phillips EH, Franklin M, Carroll BJ, Fallas MJ, Ramos R, Rosenthal D. Laparoscopic colectomy. *Ann Surg.* 1992;216:703-707.

Laparoscopic Colon Resection Trends in Utilization and Rate of Conversion to Open Procedure: A National Database Review of Academic Medical Centers
Simorov A, Shaligram A, Shostrom V, et al (Univ of Nebraska Med Ctr, Omaha)
Ann Surg 256:462-468, 2012

Objective.—This study aims to examine trends of utilization and rates of conversion to open procedure for patients undergoing laparoscopic colon resections (LCR).

Methods.—This study is a national database review of academic medical centers and a retrospective analysis utilizing the University HealthSystem Consortium administrative database—an alliance of more than 300 academic and affiliate hospitals.

Results.—A total of 85,712 patients underwent colon resections between October 2008 and December 2011. LCR was attempted in 36,228 patients (42.2%), with 5751 patients (15.8%) requiring conversion to an open procedure. There was a trend toward increasing utilization of LCR from 37.5% in 2008 to 44.1% in 2011. Attempted laparoscopic transverse colectomy had the highest rate of conversion (20.8%), followed by left (20.7%), right (15.6%), and sigmoid (14.3%) colon resections. The rate of utilization was highest in the Mid-Atlantic region (50.5%) and in medium- to large-sized hospitals (47.0%−49.0%).

Multivariate logistic regression has shown that increasing age [odds ratio (OR) = 4.8, 95% confidence interval (CI) = 3.6−6.4], male sex (OR = 1.2, 95% CI = 1.1−1.3), open as compared with laparoscopic approach (OR = 2.6, 95%, CI = 2.3−3.1), and greater severity of illness category (OR = 27.1, 95% CI = 23.0−31.9) were all associated with increased mortality and morbidity and prolonged length of hospital stay.

Conclusions.—There is a trend of increasing utilization of LCR, with acceptable conversion rates, across hospitals in the United States over the recent years. When feasible, attempted LCR had better outcomes than open colectomy in the immediate perioperative period.

▶ For some time there has been concern as to why laparoscopic surgery for colon resection was so infrequent in the United States despite excellent data confirming its efficacy for nearly all conditions. Masoomi et al have estimated that only 10% of

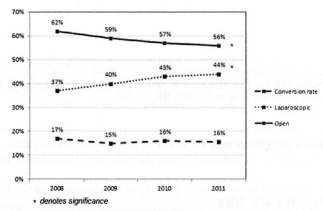

* denotes significance

FIGURE 1.—Trends of colon resections from 2008 to 2011 by approach: Laparoscopic, open, and conversion rate to an open procedure. (Reprinted from Simorov A, Shaligram A, Shostrom V, et al. Laparoscopic colon resection trends in utilization and rate of conversion to open procedure: a national database review of academic medical centers. *Ann Surg.* 2012;256:462-468, © 2012, Southeastern Surgical Congress.)

TABLE 6.—Subgroup Analysis of Outcomes of Patients Undergoing Laparoscopic Only or Laparoscopic Converted to Open Colectomy

Outcomes	Laparoscopic (n = 30,477)	Converted (n = 5,751)	P
Mortality (%)	140 (0.5)	75 (1.3)	<0.001
Morbidity (%)	2213 (7.3)	1006 (17.5)	<0.001
LOS (mean ± SD), d	6.3 ± 5.8	9.2 ± 8.9	<0.001
30-d readmission (%)	1356 (4.5)	436 (7.6)	<0.001
ICU cases (%)	2545 (8.4)	1085 (18.9)	<0.001
Cost ± SD (US$)	11,758 ± 11,124	16,785 ± 18,199	<0.001

SOI indicates severity of illness; LOS, length of stay; ICU, intensive care unit; SD, standard deviation.

resections for diverticular disease were performed with a laparoscopic technique.[1] In 2007, the reported rate of laparoscopic resection for colon cancer was 6.7%. Clearly, rolling out new operative techniques requires time for skill acquisition through retraining of practicing surgeons and the infusion of new graduates with specialized expertise. However, this study reports improved utilization of laparoscopic colon resection at university hospitals across the country (Fig 1). This trend is accompanied by a decrease in conversion rates to open operation. Left and transverse colon resections were most commonly converted to open procedures, and patients who had a converted operation had a nearly 3-fold higher mortality rate, more than twice the morbidity rate, and a longer length of stay and readmission rate (Table 6). Still, more than half of the colectomies in the United States are performed in an open fashion, but this new analysis shows that this is steadily changing.

J. Hines, MD

Reference

1. Masoomi H, Buchberg BS, Magno C, Mills SD, Stamos MJ. Trends in diverticulitis management in the United States from 2002 to 2007. *Arch Surg.* 2011;146:400-406.

Consensus Statements for Management of Barrett's Dysplasia and Early-Stage Esophageal Adenocarcinoma, Based on a Delphi Process
Bennett C, Vakil N, Bergman J, et al (Queens Univ, Belfast, UK; Univ of Wisconsin School of Medicine and Public Health, Madison; Amsterdam Med Ctr, The Netherlands; et al)
Gastroenterology 143:336-346, 2012

Background & Aims.—Esophageal adenocarcinoma (EA) is increasingly common among patients with Barrett's esophagus (BE). We aimed to provide consensus recommendations based on the medical literature that clinicians could use to manage patients with BE and low-grade dysplasia, high-grade dysplasia (HGD), or early-stage EA.

Methods.—We performed an international, multidisciplinary, systematic, evidence-based review of different management strategies for patients with BE and dysplasia or early-stage EA. We used a Delphi process to develop consensus statements. The results of literature searches were screened using a unique, interactive, Web-based data-sifting platform; we used 11,904 papers to inform the choice of statements selected. An a priori threshold of 80% agreement was used to establish consensus for each statement.

Results.—Eighty-one of the 91 statements achieved consensus despite generally low quality of evidence, including 8 clinical statements: (1) specimens from endoscopic resection are better than biopsies for staging lesions, (2) it is important to carefully map the size of the dysplastic areas, (3) patients that receive ablative or surgical therapy require endoscopic follow-up, (4) high-resolution endoscopy is necessary for accurate

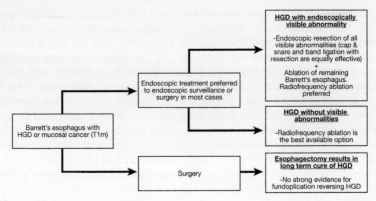

FIGURE 2.—Management of HGD and/or mucosal cancer (stage T1m) in BE. This consensus has allowed the development of a care pathway for HGD and early adenocarcinoma. (Reprinted from Gastroenterology. Bennett C, Vakil N, Bergman J, et al. Consensus statements for management of Barrett's dysplasia and early-stage esophageal adenocarcinoma, based on a Delphi process. *Gastroenterology.* 2012;143:336-346, Copyright 2012, with permission from the AGA Institute.)

TABLE 2.—Areas Ready to Be Applied to Clinical Management

Pathology
1. At least 2 experienced gastrointestinal pathologists should evaluate all Barrett's biopsies when a diagnosis of dysplasia is considered.
Endoscopy
1. The Prague C&M[a] Criteria is the best available tool for grading the endoscopic extent of BE.
2. Visible lumps in nodules consisting of HGD suggest a more advanced lesion with invasion might be present.
Populations at risk
1. Men have approximately twice the rate of developing HGD or esophageal cancer compared with women, and the rate at which EA is increasing in Western populations is twice as high in men as it is in women.
2. Non-Hispanic white patients with BE are at higher risk for development of HGD/cancer compared with other racial/ethnic groups with BE.
3. Obesity is an independent risk factor for development of EA.
Therapy
1. Endoscopic treatment should be preferred over endoscopic surveillance for management of most patients with HGD/T1m BE.
2. RFA is currently the best available ablation technique for treatment of flat HGD and for eradication of residual BE after focal EMR.
3. The operative mortality is improved if surgery is undertaken in specialist surgical centers.

NOTE. Several areas that can be applied to clinical practice now include use of Prague Criteria, recognition of subtle masses and use of ER to stage lesions.
[a]C, circumferential length, M, maximal length.

---

diagnosis, (5) endoscopic therapy for HGD is preferred to surveillance, (6) endoscopic therapy for HGD is preferred to surgery, (7) the combination of endoscopic resection and radiofrequency ablation is the most effective therapy, and (8) after endoscopic removal of lesions from patients with HGD, all areas of BE should be ablated.

Conclusions.—We developed a data-sifting platform and used the Delphi process to create evidence-based consensus statements for the management of patients with BE and early-stage EA. This approach identified important clinical features of the diseases and areas for future studies (Fig 2, Table 2).

▶ The management of Barrett's esophagus has evolved with new endoscopic modalities to ablate this metaplasia. These patients clearly need surveillance, but for many years it was clear that when high-grade dysplasia was identified, esophagectomy was recommended. This year a consensus article on the management of high-grade dysplasia and early adenocarcinoma of the esophagus was published. Surgery has become a secondary therapy for these patients according to this group, and they have stated that fundoplication is not a means to prevent progression to carcinoma (Fig 2). Many surgeons, including myself, have seen patients who have progressed to adenocarcinoma despite a fundoplication. This consensus statement recommends endoscopic resection for visible abnormalities and radiofrequency ablation for high-grade dysplasia. Additionally, the group recommends 9 areas ready for clinical application (Table 2). The field is rapidly evolving, but, in my estimation, high-grade dysplasia and early esophageal adenocarcinoma still require esophagectomy.

J. Hines, MD

Comparison Between Radical Esophagectomy and Definitive Chemoradiotherapy in Patients with Clinical T1bN0M0 Esophageal Cancer

Motoori M, Yano M, Ishihara R, et al (Osaka Med Ctr for Cancer and Cardiovascular Diseases, Japan)
Ann Surg Oncol 19:2135-2141, 2012

Background.—Esophagectomy remains the mainstay treatment for clinical T1bN0M0 esophageal cancer because pathologic lymph node metastases in these patients are not negligible. Recently, chemoradiotherapy (CRT), which can preserve the esophagus, has been reported to be a promising therapeutic alternative to esophagectomy. However, to our knowledge, no comparative studies of esophagectomy and CRT have been reported in clinical T1bN0M0 esophageal cancer.

Methods.—A total of 173 patients with clinical T1bN0M0 squamous cell carcinoma of the thoracic esophagus were enrolled in this study, 102 of whom were treated with radical esophagectomy (S group) and 71 with definitive CRT (CRT group). Treatment results of both groups were retrospectively compared.

Results.—No statistically significant difference was found in overall survival, but the S group displayed significantly better progression-free survival than the CRT group. Disease recurrence was observed in 12 S group patients and 20 CRT group patients. The incidence of distant recurrence was similar, while local recurrence and lymph node recurrence were significantly more frequent in the CRT group. In the S group, 20 patients had pathologic lymph node metastasis. The progression-free survival of patients with pathologic lymph node metastasis did not differ from those without nodal metastasis. In the CRT group, local recurrence could be

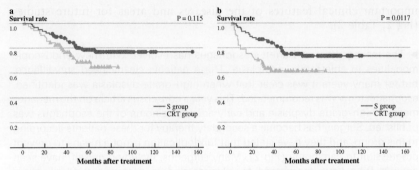

FIGURE 1.—a Overall survival curves of the S group and the CRT group. b Progression-free survival curves of the S group and the CRT group. *CRT* chemoradiotherapy. (With kind permission from Springer Science+Business Media: Motoori M, Yano M, Ishihara R, et al. Comparison between radical esophagectomy and definitive chemoradiotherapy in patients with clinical T1bN0M0 esophageal cancer. *Ann Surg Oncol*. 2012;19:2135-2141.)

controlled by salvage esophagectomy, but treatment results of lymph node recurrence were poor; only 4 of 12 patients with lymph node recurrences were cured.

Conclusions.—Selection of patients at high risk of pathologic lymph node metastasis is essential when formulating treatment decisions for clinical T1bN0M0 esophageal cancers (Fig 1).

▶ The treatment algorithms for esophageal cancer have clearly evolved over the last 5 years with the institution of more effective chemoradiation protocols. In some cases, these regimens result in complete pathologic responses, leading some to question the utility of surgical resection. Motoori et al report a case comparison investigating the use of chemoradiation alone for patients with early-stage T1bN0M0 disease. In this report, all but one patient (70 of 71) had a complete response to chemoradiation as determined by repeat endoscopy. The overall survival between the surgery and chemoradiation group was equal, but the age of the chemoradiation group was statistically older. Progression-free survival was superior, however, in the patients who underwent surgery (Fig 1). This is reflected in the fact that 28.2% of patients in the chemoradiation group were found to have recurring disease, including 12 patients with local lymph node disease. Interestingly, of the patients who had surgery, only 53.9% were found to actually be pathologic T1bN0M0, and 21 patients showed more advanced stages. Although the concept of chemoradiation alone is an appealing approach for early lesions, until reliable staging modalities are available—including improved endoscopic ultrasonography—this concept outside the context of a trial will remain experimental and should not be offered unless the patient cannot undergo resection.

J. Hines, MD

Impact of perioperative administration of synbiotics in patients with esophageal cancer undergoing esophagectomy: A prospective randomized controlled trial
Tanaka K, Yano M, Motoori M, et al (Osaka Med Ctr for Cancer and Cardiovascular Diseases, Japan; et al)
Surgery 152:832-842, 2012

Background.—The clinical value of synbiotics in patients undergoing esophagectomy remains unclear. This study investigated the effects of synbiotics on intestinal microflora and surgical outcomes in a clinical setting.

Methods.—We studied 70 patients with esophageal cancer who were scheduled to undergo esophagectomy. They were randomly allocated to 2 groups: 1 group received synbiotics before and after surgery, and the other did not. Fecal microflora and organic acid concentrations were determined. Postoperative infections, abdominal symptoms, and duration of systemic inflammatory response syndrome (SIRS) were recorded.

Results.—Of the patients, 64 completed the trial (synbiotics, 30; control, 34). The counts of beneficial bacteria and harmful bacteria in the group given synbiotics were significantly larger and smaller, respectively, than those in the control group on postoperative day (POD) 7. The concentrations of total organic acid and acetic acid were higher in the synbiotics group than in the control group $(P < .01)$, and the intestinal pH in the synbiotics group was lower than that in the control $(P < .05)$ on POD 7. The rate of infections was 10% in the synbiotics group and 29.4% in the control group $(P = .0676)$. The duration of SIRS in the synbiotics group was shorter than in the control group $(P = .0057)$. The incidence of interruption or reduction of enteral nutrition by abdominal symptoms was 6.7% in the synbiotics group and 29.4% in the control group $(P = .0259)$.

Conclusion.—Perioperative administration of synbiotics in patients with esophagectomy is useful because they suppress excessive inflammatory response and relieve uncomfortable abdominal symptoms through the adjustment of the intestinal microfloral environment.

▶ In an era when there is intense focus on postoperative complications, infections, and the pressure to shorten hospital stays, this report promises to significantly impact these issues. Esophagectomy is associated with relatively high complication rates and extended hospitalization. This group from Japan reports on the use of synbiotics to address these concerns. Synbiotics are a combination of helpful bacteria, including *Lactobacillus* and *Bifidobacterium*, along with the prebiotics, which include nondigestive food constituents that selectively alter the growth and activity of bacteria. Prebiotics comprise galacto-oligosaccharides, fructo-oligosaccharides, and inulin. This randomized study enrolled 70 patients scheduled for esophagectomy to the perioperative administration of a synbiotic (Yakult BL) vs control bacteria. Patients who received the synbiotic had lower infection rates, shorter postoperative ileus, and less perioperative inflammatory response. This was accompanied by alternations in colonic flora and fewer postoperative complaints of abdominal discomfort. Although the difference in infection rates just missed statistical significance, a 3-fold reduction was noted. The utility of synbiotics for other extensive operations like hepatobiliary surgery, liver transplantation, and colectomy has been reported. This simple intervention with synbiotics may be an important approach to address many issues with our most complex surgical patients.

J. Hines, MD

A Meta-analysis of Outcomes Following Use of Somatostatin and Its Analogues for the Management of Enterocutaneous Fistulas
Rahbour G, Siddiqui MR, Ullah MR, et al (St Mark's Hosp and Academic Inst, Harrow, Middlesex, UK)
Ann Surg 256:946-954, 2012

Objective.—Several randomized control trials (RCTs) have compared somatostatin and its analogues versus a control group in patients with enterocutaneous fistulas (ECF). This study meta-analyzes the literature and establishes whether it shows a beneficial effect on ECF closure.

Methods.—We searched MEDLINE, EMBASE, CINAHL, Cochrane, and PubMed databases according to PRISMA guidelines. Seventy-nine articles were screened. Nine RCTs met the inclusion criteria. Statistical analyses were performed using Review Manager 5.1.

Results.—Somatostatin analogues versus control

Number of fistula closed: A significant number of ECF closed in the somatostatin analogue group compared to control group, $P = 0.002$.

Time to closure: ECF closed significantly faster with somatostatin analogues compared to controls, $P < 0.0001$.

Mortality: No significant difference between somatostatin analogues and controls, $P = 0.68$.

Somatostatin versus control

Number of fistula closed: A significant number of ECF closed with somatostatin as compared to control, $P = 0.04$.

Time to closure: ECF closed significantly faster with somatostatin than controls, $P < 0.00001$.

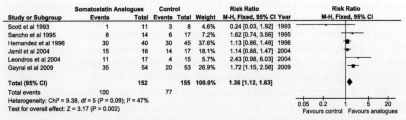

FIGURE 2.—Forest plot—Somatostatin analogues versus control. Outcome—Number of ECF closed. (Reprinted from Rahbour G, Siddiqui MR, Ullah MR, et al. A meta-analysis of outcomes following use of somatostatin and its analogues for the management of enterocutaneous fistulas. *Ann Surg.* 2012;256:946-954, © 2012, Southeastern Surgical Congress.)

	Somatostatin analogue			Control				Std. Mean Difference		Std. Mean Difference
Study or Subgroup	Mean	SD	Total	Mean	SD	Total	Weight	IV, Fixed, 95% CI Year		IV, Fixed, 95% CI
Sancho et al 1995	7	3	14	12	7	17	10.1%	-0.87 [-1.62, -0.13] 1995		
Hernandez et al 1996	18	13	40	27	13	45	29.0%	-0.69 [-1.12, -0.25] 1996		
Leondros et al 2004	16.5	16.6	17	18	5.3	15	11.5%	-0.12 [-0.81, 0.58] 2004		
Jamil et al 2004	14	5.4	16	17.7	5.4	17	11.3%	-0.67 [-1.37, 0.04] 2004		
Gayral et al 2009	17	24.5	54	26	24.5	53	38.2%	-0.36 [-0.75, 0.02] 2009		
Total (95% CI)			141			147	100.0%	-0.51 [-0.75, -0.28]		

Heterogeneity: Chi² = 3.52, df = 4 (P = 0.47); I² = 0%
Test for overall effect: Z = 4.27 (P < 0.0001)

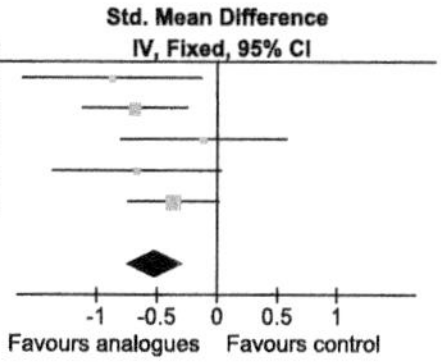

-1   -0.5   0   0.5   1
Favours analogues   Favours control

FIGURE 3.—Forest plot—Somatostatin analogues versus control. Outcome—Time to closure. (Reprinted from Rahbour G, Siddiqui MR, Ullah MR, et al. A meta-analysis of outcomes following use of somatostatin and its analogues for the management of enterocutaneous fistulas. *Ann Surg*. 2012;256:946-954, © 2012, Southeastern Surgical Congress.)

Mortality: No significant difference between somatostatin and controls, $P = 0.63$

Conclusions.—Somatostatin and octreotide increase the likelihood of fistula closure. Both are beneficial in reducing the time to fistula closure. Neither has an effect on mortality. The risk ratio (RR) for somatostatin was higher than the RR for analogues. This may suggest that somatostatin could be better than analogues in relation to the number of fistulas closed and time to closure. Further studies are required to corroborate these apparent findings (Figs 2 and 3).

▶ The utility of somatostatin or its analogues for the management of enterocutaneous fistulas has been uncertain. This meta-analysis appears to definitely clarify this issue and clearly favors the use of this approach. The authors have performed an exhaustive literature review and detailed statistical examination showing that somatostatin and somatostatin analogues (octreotide and lanreotide) speed the time to fistula closure and increase the number of fistulae closed (Figs 2 and 3). These drugs do not impact overall mortality but may make the management of electrolyte and volume replacement simpler. Even though the somatostatin appears more effective than the analogues, somatostatin requires continuous intravenous infusion. A dose of 100 µg 3 times a day subcutaneously of somatostatin analogue is more feasible. Some patients may experience abdominal cramping, but this usually resolves. Long-term analogue treatment appears to increase the formation of gallstones. Although the study also includes patients with pancreatic fistula, the results appear compelling enough to recommend this approach for all patients with enterocutaneous fistula.

J. Hines, MD

A Double-Blinded Randomized Controlled Trial of Laparoendoscopic Single-Site Access Versus Conventional 3-Port Appendectomy

Teoh AYB, Chiu PWY, Wong TCL, et al (The Chinese Univ of Hong Kong, Shatin; et al)
Ann Surg 256:909-914, 2012

Objective.—The aim of the current study was to perform a multicentered prospective double-blinded randomized controlled trial comparing

laparoendoscopic single-site access (LESS) versus conventional three-port laparoscopic appendectomy (TPLA).
Background.—The clinical benefits and disadvantages of LESS appendectomy are uncertain.
Methods.—Between October 2009 and March 2011, consecutive patients admitted with clinical or radiological evidence of appendicitis were randomly assigned to receive either LESS or TPLA. The main outcome measurement was overall pain score. Secondary outcome measurements included operative time, conversion rates, morbidity rates, activity pain scores, activity scores, patient satisfaction, and cosmesis scores.
Results.—During the study period, 200 patients were recruited to the study. There were no significant differences in the morbidity rates, operative time, conversion rates, and postoperative recovery. There were also no differences in the overall pain score and pain score at rest. However, patients in the LESS group experienced significantly more pain upon coughing or standing and required more intravenous analgesics ($P = 0.001$, 0.038, and 0.035, respectively). Wound cosmesis and satisfaction scores on the contrary were better in the LESS group ($P = 0.002$ and $P = 0.052$). No differences in the quality-of-life assessments were present at 2 weeks after operation.
Conclusions.—LESS and conventional appendectomy resulted in similar perioperative outcomes. However, LESS appendectomy resulted in worst pain scores upon exertion and required a higher dosage of intravenous analgesics when compared with TPLA. On the contrary, wound cosmesis and satisfaction scores were better in the LESS group. Hence, adoption of the technique for appendectomy will depend on patient preferences and the presence of local expertise.

▶ This group from Hong Kong presents a double-blinded, randomized, controlled trial of laparoendoscopic single-site access (LESS) compared with conventional 3-port appendectomy (TPLA). Adult patients (200) with a diagnosis of appendicitis with 5 days or less of symptoms and without a palpable right lower quadrant mass were randomized to 1 of either procedure. Reasons for exclusion from the study included previous surgery, peritonitis, extended symptoms, coagulopathy, previous pregnancy, palpable mass, shock, myocardial infarction, or refusal to enter the study. LESS was performed by making a 13-mm transumbilical incision with insertion of a 10-mm and two 5-mm trocars through separate fascial incisions. The TPLA approach included a 10-mm subumbilical port and a 5-mm port in each of the right and left lower quadrants. The mesoappendix was divided with ultrasonic dissection and the appendix ligated with 2 endoloop sutures. The fascial defects of the 10-mm ports were closed along with the skin, and 3 wound dressings were left in place simulating the wound coverage for the TPLA. This clever approach, therefore, blinded the patient and the data collection staff to the surgical technique. Evaluation of the efficacy of either procedure revealed no advantage to either approach with regard to morbidity, operative time (63 vs 60 minutes), conversion rate (8 vs 3%), or hospital stay. Overall, LESS patients reported improved cosmesis with the single-site approach and overall satisfaction with the operation. Although total pain scores were equal, patients undergoing LESS had more pain with standing and extended coughing, which correlated with higher pain medication usage. This also correlated with less activity in the LESS group early in the postoperative period. The authors surmise that the difference in pain may be explained by the fact that the total fascial incision distance is the same with each procedure, and that the pelvic peritoneum where the 5-mm TPLA trocars were introduced is less sensitive to pain triggers than the peritoneum in the rest of the abdominal cavity. However, most surgeons performing laparoscopic procedures recognize that patients complain most commonly about the umbilical trocar site, and in the LESS group all 3 ports were placed through the umbilicus. Whether single-site appendectomy ultimately becomes the newest standard is unknown. This well-executed study does demonstrate, though, that single-site appendectomy can be safely performed with little additional time over that of a traditional laparoscopic approach. Also, supply cost-savings may be realized with the described procedures in this study. The appendiceal stump can be safely controlled with an endoloop rather than an endoGIA, and a single-port approach does not require special access devices. The same trocars used for a laparoscopic appendectomy can be used for a LESS procedure.

J. Hines, MD

Irrigation Versus Suction Alone During Laparoscopic Appendectomy for Perforated Appendicitis: A Prospective Randomized Trial
St Peter SD, Adibe OO, Iqbal CW, et al (The Children's Mercy Hosp, Kansas City, MO)
Ann Surg 256:581-585, 2012

Background.—The efficacy of irrigating the peritoneal cavity during appendectomy for perforated appendicitis has been debated extensively. To date, prospective comparative data are lacking. Therefore, we conducted a prospective, randomized trial comparing peritoneal irrigation to suction alone during laparoscopic appendectomy in children.

Methods.—Children younger than 18 years with perforated appendicitis were randomized to peritoneal irrigation with a minimum of 500 mL normal saline, or suction only during laparoscopic appendectomy. Perforation was defined as a hole in the appendix or fecalith in the abdomen. The primary outcome variable was postoperative abscess. Using a power of 0.8 and alpha of 0.05, a sample size of 220 patients was calculated. A battery-powered laparoscopic suction/irrigator was used in all cases. Pre- and postoperative management was controlled. Data were analyzed on an intention-to-treat basis.

Results.—A total of 220 patients were enrolled between December 2008 and July 2011. There were no differences in patient characteristics at presentation. There was no difference in abscess rate, which was 19.1% with suction only and 18.3% with irrigation ($P = 1.0$). Duration of hospitalization was 5.5 ± 3.0 with suction only and 5.4 ± 2.7 days with group ($P = 0.93$). Mean hospital charges was \$48.1K in both groups ($P = 0.97$).

No irrigation   Irrigation

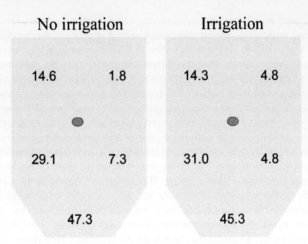

FIGURE 2.—Distribution of abscesses as percentage of abscesses per region. Comparing the percentage of abscesses per region between groups, $P = 1$ for right upper quadrant, $P = 0.80$ for left upper quadrant, $P = 1$ for right lower quadrant, $P = 0.95$ for left lower quadrant, and $P = 1$ for pelvis. (Reprinted from St Peter SD, Adibe OO, Iqbal CW, et al. Irrigation versus suction alone during laparoscopic appendectomy for perforated appendicitis: a prospective randomized trial. *Ann Surg.* 2012;256:581-585, © 2012, Southeastern Surgical Congress.)

Mean operative time was 38.7 ± 14.9 minutes with suction only and 42.8 ± 16.7 minutes with irrigation $(P = 0.056)$. Irrigation was felt to be necessary in one case (0.9%) randomized to suction only. In the patients who developed an abscess, there was no difference in duration of hospitalization, days of intravenous antibiotics, duration of home health care, or abscess-related charges.

Conclusions.—There is no advantage to irrigation of the peritoneal cavity over suction alone during laparoscopic appendectomy for perforated appendicitis. The study was registered with clinicaltrials.gov at the inception of enrollment (NCT00981136) (Fig 2).

▶ Is the solution to pollution dilution? Every surgery resident learns or has heard this statement, and intuitively it makes sense. Over the last decade however, high-quality studies have questioned this dogma. We certainly know now that antibiotic irrigation does not seem to lower infectious complications. The Children's Mercy Hospital Group in Kansas City and their Center for Prospective Clinical Trials reports a large randomized study examining the utility of irrigation for perforated appendicitis in children undergoing laparoscopic appendectomy. The study groups were well matched and the outcomes nearly the same. The abscess rate was nearly 20% and located most commonly in the pelvis and right lower quadrant (Fig 2). Despite the irrigation, the location of the abscesses did not differ between the groups. It will be hard to resist the urge to irrigate and wash out the muck associated with perforated appendicitis, but if we can simply aspirate, then we may save some time (4 minutes in the study) and resources (1 L bag of saline and a battery-powered suction/irrigation device) all the while anticipating the same outcome.

J. Hines, MD

Laparoscopic versus open adhesiolysis in patients with adhesive small bowel obstruction: A systematic review and meta-analysis

Li M-Z, Lian L, Xiao L-B, et al (Sun Yat-sen Univ, Guangzhou, China)
Am J Surg 204:779-786, 2012

Background.—The objective of this study was to evaluate whether surgical outcomes differ between laparoscopy versus the open approach for adhesive small bowel obstruction.

Methods.—PubMed, MEDLINE, Embase, and the Cochrane Library databases were electronically searched from 1985 to 2010. The study pooled the effects of outcomes of a total of 334 patients enrolled into 4 retrospective comparative studies using meta-analytic methods.

Results.—Laparoscopic adhesiolysis was associated with a reduced overall complication rate (odds ratio = .42, .25−.70, *P* < .01), prolonged ileus rate (odds ratio = .28, .10−.73, *P* = .01) and pulmonary complication rate (odds ratio = .20, .04−.94, *P* = .04) compared with the open approach. No significant differences were noted for intraoperative injury to bowel rates (odds ratio = 1.93, .76−4.89, *P* = .17), wound infection rates (odds ratio = .44, .17−1.12, *P* = .08), and mortality (odds ratio = .81, .12−.49, *P* = .83).

Conclusions.—Laparoscopic adhesiolysis is advantageous in most of the analyzed outcomes. Laparoscopic treatment of small bowel obstruction is recommended by experienced laparoscopic surgeons in selected patients (Fig 6).

▶ Lysis of adhesions for small bowel obstruction is a common procedure by general surgeons. These cases often are some of the most challenging, lasting hours and sometimes result in worse conditions like enterocutaneous fistula. Another concern is adhesions that will form postoperatively resulting in recurrent obstruction. There is no doubt that laparoscopic surgery results in fewer

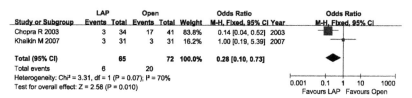

FIGURE 6.—A forest plot showing prolonged ileus between laparoscopy and open adhesiolysis for patients with adhesive small bowel obstruction requiring surgery. LAP, laparoscopic group. (Reprinted from The American Journal of Surgery. Li M-Z, Lian L, Xiao L-B, et al. Laparoscopic versus open adhesiolysis in patients with adhesive small bowel obstruction: a systematic review and meta-analysis. *Am J Surg.* 2012;204:779-786, Copyright 2012, with permission from Elsevier.)

adhesions and, therefore, may offer advantages over an open approach. However, the safety and practical realities of a laparoscopic lysis of adhesions can be daunting. Who wants to extend the operating time of an already lengthy procedure? Li et al have attempted to provide some clarification with this meta-analysis. From 105 studies identified, only 4 retrospective case-controlled reports were acceptable for analysis. From this they surmise that laparoscopic lysis of adhesions offers advantages with regard to complication rates and post-operative ileus (Fig 6). No data are available regarding the likelihood of the recurrent small bowel obstruction between these 2 approaches. Although not significant, the risk of intraoperative bowel injury was nearly twice as high in the laparoscopic group. This report suggests that there may be some advantages with a laparoscopic approach, but we are left making this decision on a case-by-case basis until better data are available.

J. Hines, MD

Comparison of open preperitoneal and Lichtenstein repair for inguinal hernia repair: a meta-analysis of randomized controlled trials
Li J, Ji Z, Cheng T (Southeast Univ, Nanjing, Jiangsu, China)
Am J Surg 204:769-778, 2012

Background.—The aim of this article was to compare the outcomes of the open preperitoneal approaches and the Lichtenstein technique in the repair of inguinal hernias.

Methods.—A systematic literature review was undertaken to identify studies comparing the outcomes of open preperitoneal and Lichtenstein techniques in the repair of inguinal hernias.

Results.—The present meta-analysis pooled the effects of outcomes of a total of 2,860 patients enrolled into 10 randomized controlled trials and 2 comparative studies. The preperitoneal technique was associated with a lesser incidence of recurrence (odds ratio = .51; 95% confidence interval, .28–.92). However, statistically there was no difference in the incidence of chronic pain, hematoma, wound infection, testicular problem, urinary problem, numbness, inguinal parenthesis, and operative time.

Conclusions.—The open preperitoneal approach is a feasible alternative for the standard Lichtenstein procedure with similar complication rates and potentially less postoperative recurrence (Fig 2A).

▶ We now know that not all inguinal hernias require repair and that watchful waiting for asymptomatic hernias is acceptable. Regardless, inguinal hernia repair is one of the most common operations, and, to date, more than 80 different operative techniques have been described. Modern open techniques include the anterior (Lichtenstein) and posterior or preperitoneal (Kugel patch, prolene hernia system, and transinguinal preperitoneal technique with memory ring patch) approaches. The preperitoneal approach may have an advantage because the mesh is held in place with intra-abdominal pressure and, therefore, requires relatively little or no fixation. The superiority of these techniques has been compared

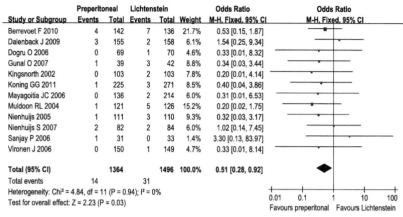

Study or Subgroup	Preperitoneal Events	Total	Lichtenstein Events	Total	Weight	Odds Ratio M-H, Fixed, 95% CI
Berrevoet F 2010	4	142	7	136	21.7%	0.53 [0.15, 1.87]
Dalenback J 2009	3	155	2	158	6.1%	1.54 [0.25, 9.34]
Dogru O 2006	0	69	1	70	4.6%	0.33 [0.01, 8.32]
Gunal O 2007	1	39	3	42	8.8%	0.34 [0.03, 3.44]
Kingsnorth 2002	0	103	2	103	7.8%	0.20 [0.01, 4.14]
Koning GG 2011	1	225	3	271	8.5%	0.40 [0.04, 3.86]
Mayagoitia JC 2006	0	136	2	214	6.0%	0.31 [0.01, 6.53]
Muldoon RL 2004	1	121	5	126	15.2%	0.20 [0.02, 1.75]
Nienhuijs 2005	1	111	3	110	9.3%	0.32 [0.03, 3.17]
Nienhuijs S 2007	2	82	2	84	6.0%	1.02 [0.14, 7.45]
Sanjay P 2006	1	31	0	33	1.4%	3.30 [0.13, 83.97]
Vironen J 2006	0	150	1	149	4.7%	0.33 [0.01, 8.14]
Total (95% CI)		1364		1496	100.0%	0.51 [0.28, 0.92]
Total events	14		31			

Heterogeneity: Chi² = 4.84, df = 11 (P = 0.94); I² = 0%
Test for overall effect: Z = 2.23 (P = 0.03)

0.01 0.1 1 10 100
Favours preperitonal Favours Lichtenstein

FIGURE 2.—(A) Postoperative inguinal hernia recurrence. (Reprinted from The American Journal of Surgery. Li J, Ji Z, Cheng T. Comparison of open preperitoneal and Lichtenstein repair for inguinal hernia repair: a meta-analysis of randomized controlled trials. *Am J Surg.* 2012;204:769-778, Copyright 2012, with permission from Elsevier.)

in various studies with no clear champion. This large meta-analysis includes 12 high-quality randomized studies comparing the Lichtenstein and the preperitoneal approaches listed above. The study included more than 2800 patients and determined that the preperitoneal approaches result in a nearly 2-fold lower recurrence rate (Fig 2A). Other morbidity, including chronic pain and overall operating time, was no better with either approach. Every surgeon has their preferred technique, but this study has compelling results for our patients.

J. Hines, MD

11 Oncology

Breast

Factors Associated With Local-Regional Recurrence After a Negative Sentinel Node Dissection: Results of the ACOSOG Z0010 Trial

Hunt KK, Ballman KV, McCall LM, et al (MD Anderson Cancer Ctr, Houston, TX; Division of Biomedical Statistics and Informatics, Rochester, MN; Duke Cancer Inst, Durham, NC; et al)

Ann Surg 256:428-436, 2012

Objective.—To determine factors important in local-regional recurrence (LRR) in patients with negative sentinel lymph nodes (SLNs) by hematoxylin and eosin (H&E) staining.

Background.—Z0010 was a prospective multicenter trial initiated in 1999 by the American College of Surgeons Oncology Group to evaluate occult disease in SLNs and bone marrow of early-stage breast cancer patients. Participants included women with biopsy-proven T1–2 breast cancer with clinically negative nodes, planned for lumpectomy and whole breast irradiation.

Methods.—Women with clinical T1–2,N0,M0 disease underwent lumpectomy and SLN dissection. There was no axillary-specific treatment for H&E-negative SLNs, and clinicians were blinded to immunohistochemistry results. Systemic therapy was based on primary tumor factors. Univariable and multivariable analyses were performed to determine clinicopathologic factors associated with LRR.

Results.—Of 5119 patients, 3904 (76.3%) had H&E-negative SLNs. Median age was 57 years (range 23–95). At median follow-up of 8.4 years, there were 127 local, 20 regional, and 134 distant recurrences. Factors associated with local-regional recurrence were hormone receptor-negative disease ($P = 0.0004$) and younger age ($P = 0.047$). In competing risk-regression models, hormone receptor-positive disease and use of chemotherapy were associated with reduction in local-regional recurrence. When local recurrence was included in the model as a time-dependent variable, older age, T2 disease, high tumor grade, and local recurrence were associated with reduced overall survival.

Conclusions.—Local-regional recurrences are rare in early-stage breast cancer patients with H&E-negative SLNs. Younger age and hormone receptor-negative disease are associated with higher event rates, and local recurrence is associated with reduced overall survival.

▶ Several recent randomized trials in treatment of early-stage breast cancer have revealed the value of sentinel lymph node biopsy and that axillary dissection is often not necessary in patients with a positive sentinel node. Few studies have looked at risk factors for local or regional recurrence in patients with negative sentinel lymph nodes. Another American College of Surgeons Oncology Group breast trial, the Z0010 trial, set out to prospectively evaluate patients with T1 and T2, clinically node-negative breast cancer, who underwent sentinel lymph node biopsy and breast-conserving surgery with radiation. The current study specifically examined risk factors for local and regional recurrence. This trial included 5539 patients, and this study focused on 3904 patients with H + E negative lymph nodes with a mean follow-up of 8.4 years. In this group, there were 317 deaths, and the number of recurrences included 127 local (2.4%), 20 regional (0.5%), and 134 distant recurrences (2.8%). In a multivariate analysis, the only risk factors for both local and regional recurrence were age less than 50 years and negative hormone receptor status. For distant recurrences, the risk was increased by lymphovascular invasion or grade 2 to 3 lesions. With respect to overall survival, the important risk factors were age greater than 50, increase in tumor size, and grade 3 disease. The significance of this study was that it showed a low local recurrence rate along with the associated risk factors, and it confirmed the low incidence of regional lymph node metastases in patients with sentinel node negative disease. This was only 0.5% at 5 years, which speaks to the potential beneficial effects of adjuvant chemotherapy or hormonal therapy. Because of these findings, future trials propose to examine breast-conserving therapy with sentinel lymph node biopsy vs no treatment of the axilla at all.

J. Howe, MD

Characteristics and Outcomes of Sentinel Node–Positive Breast Cancer Patients after Total Mastectomy without Axillary-Specific Treatment
Milgrom S, Cody H, Tan L, et al (Memorial Sloan-Kettering Cancer Ctr, NY)
Ann Surg Oncol 19:3762-3770, 2012

Purpose.—Regional failure rates are low in patients with a positive sentinel lymph node biopsy (SLNB) who undergo breast-conserving therapy without axillary lymph node dissection (ALND). The applicability of these findings to total mastectomy (TM) patients is not established. Our aims were to evaluate the characteristics and outcomes of SLNB-positive TM patients who did not receive axillary-specific treatment and to compare them to similar patients who underwent breast-conserving surgery (BCS).

Methods.—A total of 535 patients with early-stage breast cancer who underwent definitive breast surgery (210 TM, 325 BCS), had a positive SLNB and did not receive ALND between 1997 and 2009 were identified from an institutional database. Characteristics and outcomes were compared between the TM and BCS groups.

Results.—Most patients had stage I to IIA, estrogen receptor−positive, progesterone receptor−positive, Her2-negative invasive ductal carcinoma, with minimal nodal disease. Compared to the BCS group, TM patients were younger, had larger tumors, had higher nomogram scores predicting additional axillary disease and were more likely to receive chemotherapy. Ninety-four percent of the BCS cohort and 5 % of the TM cohort received adjuvant radiotherapy. At a median follow-up of 57.8 months, the 4-year local, regional and distant failure rates were 1.7, 1.2 and 0.7% in the TM group and 1.4, 1.0 and 3.7% in the BCS group. The 4-year disease-free and overall survival rates were 94.8 and 97.8% in the TM group and 90.1 and 92.6% in the BCS group.

Conclusions.—Early-stage breast cancer patients with minimal sentinel node disease experience excellent outcomes without ALND, whether they undergo BCS or TM.

▶ The ACOSOG Z0011 trial randomly assigned patients with up to 2 positive sentinel lymph nodes who had had breast-conserving surgery (BCS) to receive either axillary lymph node dissection or observation. The results showed very low regional recurrence rates in both arms of less than 1%. One hypothesis for the low risk of regional recurrence was that radiation therapy (RT) of the breast might have treated the level 1 and low level 2 nodes, thereby killing micrometastases. This study from Memorial Sloan-Kettering looked at this question by evaluating patients at their institution who had T1 and T2 breast cancers (who had not received neoadjuvant chemotherapy) and had either total mastectomy or BCS performed, during which they were found to have a positive axillary sentinel node but did not go on to receive axillary dissection. This was a retrospective chart review of 535 patients, 210 who had a total mastectomy and 325 who had BCS. The findings were of interest in that there is no significant difference in the incidence of local or regional failure between the 2 groups, of whom only 5% of the total mastectomy patients had received RT, whereas 94% of the BCS arm received RT. The rates of adjuvant chemotherapy and hormonal therapy were similar in the 2 groups. There was a slightly higher risk of distant metastases in the BCS arm, which was statistically significant, and a small decrease in overall survival. The disease-free survival rate was 95% for total mastectomy and 90% for BCS, and the overall survival rate was 98% for total mastectomy vs 93% for BCS. When patients with just immunohistochemistry-positive nodal disease were excluded, the same trends were seen, but the statistical significance was lost. The results of the study are intriguing because they show that the addition of RT to the local treatment of the breast does not influence regional or local failure rates when comparing total mastectomy vs BCS; therefore, RT alone is probably not responsible for the lower risk of axillary recurrence. This study helps confirm that completion axillary nodal dissection is not necessary in breast cancer patients with positive sentinel lymph nodes. Because this study was retrospective, there are certain biases, including the fact that patients undergoing total mastectomy had larger tumors and more often had multicentric disease and higher nomogram scores and, therefore, would be expected to have potentially even worse outcomes than observed in the study. Furthermore, 68% of total mastectomy patients had chemotherapy, whereas this was even less in the BCS group at 56%, which may explain why there was a higher rate of distant metastases in patients in the BCS arm. The authors also caution that there may be a role for RT in some patients undergoing total mastectomy, because all of the regional failures in this group had not received RT, and all 3 of these patients had microscopic disease found in the sentinel node rather than being detected by the immunohistochemistry.

J. Howe, MD

Complete Axillary Lymph Node Dissection Versus Clinical Follow-up in Breast Cancer Patients With Sentinel Node Micrometastasis: Final Results from the Multicenter Clinical Trial AATRM 048/13/2000

Solá M, Alberro JA, Fraile M, et al (Hospital Universitari Germans Trias i Pujol de Badalona, Barcelona, Spain; Instituto Oncológico de San Sebastian, Spain; et al)
Ann Surg Oncol 20:120-127, 2013

Background.—It has been suggested that selective sentinel node (SN) biopsy alone can be used to manage early breast cancer, but definite evidence to support this notion is lacking. The aim of this study was to investigate whether refraining from completion axillary lymph node dissection (ALND) suffices to produce the same prognostic information and disease control as proceeding with completion ALND in early breast cancer patients showing micrometastasis at SN biopsy.

Methods.—This prospective, randomized clinical trial included patients with newly diagnosed early-stage breast cancer ($T < 3.5$ cm, clinical N0, M0) who underwent surgical excision as primary treatment. All had micrometastatic SN. Patients were randomly assigned to one of the two study arms: complete ALND (control arm) or clinical follow-up (experimental arm). Median follow-up was 5 years, recurrence was assessed, and the primary end point was disease-free survival.

Results.—From a total sample of 247 patients, 14 withdrew, leaving 112 in the control arm and 121 in the experimental arm. In 15 control subjects (13%), completion ALND was positive, with a low tumor burden. Four patients experienced disease recurrence: 1 (1%) of 108 control subjects and 3 (2.5%) of 119 experimental patients. There were no differences in disease-free survival ($p = 0.325$) between arms and no cancer-related deaths.

Conclusions.—Our results strongly suggest that in early breast cancer patients with SN micrometastasis, selective SN lymphadenectomy suffices to control locoregional and distant disease, with no significant effects on survival.

▶ Another effort to determine the importance of completion axillary nodal dissection after positive sentinel lymph node biopsy in breast cancer came from Northern Spain. The authors analyzed patients who had micrometastases within sentinel lymph nodes, defined as being in the size range of 0.2 to 2 mm, with at least 1 metastatic cell deposit. They randomized patients with primary tumors less than

3.5 cm in size with clinically negative nodes and micrometastatic deposits in sentinel lymph nodes to receive either completion axillary lymph node dissection or observation. The groups were similar in terms of demographics and tumor factors. The majority of patients in both groups received breast conservation surgery (91% to 93%). The groups were also similar in that 90% of patients also received chemotherapy and the majority also underwent radiation therapy (91% to 93%). There were 233 patients enrolled in the study, and there were 4 recurrences in all. In the axillary dissection group, there was one cutaneous recurrence treated by local excision, and in the observation arm there were 3 recurrences (one was distant with lung metastases, and the other two were nodal metastases). There was no overall difference in survival. Interestingly, of those patients who underwent axillary dissection, 13% had additional positive non—sentinel lymph nodes. The authors suggested that the reason that the relapse rate was not higher in the breast conservation arm was that the use of adjuvant chemotherapy with radiation in most cases probably was adequate to treat the low disease burden in these non—sentinel lymph nodes and, therefore, the relapse rate was reduced from the expected 13% (additional non—sentinel lymph nodes positive in axillary dissection arm) down to approximately 2.5%. One limitation of the study is that the authors did not meet their accrual goals; they also stated that one of the disadvantages of not doing axillary nodal dissection is that the number of positive nodes has been used for decision-making for adjuvant radiotherapy (whether to use additional supraclavicular and infraclavicular ports is based on 4 or more positive nodes). The authors contend that the findings of low recurrence rate in the observation arm suggested that current radiation therapy and adjuvant chemotherapy regimens appear to be adequate to maintain regional control.

J. Howe, MD

Axillary Dissection Versus No Axillary Dissection in Older Patients With T1N0 Breast Cancer: 15-Year Results of a Randomized Controlled Trial
Martelli G, Boracchi P, Ardoino I, et al (Fondazione IRCCS Istituto Nazionale Dei Tumori, Milan, Italy; Univ of Milan, Melegnano, Italy; et al)
Ann Surg 256:920-924, 2012

Objective.—To assess the role of axillary dissection in older breast cancer patients with a clinically clear axilla.

Background.—Axillary dissection, once standard treatment for breast cancer, is associated with considerable morbidity. It has been substituted by sentinel node biopsy with dissection only if the sentinel node is positive. We aimed to determine whether axillary surgery can be omitted in older women, thereby sparing them morbidity, without compromising long-term disease control.

Methods.—We carried out a randomized clinical trial on 238 older (65—80 years) breast cancer patients, with clinically N0 disease of radiographic diameter 2 cm or less. Patients were randomized to quadrantectomy with or without axillary dissection. All received radiotherapy to the residual breast but not the axilla; all were prescribed tamoxifen for 5 years. Main outcome measures were overall survival and breast cancer mortality. We also assessed overt axillary disease in those who did not receive axillary dissection.

Results.—After 15 years of follow-up, distant metastasis rate, overall survival, and breast cancer mortality in the axillary dissection and no axillary dissection arms were indistinguishable. The 15-year cumulative incidence of overt axillary disease in the no axillary dissection arm was only 6%.

Conclusions.—Older patients with early breast cancer and a clinically clear axilla treated by conservative surgery, postoperative radiotherapy, and adjuvant tamoxifen do not benefit from axillary dissection. This study was registered at clinicaltrials.gov (ID NCT00002720).

▶ The question of what to do with regional lymph nodes in patients with early breast cancer has been a subject of increasing focus in the past decade. The American College of Surgeons Oncology Group (ACOSOG) Z0011 trial showed that patients with early breast cancer who were randomized to axillary dissection vs no further axillary treatment with positive sentinel lymph nodes revealed no significant difference in disease-free or overall survival. The current study by Martelli et al looks at a European cohort that randomized patients between the ages of 65 and 80 years of age with clinical T1N0 breast cancers to either lumpectomy with axillary dissection vs lumpectomy without axillary dissection in 1996. These patients were all treated with radiation to the breast as well as with adjuvant tamoxifen. This is a 15-year follow-up study looking at this subgroup of patients; interestingly, 23% of patients who had axillary dissection had involvement of axillary lymph nodes. However, in those patients who did not undergo axillary dissection, only 6% developed axillary nodal metastases and subsequently underwent axillary dissection. The overall findings showed that there was no significant difference in breast cancer death or rate of distant metastases in the 2 groups. The conclusions of this study were that older women with clinical T1N0 breast cancers can be treated with lumpectomy, radiation, and adjuvant tamoxifen and do not need to undergo axillary dissection. The limitations of the study were that it was somewhat underpowered with 238 patients who showed no significant difference between treatments; however, it does seem to confirm the findings of the ACOSOG Z0011 trial, and, therefore, these elderly patients may not only avoid axillary dissection, but the authors also conclude that sentinel node biopsy may also be unnecessary.

J. Howe, MD

Effect of Introducing Hematoma Ultrasound-Guided Lumpectomy in a Surgical Practice

Larrieux G, Cupp JA, Liao J, et al (Univ of Iowa, Iowa City)

J Am Coll Surg 215:237-243, 2012

Background.—Preoperative needle localization (NL) is the gold standard for lumpectomy of nonpalpable breast cancer. Hematoma ultrasound-guided (HUG) lumpectomy can offer several advantages. The purpose of this study was to compare the use of HUG with NL lumpectomy in a single surgical practice.

Study Design.—Patients with nonpalpable lesions who underwent NL or HUG lumpectomy from January 2007 to December 2009 by a single surgeon were identified from a breast surgery database. Ease of scheduling, volume excised, re-excision rates, operating room time, and health care charges were the main outcomes variables. Univariate and multivariate analyses were performed to compare the 2 groups.

Results.—Lumpectomy was performed in 110 patients, 55 underwent HUG and 55 underwent NL. Hematoma ultrasound-guided lumpectomy was associated with a nearly 3-fold increase in the odds ratio of additional tissue being submitted to pathology ($p = 0.039$), but neither the total amount of breast tissue removed, nor the need for second procedure were statistically different between the 2 groups. Duration of the surgical procedure did not vary between the 2 groups; however, the time from biopsy to surgery was shorter for HUG by an expected 9.7 days ($p = 0.019$), implying greater ease of scheduling. Mean charges averaged $250 less for HUG than for NL, but this difference was not statistically significant.

Conclusions.—Hematoma ultrasound-guided is equivalent to NL with regard to volume of tissue excised, need for operative re-excision, and operating room time. Adoption of HUG in our practice allowed for more timely surgical care.

▶ Screening mammography has led to an increased identification of small, non-palpable breast lesions. Typically when these are identified, stereotactic core needle biopsy is performed and a clip is left at the site of biopsy. Conventional treatment after this will involve needle localization followed by lumpectomy. The authors of this study employ a different technique: They perform a lumpectomy around the site of the biopsy using ultrasound-guided excision of the hematoma resulting from the previous biopsy as a guide. This study looked at 110 patients who had hematoma ultrasound-guided (HUG) lumpectomy vs standard needle localization performed by a single surgeon. It found that HUG was equally successful as needle localization at removing the lesion, and there was no difference in the number of patients requiring reexcision in the 2 groups. HUG did result in shorter scheduling times until surgery than needle localization with slightly reduced charges. This study introduces a novel and effective means of treating patients with early breast cancer that simplifies operative scheduling, but it is not appropriate in all circumstances: This includes those patients who have undergone neoadjuvant chemotherapy because the hematoma will not be present, and patients with multiple calcifications because of potential fear of missing the lesions. It simplifies the procedure by not requiring radiology because it can be performed by surgeons as long as they are skilled in breast ultrasonography.

J. Howe, MD

Long-Term Results of Excision Followed by Radiofrequency Ablation as the Sole Means of Local Therapy for Breast Cancer

Wilson M, Korourian S, Boneti C, et al (Univ of Arkansas for Med Sciences, Little Rock)
Ann Surg Oncol 19:3192-3198, 2012

Introduction.—Clinical trials have yet to find a size or grade of invasive cancer which can be treated with lumpectomy alone due to the higher local recurrence (LR) rate without radiation (XRT). Excision followed by radiofrequency ablation (eRFA) is an intraoperative method which utilizes heat to create an additional tumor-free zone around the lumpectomy cavity. We hypothesized that eRFA after lumpectomy for invasive breast cancer could reduce the need for re-excision in close margins and potentially maintain local control without the need for XRT.

Methods.—This institutional review board-approved study from July 2002 to December 2010 involved patients undergoing eRFA. A standard lumpectomy was performed and then the RFA probe was deployed 1 cm circumferentially into the walls of the lumpectomy cavity and maintained at 100 °C for 15 min. Validated doppler sonography was used to determine final ablation size.

Results.—Seventy-three patients (mean age of 68.8 ± 10.9 years) with invasive cancer who had an average tumor size of 1.0 ± 0.54 cm (range of 0.2-2.6 cm) underwent eRFA. Margins were negative in 54, close in 10, focally positive in 6, and grossly positive in 3 patients. Sixteen out of 19 (84%) of patients with close or positive margins were spared of re-excision. Median follow-up was 55 ± 21 months. Only one patient (1.3%) developed an in site recurrence. There were three recurrences, elsewhere.

Conclusions.—Long-term follow-up suggests that eRFA may reduce the need for re- excision as well as reduce LR for invasive breast cancer treated without XRT.

▶ Lumpectomy followed by breast irradiation has been shown be an alternative to mastectomy for the local treatment of breast cancers since the NSABP B06 trial in 1985. However, a certain percentage of women, especially those older than 70 years of age and with smaller tumors, may not require radiation therapy in order to reduce the risk of local recurrence. Klimberg et al have studied performing lumpectomy followed by radiofrequency ablation of the biopsy cavity to margins of 1 cm in carefully selected patients to determine whether this modality can reduce the risk of local recurrence without the need for radiation therapy. They selected patients older than 50 years of age with tumors ≤ 3 cm in size and clinically negative nodes to enter the study. These patients had excision performed, followed by radiofrequency ablation at the same sitting using a purse-string suture to reduce the cavity size, and deployment 1 cm into the adjacent excision bed. A total of 73 patients were followed for a mean of 52 months. Their study revealed a very low recurrence rate (1 patient developing a local recurrence; 3 patients developing recurrences elsewhere in the breast). They also found that in this group of 73 patients that 54 had negative margins, 10 had close margins,

6 were focally positive, and 3 were grossly positive. The latter 3 patients had repeat excisions. Most importantly from this study, 16 of 19 patients with close or positive margins did not require reexcision. Long-term follow-up revealed that the recurrence in the breast was 5%, which was comparable to that seen in patients who undergo lumpectomy and radiation to the breast. Complications were that 5% of patients developed wound infection, and cosmesis was deemed good or excellent in 90% of the patients. This study, therefore, revealed that radiofrequency ablation after lumpectomy may be a useful means of avoiding radiation therapy in carefully selected patients.

J. Howe, MD

Colon

Primary mFOLFOX6 Plus Bevacizumab Without Resection of the Primary Tumor for Patients Presenting With Surgically Unresectable Metastatic Colon Cancer and an Intact Asymptomatic Colon Cancer: Definitive Analysis of NSABP Trial C-10

McCahill LE, Yothers G, Sharif S, et al (Natl Surgical Adjuvant Breast and Bowel Project, Pittsburgh, PA; et al)

J Clin Oncol 30:3223-3228, 2012

Purpose.—Major concerns surround combining chemotherapy with bevacizumab in patients with colon cancer presenting with an asymptomatic intact primary tumor (IPT) and synchronous yet unresectable metastatic disease. Surgical resection of asymptomatic IPT is controversial.

Patients and Methods.—Eligibility for this prospective, multicenter phase II trial included Eastern Cooperative Oncology Group (ECOG) performance status 0 to 1, asymptomatic IPT, and unresectable metastases. All received infusional fluorouracil, leucovorin, and oxaliplatin (mFOLFOX6) combined with bevacizumab. The primary end point was major morbidity events, defined as surgical resection because of symptoms at or death related to the IPT. A 25% major morbidity rate was considered acceptable. Secondary end points included overall survival (OS) and minor morbidity related to IPT requiring hospitalization, transfusion, or nonsurgical intervention.

Results.—Ninety patients registered between March 2006 and June 2009: 86 were eligible with follow-up, median age was 58 years, and 52% were female. Median follow-up was 20.7 months. There were 12 patients (14%) with major morbidity related to IPT: 10 required surgery (eight, obstruction; one, perforation; and one, abdominal pain), and two patients died. The 24-month cumulative incidence of major morbidity was 16.3% (95% CI, 7.6% to 25.1%). Eleven IPTs were resected without a morbidity event: eight for attempted cure and three for other reasons. Two patients had minor morbidity events only: one hospitalization and one nonsurgical intervention. Median OS was 19.9 months (95% CI, 15.0 to 27.2 months).

Conclusion.—This trial met its primary end point. Combining mFOL-FOX6 with bevacizumab did not result in an unacceptable rate of obstruction, perforation, bleeding, or death related to IPT. Survival was not compromised. These patients can be spared initial noncurative resection of their asymptomatic IPT.

▶ One dilemma that has long faced general surgeons is how to approach the primary tumor in somebody with colorectal cancer and distant metastases. About 20% of patients with colorectal cancer will have distant disease, and about 80% of these will be unresectable. Should all patients in this situation have resection of the primary tumor because of the risk of obstruction and bleeding? This approach has a 10% mortality rate and a 30% to 50% major morbidity rate. This prospective study looked at using 5-fluorouracil, leucovorin, and oxaliplatin with bevacizumab to treat patients with an intact primary tumor and metastatic disease to determine the rate of major morbidity resulting from leaving the primary tumor in place with this therapy. Concerns have been raised previously about the risk of perforation with bevacizumab. This study accrued 86 patients from 29 centers, and patients were given 5-fluorouracil, leucovorin, oxaliplatin, and bevacizumab if they had colon cancers with metastases considered to be unresectable. Chemotherapy was continued until toxicity or disease progression was seen. This study found that of these 86 patients, 12 had major events. Ten patients required surgery for symptoms related to the primary tumor, of which, 8 were performed for obstruction, 1 for perforation, and 1 for abdominal pain. The other 2 events were patient deaths, one of which was likely caused by a perforation after the first cycle of chemotherapy, while the other was caused by a bowel obstruction in a patient treated palliatively after progression of disease. Two other patients had minor morbidity, including hospitalization for bowel obstruction, which resolved in one and required endoscopic colonic stent placement in another. Eight patients had surgery with the intent to remove the primary and metastatic lesions, but in 3 of those patients the liver lesions were unresectable. One had complete response in the liver and only the primary tumor was removed, and in 4 patients combined resection of both the primary tumor and metastases was carried out (1 at 2 operations). Two of the 3 combined resection patients died of postoperative complications. There were also 4 deaths potentially related to the chemotherapy alone and 4 others within 3 months of chemotherapy, but these were thought to be unrelated to the chemotherapy itself. The overall risk of major morbidity was 16%. The conclusions of this study were that perforation was a rare event and, therefore, the use of bevacizumab in this setting seemed reasonable. The mortality rate of a nonoperative approach appeared to be just less than 4%, and 84% of all patients were able to receive systemic therapy and avoid surgical resection. The most common complication was obstruction. This ultimately led to surgery, which, in more than half of the cases, was nonemergent. Therefore, it appears that in the setting of distant metastases, leaving the primary colon tumor intact and treating both with chemotherapy and bevacizumab is a reasonable approach, and surgery can be avoided in most cases.

J. Howe, MD

Colonoscopic Polypectomy and Long-Term Prevention of Colorectal-Cancer Deaths

Zauber AG, Winawer SJ, O'Brien MJ, et al (Memorial Sloan-Kettering Cancer Ctr, NY; Boston Univ School of Medicine, MA; et al)
N Engl J Med 366:687-696, 2012

Background.—In the National Polyp Study (NPS), colorectal cancer was prevented by colonoscopic removal of adenomatous polyps. We evaluated the long-term effect of colonoscopic polypectomy in a study on mortality from colorectal cancer.

Methods.—We included in this analysis all patients prospectively referred for initial colonoscopy (between 1980 and 1990) at NPS clinical centers who had polyps (adenomas and nonadenomas). The National Death Index was used to identify deaths and to determine the cause of death; follow-up time was as long as 23 years. Mortality from colorectal cancer among patients with adenomas removed was compared with the expected incidence-based mortality from colorectal cancer in the general population, as estimated from the Surveillance Epidemiology and End Results (SEER) Program, and with the observed mortality from colorectal cancer among patients with nonadenomatous polyps (internal control group).

Results.—Among 2602 patients who had adenomas removed during participation in the study, after a median of 15.8 years, 1246 patients had died from any cause and 12 had died from colorectal cancer. Given an estimated 25.4 expected deaths from colorectal cancer in the general population, the standardized incidence-based mortality ratio was 0.47 (95% confidence interval [CI], 0.26 to 0.80) with colonoscopic polypectomy, suggesting a 53% reduction in mortality. Mortality from colorectal cancer was similar among patients with adenomas and those with nonadenomatous polyps during the first 10 years after polypectomy (relative risk, 1.2; 95% CI, 0.1 to 10.6).

Conclusions.—These findings support the hypothesis that colonoscopic removal of adenomatous polyps prevents death from colorectal cancer. (Funded by the National Cancer Institute and others.)

▶ Screening colonoscopy may detect cancers at an earlier, more curable, stage or allow for removal of adenomas that may later go on to become cancerous. Long-term studies with large numbers of patients would be required to determine whether removing adenomas leads to a decrease in colorectal cancer deaths relative to the general population. This National Polyp Study examined this question in patients from 7 centers over a 10-year period, including 2602 patients with adenomas removed. These results were compared to matched patients from the Surveillance Epidemiology and End Results (SEER) database. The adenoma group had 12 deaths at a mean of 15.8 years of follow-up, whereas the SEER population had 25 deaths, indicating that removal of adenomas colonoscopically significantly reduced colorectal cancer mortality. The benefits may have been understated because all the treated patients had adenomas, whereas not all patients in the normal population did. However, one must also ponder whether performing 200 colonoscopies (plus continued surveillance) for each life saved is justified, and whether the results could be influenced by better access to health care for patients enrolled in the study, all of whom had the opportunity to change their lifestyle after the discovery of an adenoma.

J. Howe, MD

Comparative Genomic Analysis of Primary Versus Metastatic Colorectal Carcinomas

Vakiani E, Janakiraman M, Shen R, et al (Memorial Sloan-Kettering Cancer Ctr, NY)
J Clin Oncol 30:2956-2962, 2012

Purpose.—To compare the mutational and copy number profiles of primary and metastatic colorectal carcinomas (CRCs) using both unpaired and paired samples derived from primary and metastatic disease sites.

Patients and Methods.—We performed a multiplatform genomic analysis of 736 fresh frozen CRC tumors from 613 patients. The cohort included 84 patients in whom tumor tissue from both primary and metastatic sites was available and 31 patients with pairs of metastases. Tumors were analyzed for mutations in the *KRAS, NRAS, BRAF, PIK3CA,* and *TP53* genes, with discordant results between paired samples further investigated by analyzing formalin-fixed, paraffin-embedded tissue and/or by 454 sequencing. Copy number aberrations in primary tumors and matched metastases were analyzed by comparative genomic hybridization (CGH).

Results.—*TP53* mutations were more frequent in metastatic versus primary tumors (53.1% *v* 30.3%, respectively; *P* < .001), whereas *BRAF* mutations were significantly less frequent (1.9% *v* 7.7%, respectively; *P* = .01). The mutational status of the matched pairs was highly concordant (> 90% concordance for all five genes). Clonality analysis of array CGH data suggested that multiple CRC primary tumors or treatment-associated effects were likely etiologies for mutational and/or copy number profile differences between primary tumors and metastases.

Conclusion.—For determining *RAS, BRAF,* and *PIK3CA* mutational status, genotyping of the primary CRC is sufficient for most patients. Biopsy of a metastatic site should be considered in patients with a history of multiple primary carcinomas and in the case of *TP53* for patients who have undergone interval treatment with radiation or cytotoxic chemotherapies.

▶ The development of biologic therapies for adjuvant treatment of colon cancer has made sequence analysis of colorectal cancers more commonplace. Specifically, patients who have KRAS wild-type tumors are likely to respond to epidermal growth factor receptor inhibition (Cetuximab). However, there has been doubt whether the primary tumor itself should be sequenced or whether metastatic foci such as liver biopsies can be sequenced and, related to this, whether there is concordance between the primary tumor and metastatic sites. This ambitious study set out to answer the question of concordance for 5 different genes, including *KRAS, NRAS, BRAF, PIK3CA*, and *TP53*. This study examined 406 primary tumors and 291 metastases (the vast majority from the liver followed by lung and other sites). In the primary tumors vs metastases, the concordance rate was more than 90% for each of the genes. *KRAS* mutations were about the same in primary tumor and their metastases, whereas *TP53* mutations were more common in metastases and *BRAF* mutations were less common in metastases than primary tumors. Cases of discordance raised the question of whether there were possibly multiple primaries that could result from the treatment effect of chemotherapy or radiation. The recommendation of the study is to sequence the primary tumor first, but in patients with more than 1 primary, or in those with potential *TP53* mutations after receiving chemotherapy or radiation, then analysis of the metastatic site is recommended.

J. Howe, MD

Gallbladder

An Often Overlooked Diagnosis: Imaging Features of Gallbladder Cancer
Pilgrim CHC, Groeschl RT, Pappas SG, et al (Med College of Wisconsin, Milwaukee)
J Am Coll Surg 216:333-339, 2013

Background.—Up to 50% of patients with gallbladder carcinoma (GBCA) are not diagnosed on initial imaging and undergo simple cholecystectomy, yet a more careful evaluation of imaging findings may identify the cancer preoperatively. Certain features seen on computed tomography (CT), ultrasound (US), or other modalities should raise the suspicion for malignancy and lead to better treatment planning. Certain commonly accepted indicators of disease not well supported by evidence should be reconsidered.

Indicators.—Currently it is accepted that gallbladder polyps over 10 mm warrant cholecystectomy to reduce the incidence of malignancy. Removing such polyps is believed to remove adenoma and minimizes progression to GBCA, but most polyps are not adenoma and most GBCA arise from dysplastic lesions, not adenoma. If polyps features suggest malignancy, such as local invasion, vascularity, or sessile shape, or are accompanied by enlarged regional lymph nodes, they should be considered cancer, with additional imaging studies and oncologic surgery as appropriate. Removing all polyps does not appreciably affect GBCA incidence. Polypoid lesions of the gallbladder warrant cholescystectomy with abdominal symptoms or concurrent gallstones.

Studies show GBCA usually appears as nonspecific gallbladder wall thickening, yet this diagnosis is seldom considered with this finding. Further imaging is usually needed to identify the specific nature of the gallbladder wall thickening, but this is rarely done. Finding 10-mm wall thickening is at least as important an indicator of malignancy as finding a 10-mm polyp. Simple thickness is an important but overlooked feature helpful in identifying GBCA.

The most useful modality for assessing gallbladder wall thickening is multidetector CT. This may also differentiate benign from malignant causes and accurately assign T stage preoperatively. Five patterns of wall enhancement on CT correlate well with the differential diagnoses of GBCA, adenomyomatosis, and acute and chronic cholecystitis, including a heterogeneously enhancing thick, one-layer pattern and a strongly enhancing thick inner layer with a weakly enhancing or nonenhancing thin outer layer, which are indicative of GBCA. Magnetic resonance Half-Fourier Acquisition Singleshot Turbo spinEcho sequences reveals four distinct layered patterns and is widely available, but its advantages over CT remain to be identified.

A mean gallbladder wall thickness of 19.4 mm on endoscopic US (EUS) is considered neoplastic. EUS allows one to perform fine-needle aspiration at the same sitting as the scan, which can provide a tissue diagnosis for patients with unresectable GBCA. It does not offer the same breadth of information about metastases and is insufficient as a single diagnostic method preoperatively.

Differentiating GBCA from xanthogranulomatous cholecystitis (XGC) and adenomyomatosis may require the use of magnetic resonance imaging (MRI). XGC is seen predominantly in the gallbladder wall, leaving the mucosal surface overlying the lesion either intact or focally denuded. In contrast, the mucosal line in GBCA is often disrupted as malignancy progresses, a change visible on CT. Five CT features suggesting XGC are diffuse gallbladder wall thickening, a continuous mucosal line, intramural hypoattenuated nodules, and no macroscopic hepatic invasion or intrahepatic bile duct dilation. If any three of these five findings are present, it is highly likely that XGC is the correct diagnosis. GBCA may be diagnosed earlier by paying closer attention to the results of the initial US imaging and moving to more detailed axial scanning when the clinician suspects a malignancy is present. Surgeons can perform an open operation with planned intraoperative frozen section to confirm the diagnosis.

Established GBCA.—When GBCA is diagnosed preoperatively, T, N, and M stage assessment is critical in planning treatment and surgery. US is highly sensitive for detecting advanced stages, but limited for use in early lesions and unreliable for staging. CT is better, and multiplanar reconstruction can increase the value of standard axial CT images. However, T1 and T2 lesions can be hard to differentiate. In addition, the significance of local nodal disease on postoperative scanning is difficult to determine after cholecystectomy. Finding enlarged nodes before surgery is highly suspicious for malignancy. For some patients, involved nodal groups beyond the hepatoduodenal ligament may be a contraindication to surgery, with very few long-term survivors in patients with N2 nodal disease. Although the value of positron emission tomography (PET) in GBCA is not conclusively supported by evidence, postoperatively after incidental GBCA, PET may help find metastatic disease and contraindicate additional surgery. CT is more useful in identifying residual locoregional disease.

Conclusions.—The detection of early-stage GBCA before cholecystectomy may be increased by considering gallbladder wall thickening as an important indicator of disease. Polyps rarely become malignant. The mainstay for workup of patients is CT. Certain CT and MRI wall changes differentiate malignant disease from acute and chronic cholecystitis and adenomyomatosis.

▶ Gallbladder carcinoma is a particularly lethal form of cancer if it cannot be picked up in its earliest stages. Careful attention to ultrasonographic findings in patients being worked up for acute cholecystitis may show the presence of polyps or wall thickening, which can lead to concern regarding the potential for malignancy. This study reviews important ultrasonographic, computed tomography (CT), magnetic resonance imaging, and positron emission tomography scanning results that help differentiate gallbladder carcinomas from other lesions. A particularly important point made by the article is that the previous concern regarding gallbladder polyps may be unwarranted. Certainly, those polyps greater than 2 cm are worrisome, but those just greater than 10 mm are of less concern despite having previously been recommended as an indication for cholecystectomy because of the risk of malignancy. Large studies looking at this have found that very few polyps will progress to cancer when followed up with over the long term. Clearly, polyps less than 10 mm do not warrant cholecystectomy for this alone. More important than the presence of a polyp is the assessment of gallbladder wall thickening. When gallbladder wall thickening greater than 10 mm is seen, further evaluation by CT scan is indicated. Here, a heterogeneously enhancing, thick, one-layer gallbladder wall is suspicious for gallbladder cancer, as is a strongly enhancing inner layer greater than 2.6 mm and a weakly enhancing thinner outer layer less than 3.4 mm. Other diagnoses that can introduce confusion would be those of adenomyomatosis and xanthogranulomatous cholecystitis. The former is difficult to determine by imaging, whereas the latter may be easier to differentiate and may have inflammation extending to within the liver or surrounding bowel. Differentiation from acute cholecystitis can also be difficult; however, the degree of thickening in acute cholecystitis is generally less than that in gallbladder carcinoma, which in one study was a mean of 8.9 mm. The finding of nodal enlargement may also be suggestive of gallbladder carcinoma in this setting. Twenty-five percent of patients with gallbladder carcinoma may present with cholecystitis, whereas only about 1% of patients with cholecystitis will have gallbladder carcinoma. This article gives nice pointers on how to pay specific attention to features that may tip one off to diagnose a gallbladder cancer preoperatively, so that cholecystectomy with adjacent gallbladder bed liver resection with lymphadenectomy can be performed instead of simple cholecystectomy.

J. Howe, MD

Gastric

Updated Analysis of SWOG-Directed Intergroup Study 0116: A Phase III Trial of Adjuvant Radiochemotherapy Versus Observation After Curative Gastric Cancer Resection

Smalley SR, Benedetti JK, Haller DG, et al (Radiation Oncology Ctr of Olathe, KS; SWOG Statistical Ctr, Seattle, WA; Univ of Pennsylvania Cancer Ctr, Philadelphia; et al)

J Clin Oncol 30:2327-2333, 2012

Purpose.—Surgical resection of gastric cancer has produced suboptimal survival despite multiple randomized trials that used postoperative chemotherapy or more aggressive surgical procedures. We performed a randomized phase III trial of postoperative radiochemotherapy in those at moderate risk of locoregional failure (LRF) following surgery. We originally reported results with 4-year median follow-up. This update, with a more than 10-year median follow-up, presents data on failure patterns and second malignancies and explores selected subset analyses.

Patients and Methods.—In all, 559 patients with primaries ≥ T3 and/or node-positive gastric cancer were randomly assigned to observation versus radiochemotherapy after R0 resection. Fluorouracil and leucovorin were administered before, during, and after radiotherapy. Radiotherapy was given to all LRF sites to a dose of 45 Gy.

Results.—Overall survival (OS) and relapse-free survival (RFS) data demonstrate continued strong benefit from postoperative radiochemotherapy. The hazard ratio (HR) for OS is 1.32 (95% CI, 1.10 to 1.60; $P = .0046$). The HR for RFS is 1.51 (95% CI, 1.25 to 1.83; $P < .001$). Adjuvant radiochemotherapy produced substantial reduction in both overall relapse and locoregional relapse. Second malignancies were observed in 21 patients with radiotherapy versus eight with observation ($P = .21$). Subset analyses show robust treatment benefit in most subsets, with the exception of patients with diffuse histology who exhibited minimal nonsignificant treatment effect.

Conclusion.—Intergroup 0116 (INT-0116) demonstrates strong persistent benefit from adjuvant radiochemotherapy. Toxicities, including second malignancies, appear acceptable, given the magnitude of RFS and OS improvement. LRF reduction may account for the majority of overall relapse reduction. Adjuvant radiochemotherapy remains a rational standard therapy for curatively resected gastric cancer with primaries T3 or greater and/or positive nodes.

▶ Survival from gastric cancer has been disappointing, mostly owing to the high locoregional failure rate. Clinical trials with neoadjuvant chemotherapy, postoperative chemoradiation, and adjuvant chemotherapy have been performed in an attempt to improve these results. One of the most conclusive trials performed was the Intergroup 0116 trial, which was a phase 3, randomized trial comparing surgical treatment of gastric cancer followed by observation or adjuvant radioche-motherapy (with 5-fluorouracil and leucovorin before, during, and after 45 Gy of radiation). Preliminary results revealed a significant improvement in overall survival and disease-free survival in the treatment group. The current study repre-sents the 10-year follow-up of this trial. This revealed similar hazard ratios, as seen earlier for patients in the observation arm, of 1.32 for overall survival and 1.51 for relapse-free survival. Other interesting findings were that there was little effect for multiple treatment variables, such as T stage, N stage, extent of resection, and tumor location. Also, patients with diffuse histology did not appear to benefit from radiochemotherapy. There did not appear to be a benefit with more extensive nodal dissection, which is supported by other Western trials (which revealed no survival benefit, but increased morbidity or mortality). Therefore, this study confirms the significant survival benefit in patients with moderate risk gastric cancer when receiving postoperative radiochemotherapy. Another contemporary trial in gastric cancer was the MAGIC trial, in which patients had preoperative epi-rubicin, cisplatinum, and fluorouracil, which showed similar improvements in survival to the current study. However, the authors note that the MAGIC trial had double the incidence of node-negative disease and, therefore, these 2 trials may not be comparable. Both of these trials represent significant steps forward for patients with this lethal disease.

J. Howe, MD

Guidelines for Extended Lymphadenectomy in Gastric Cancer: A Prospective Comparative Study
Asoglu O, Matlim T, Kurt A, et al (Istanbul Univ, Turkey; Cumhuriyet Univ, Sivas Merkez, Turkey; et al)
Ann Surg Oncol 20:218-225, 2013

Aims.—To assess the efficacy of extended lymph node dissection in gastric cancer and to identify factors affecting lymph node detection.

Methods.—A prospective study of 126 gastric cancer patients was con-ducted. Patients eligible for curative resection received total gastrectomy and extended lymphadenectomy (D2) and paraaortic lymph node sampling as the standard of care (study group). Supramesocolic total lymphadenec-tomy of the upper gastrointestinal tract was performed on 23 autopsy cases as a control group.

Results.—Fifty-five gastric carcinoma patients were included in the study group. Median age was 58 years (range 31—80 years); 14 patients were female (25%), and 41 were male (75%). The median number of lymph nodes harvested from the specimen was 47 (24—95), and the median number of metastatic lymph nodes was 15 (1—71). In contrast, in the autopsy comparative group, the median number of harvested lymph nodes was 72 (50—91). The median number of stational lymph nodes excised (lymph nodes excised from stations 4, 5, 10, 11, 12, and 16) was significantly higher in the control group than in the study group ($P < 0.05$). Lymph node detec-tion was adversely affected by body mass index (BMI) ($P < 0.03$). In the study group, stations 5, 12, 11, and 10 had the highest lymph node absence (LNA) (noncompliance) ratio with percentages of 53, 36, 33, and 22%, respectively. In the autopsy group, LNA (noncompliance) was not detected.

Conclusions.—Lymph nodes should be dissected by surgeons with sufficient technical and anatomical experience, and then examined and counted by experienced pathologists to reduce the occurrence of LNA. The results of this anatomical study can serve as a guideline to assess the success of lymph node dissection during gastric cancer surgery. Similar studies should be conducted in every country to establish national guidelines.

▶ Gastric cancers are one of the few cancers that have been decreasing in incidence over the past century; however, survival still remains poor in the Western world, with 5-year survivals of 20% to 40%. In Japan, however, early diagnosis and systematic lymph node dissection seem to be factors that have resulted in improved 5-year survivals of up to 70%. Operations done for gastric cancer vary, with the Japanese continuing to adhere to extended lymphadenectomy, whereas in Western countries this is not as routinely performed. The current study, from Istanbul, Turkey, set out to look at the number of lymph nodes harvested in patients undergoing extended lymphadenectomy for gastric cancer and to determine the number of lymph nodes present at various lymph node stations. A single surgeon performed operations on 55 patients as well as in 23 autopsy cases. In each case, the lymph node stations were coded and then assessed pathologically. The operations included total gastrectomy and extended lymphadenectomy, which included sampling of the periaortic lymph nodes, celiac, superior mesenteric artery (SMA), right gastric pyloric station 6 nodes, right gastric station 5 nodes, common hepatic arteries station 8 nodes, splenic artery nodes in station 11, celiac trunk nodes in station 9, splenic hilum nodes in station 10, and stations 1 and 2 lymph nodes at the crura. In autopsy specimens, en bloc resection of celiac, SMA, splenic arteries with spleen, and the hepatoduodenal ligament with division of the liver hilus were all taken for more extensive analyses. The end points for the study were the absence of lymph nodes identified at the various stations, with minor lymph node absence being defined when this was found in 1 or 2 stations and major when it was found in 3 or more stations. Overall, the median number of nodes removed from the 55 patients with cancer was 47, and the median number of involved nodes was 15. In the 23 patients undergoing autopsy, the median number of nodes was 72. The nodal stations with highest lymph node absence were station 5 with 53% having absent nodes, followed by a splenic hilum in station 10 with 33% absence, station 12 with 36% absence, and, finally, station 11 along the splenic artery with 22% absence. In autopsy cases, higher counts were seen in stations 10, 11, 12, and 16; however, the difference here was that the vascular supply could be completely removed. When examined for various patient factors and tumor factors, no relationship could be found between these lymph node absence rates. However, increased body mass index (BMI) was associated with increasing absence of lymph nodes at various nodal stations. The authors make the point that important factors for harvesting lymph nodes include surgeon experience, attention to detail of the pathologist, and that the excess fatty tissue associated with higher BMI may also result in missing lymph nodes. The finding of this study was that nodal stations 5, 10, 11, and 12 are frequently missing nodes. Limitations of the study include that it was a single institutional study from Turkey, and that the patient population may be different from the classic Western and Eastern populations.

J. Howe, MD

Hepatic Colorectal

Patterns of Recurrence After Ablation of Colorectal Cancer Liver Metastases
Kingham TP, Tanoue M, Eaton A, et al (Memorial Sloan-Kettering Cancer Ctr, NY; Creighton Univ School of Medicine, Omaha, NE)
Ann Surg Oncol 19:834-841, 2012

Purpose.—To determine the local recurrence rate and factors associated with recurrence after intraoperative ablation of colorectal cancer liver metastases.

Methods.—A retrospective analysis of a prospectively maintained database was performed for patients who underwent ablation of a hepatic colorectal cancer metastasis in the operating room from April 1996 to March 2010. Kaplan-Meier survival curves and Cox models were used to determine recurrence rates and assess significance.

Results.—Ablation was performed in 10% ($n = 158$ patients) of all cases during the study period. Seventy-eight percent were performed in conjunction with a liver resection. Of the 315 tumors ablated, most tumors were ≤ 1 cm in maximum diameter (53%). Radiofrequency ablation was used to treat most of the tumors (70%). Thirty-six tumors (11%) had local recurrence as part of their recurrence pattern. Disease recurred in the liver or systemically after 212 tumors (67%) were ablated. On univariate analysis, tumor size greater than 1 cm was associated with a significantly increased risk of local recurrence (hazard ratio 2.3, 95% confidence interval 1.2– 4.5, $P = 0.013$). The 2 year ablation zone recurrence-free survival was 92% for tumors ≤ 1 cm compared to 81% for tumors > 1 cm. On multivariate analysis, tumor size of > 1 cm, lack of postoperative chemotherapy, and use of cryotherapy were significantly associated with a higher local recurrence rate.

Conclusions.—Intraoperative ablation appears to be highly effective treatment for hepatic colorectal tumors ≤ 1 cm.

▶ The use of radiofrequency ablation of colorectal cancer liver metastases is still being defined. This modality has been shown to be useful in small hepatocellular carcinomas and plays a role in patients with bilobar liver metastases, and those who are undergoing resection that may have additional lesions that would be better treated with preservation of the parenchyma. This study from Memorial Sloan-Kettering Cancer Center examined patients undergoing ablation over a 14-year period, which comprised 10% of all patients treated over that interval. The majority underwent resection, but ablation was used either by itself in 38 patients or in conjunction with resection for 136 patients, for a total of 315 lesions.

The significance of this study is that it helped to confirm several things previously seen in other studies. Most importantly, the recurrence-free survival rate for lesions <1 cm in size was 92% at 2 years compared with 81% for tumors >1 cm in size. When tumors exceeded 3 cm, 2-year recurrence-free survival was only 49%. Of 315 ablated tumors, 36 recurred at the site of ablation, whereas 195 saw new intrahepatic lesions develop elsewhere and 160 had systemic recurrences. The patients receiving postoperative chemotherapy had lower recurrences, and patients who were treated early in the series with cryotherapy had higher recurrence rates than those treated with radiofrequency ablation or later, microwave ablation (which was found to have similar recurrence rates to radiofrequency ablation). This study shows once again that radiofrequency ablation can be a useful tool in the treatment of metastatic lesions to the liver; however, one must accept a higher recurrence rate with this over resection, especially in those tumors >1 cm. This modality may also allow for hepatic parenchymal preservation in 1 lobe, when resection of the other lobe is carried out.

J. Howe, MD

Ablation of Perivascular Hepatic Malignant Tumors with Irreversible Electroporation
Kingham TP, Karkar AM, D'Angelica MI, et al (Memorial Sloan-Kettering Cancer Ctr, NY)
J Am Coll Surg 215:379-387, 2012

Background.—Ablation is increasingly used to treat primary and secondary liver cancer. Ablation near portal pedicles and hepatic veins is challenging. Irreversible electroporation (IRE) is a new ablation technique that does not rely on heat and, in animals, appears to be safe and effective when applied near hepatic veins and portal pedicles. This study evaluated the safety and short-term outcomes of IRE to ablate perivascular malignant liver tumors.

Study Design.—A retrospective review of patients treated with IRE between January 1, 2011 and November 2, 2011 was performed. Patients were selected for IRE when resection or thermal ablation was not indicated due to tumor location. Treatment outcomes were classified by local, regional, and systemic recurrence and complications. Local failure was defined as abnormal enhancement at the periphery of an ablation defect on post-procedure contrast imaging.

Results.—Twenty-eight patients had 65 tumors treated. Twenty-two patients (79%) were treated via an open approach and 6 (21%) were treated percutaneously. Median tumor size was 1 cm (range 0.5 to 5 cm). Twenty-five tumors were < 1 cm from a major hepatic vein; 16 were < 1 cm from a major portal pedicle. Complications included 1 intraoperative arrhythmia and 1 postoperative portal vein thrombosis. Overall morbidity was 3%. There were no treatment-associated mortalities. At median follow-up of 6 months, there was 1 tumor with persistent disease (1.9%) and 3 tumors recurred locally (5.7%).

Conclusions.—This early analysis of IRE treatment of perivascular malignant hepatic tumors demonstrates safety for treating liver malignancies. Larger studies and longer follow-up are necessary to determine long-term efficacy.

▶ There have been several advances in ablative therapies over the past few decades, beginning with cryotherapy, followed by radiofrequency ablation for metastatic tumors to the liver and primary hepatocellular cancers. In the past several years, microwave ablation has gained favor because radiofrequency ablation will not adequately destroy tumors along blood vessels because of the heat sink. However, microwave ablation can injure these same blood vessels and bile ducts if the lesion is too close to major branches. Even more recently, irreversible electroporation has been introduced as yet another way to eradicate liver lesions. Electroporation causes permeability in cell membranes, which leads to cell death. This will occur right up and into hepatic veins and portal veins, but evidence from porcine models indicates that the endothelium of these structures will renew themselves after treatment. The growing interest in electroporation has come because of the difficulty of either completely ablating a lesion on a major vein branch or the potential of injuring it using microwaves. This study looked at the experience at Memorial Sloan-Kettering Cancer Center, where they tested electroporation on 65 tumors in 28 patients. These tumors were generally small with a median size of 1 cm, but they tried to pick tumors that were within ½ to 1 cm of a major hepatic vein or portal pedicle. This study showed that it could be done with a low complication rate, which included an arrhythmia during one procedure and a portal vein thrombus. The recurrence rate at 6 months was a combined 7.5%. Interestingly, the ablation zones shrunk with time between 3 and 6 months of follow-up. The authors showed that electroporation is relatively safe with a reasonably low local recurrence rate, considering that most of these tumors were not deemed ablatable and were not resected because of their location along major vascular structures.

J. Howe, MD

Laparoscopic Segmentectomy of the Liver: From Segment I to VIII
Ishizawa T, Gumbs AA, Kokudo N, et al (Univ Paris V, France; Summit Med Group, Berkeley Heights, NJ; Univ of Tokyo, Japan)
Ann Surg 256:959-964, 2012

Objective.—To evaluate the surgical techniques necessary to complete total laparoscopic segmentectomy (LS) of all liver segments (I–VIII).
Background.—When compared to open surgery, preservation of functional hepatic volume may be more difficult during laparoscopic hepatectomy. LS is a possible alternative to hemihepatectomy, but laparoscopic surgical techniques to complete anatomically accurate segmentectomy have not yet been well established.
Methods.—Data of a total of 342 consecutive patients who underwent laparoscopic hepatectomy were reviewed. LS was defined as complete removal of the Couinaud's segment, in which the corresponding hepatic

veins are exposed on the raw surface. The laparoscopic approach was facilitated by using intraoperative ultrasonography for each segment and by placing intercostal trocars to expose the root of the right hepatic vein for segmentectomy VII and VIII.

Results.—LS was completed in 62 patients: 36 segmentectomies (from I–VIII), 16 bisegmentectomies of the right lobe, and 10 subsegmentectomies were performed. Conversion to open surgery was required in 3 patients (IVa, VI, and VII). When 26 LS of the superior/posterior hepatic (sub)segments (I, IVa, VII, and VIII) were compared with the remaining 36 LS, the former group required a longer operation time (240 [132–390] minutes vs 155 [90–360]) minutes, $P < 0.01$) and showed an increased amount of blood loss (350 [20–1500] mL vs 100 [10–1100] mL, $P = 0.02$).

Conclusions.—LS is feasible and has become an essential surgical technique that can minimize the loss of functional liver volume without reducing curability, although further technical advancements are needed to enhance the accuracy of the resection, especially for the superior/posterior segments.

▶ Laparoscopic hepatectomy is being performed with increasing frequency. The advantages of this procedure are smaller incisions, less postoperative pain, and quicker recovery; however, there are some concerns about the oncologic equivalency of this procedure. This article describes some of the technical considerations for individual segmentectomies for segments 1-8. Tips for each segment are given, and the major points made are that the hepatic veins should be fully exposed and visualized while doing these segmentectomies, which requires use of intraoperative ultrasonography. The segments should be defined by their location relative to the hepatic veins, and demarcation of the particular segment can be accomplished by cutting down onto the portal blood supply and ligating it. This series describes performing 46 segmentectomies and 16 bisegmentectomies laparoscopically. Twenty-six percent of these patients required repeat hepatectomy for recurrence, there were no mortalities, and 6 patients had complications. The authors show that this is a procedure that can be performed safely with reasonable oncologic outcomes, and they provide valuable technical tips for accomplishing these resections.

J. Howe, MD

Hepatocellular

Resection or Transplantation for Early Hepatocellular Carcinoma in a Cirrhotic Liver: Does Size Define the Best Oncological Strategy?

Adam R, Bhangui P, Vibert E, et al (AP-HP Hôpital Paul Brousse, Villejuif, France)

Ann Surg 256:883-891, 2012

Background.—Resection and liver transplantation (LT) are the only curative options for hepatocellular carcinoma in cirrhotic patients (HCC-cirr).

Objective.—We tried to define the best primary intention-to-treat strategy in patients undergoing either resection or LT for early single HCC-cirr (≤ 5 cm).

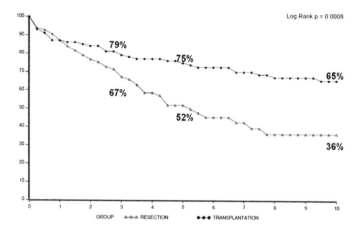

FIGURE 1.—A, OS for solitary HCC-cirr (≤5 cm), resection versus transplantation. (Reprinted from Adam R, Bhangui P, Vibert E, et al. Resection or transplantation for early hepatocellular carcinoma in a cirrhotic liver: does size define the best oncological strategy? *Ann Surg.* 2012;256:883-891, © 2012, Southeastern Surgical Congress.)

Methods.—From 1990 to 2010, 198 patients with early HCC-cirr underwent either resection (group R, n = 97) or LT (group T, n = 101) as the primary procedure. Our policy was to prioritize Childs A patients with peripheral lesions for resection rather than LT. Patient and tumor characteristics, and outcomes (recurrence-free survival [RFS] and overall survival [OS]), were studied.

Results.—A longer diagnosis-to-surgery interval, more Child Pugh B/C patients, and more tumor nodules (on histopathological examination) were found in group T patients. The postoperative mortality (4.1% vs 3.0%, $P = 0.72$) and rate of major complications (19.1% vs 24.7%, $P = 0.35$) were similar in groups R and T, respectively, whereas tumor recurrence was higher in group R (62% vs 10% in group T, $P < 0.0001$). The 5-year OS (75% vs 52%, $P = 0.0008$) and RFS (72% vs 20%, $P < 0.0001$) were better in group T; similarly, more patients were disease free at last follow-up (27% vs 62%, $P < 0.0001$). Resection as the surgical procedure, tumor diameter 3 cm or more on histology, and microvascular tumor invasion were poor prognostic factors for OS and RFS. Including dropout patients from LT list in the analysis, the outcomes in group T were still better (70% and 61% vs 51% and 36% at 5 and 10 years, $P = 0.01$).

Conclusions.—On an intention-to-treat basis, LT is associated with the best survival outcomes in patients with early HCC-cirr. Resection may achieve comparable OS in patients with single HCC-cirr of size smaller than 3 cm; however, the RFS still remains lower than that in patients of group T. This study could serve as a guide for HCC-cirr patients who are candidates for either resection or LT (Fig 1A).

▶ The decision to resect vs transplant in cases of hepatocellular cancers continues to be an area of contention. Previous studies have suggested that patients with cirrhotic livers and tumors less than 3 cm in size will benefit more from transplantation than from resection; however, these same patients also seem to be the ones most ideally suited for resection. This study from a large-volume center in France that performs both resection and transplantation evaluated cirrhotic patients with tumors less than 5 cm in size for outcomes with either resection or transplantation. This was not a prospective, randomized study, but rather was retrospective in nature. The authors stated up front that patients are more likely to undergo resection when they are Child's class A and have peripheral lesions, whereas deeper-seated tumors and more advanced cirrhosis would more likely lead to liver transplantation. In all, there were 97 patients who underwent resection vs 101 who underwent transplantation. There was a significant difference in 5-year overall survival (Fig 1A) and recurrence-free survival favoring the transplantation group, despite having patients with more advanced cirrhosis. Factors that negatively impacted prognosis were being treated by resection, a tumor diameter greater than 3 cm, and vascular invasion. In the subgroup of tumors less than 3 cm, comparable results were obtained with transplantation and resection. However, in the overall group of those less than 5 cm, it clearly appeared there was a survival benefit to having transplantation rather than resection in patients with cirrhosis and a solitary tumor. The problem with resection was a high incidence of recurrence, which ranged from 80% to 100% at 5 years. One of the reasons transplantation may be superior to resection is that cirrhotic livers can be a fertile ground for the development of new hepatocellular cancers, and transplantation introduces a noncirrhotic liver into the equation. It was also noted that examination of explanted livers found that up to 39% of hepatocellular cancers less than 3 cm in size will have other foci of hepatocellular carcinoma, another explanation for the high recurrence rates in patients undergoing resection.

J. Howe, MD

Is Surgical Resection Superior to Transplantation in the Treatment of Hepatocellular Carcinoma?
Koniaris LG, Levi DM, Pedroso FE, et al (Univ of Miami Miller School of Medicine, FL)
Ann Surg 254:527-538, 2011

Objective.—To compare outcomes for patients with hepatocellular carcinoma (HCC) treated with either liver resection or transplantation.

Methods.—A retrospective, single-institution analysis of 413 HCC patients from 1999 to 2009.

Results.—A total of 413 patients with HCC underwent surgical resection (n = 106) and transplantation (n = 270) or were listed without receiving transplantation (n = 37). Excluding transplanted patients with incidental

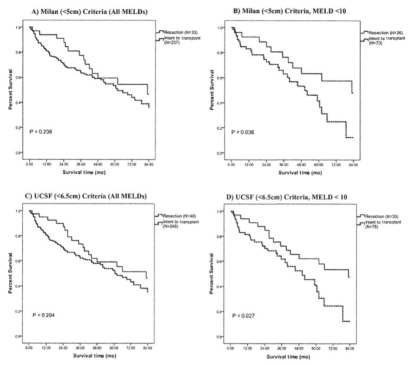

FIGURE 4.—Resection versus intent to transplant overall survival using the Kaplan-Meier method. P values via log rank (Mantel Cox) method. A, Restricted to patients meeting the Milan criteria. B, Patients meeting the Milan criteria with MELD score less than 10. C, Restricted to patients meeting the UCSF criteria. D, Patients meeting the UCSF criteria with MELD score less than 10. (Reprinted from Koniaris LG, Levi DM, Pedroso FE, et al. Is surgical resection superior to transplantation in the treatment of hepatocellular carcinoma? *Ann Surg*. 2011;254:527-538. © Southeastern Surgical Congress.)

tumors (n = 50), 257 patients with suspected HCC were listed with the intent to transplant (ITT). The median diameter of the largest tumor by radiography was 6.0 cm in resected, 3.0 cm in transplanted, and 3.4 cm in the listed-but-not-transplanted patients. Median time to transplant was 48 days. Recurrence rates were 19.8% for resection and 12.1% for all ITT patients. Overall, patient survival for resection versus ITT patients was similar (5-year survival of 53.0% vs 52.0%, not significant). However, for HCC patients with model end-stage liver disease (MELD) scores less than 10 and who radiologically met Milan or UCSF (University of California, San Francisco) criteria, 1-year and 5-year survival rates were significantly improved in resected patients. For patients with MELD score less than 10 and who met Milan criteria, 1-year and 5-year survival were 92.0% and 63.0% for resection (n = 26) versus 83.0% and 41.0% for ITT (n = 73, P = 0.036). For those with MELD score less than 10 and met UCSF criteria, 1-year and 5-year survival was 94.0% and 62.0% for resection (n = 33) versus 81.0% and 40.0% for ITT (n = 78, P = 0.027).

Conclusions.—Among known HCC patients with preserved liver function, resection was associated with superior patient survival versus transplantation. These results suggest that surgical resection should remain the first line therapy for patients with HCC and compensated liver function who are candidates for resection (Fig 4).

▶ Hepatocellular cancer (HCC) is the most common cause of cancer death in Africa and Asia and is increasing in incidence in Western countries. Current treatments for HCC include resection, transplantation, and ablative therapies. This study retrospectively reviewed the authors' experience with HCC over a 10-year period and compared outcomes in 413 patients undergoing resection (106 patients) or transplantation (270 patients plus 37 listed who did not get transplants). The groups differed in that the mean tumor size was larger in the resection group (6 vs 3 cm), more of the transplant patients had hepatitis C (74% vs 28%), and Model for End-Stage Liver disease (MELD) scores were higher in the transplant group (11 vs 6). They found that few patients were candidates for both therapies: transplant patients had to adhere to the Milan or University of California San Francisco (UCSF) criteria (tumor < 6.5 cm, multiple lesions < 3 cm, largest tumor if multiple < 4.5 cm, no vascular or extrahepatic invasion), and resections were not commonly performed on those with MELD scores above 10. There was no difference in survival in the 2 groups if the patients met the Milan or UCSF criteria for transplantation for HCC; the resection group were found to have significantly improved survival if they met these criteria and had MELD scores < 10. The recurrence-free survival rates were equivalent between these groups at 5 years, however, and the benefit was lost when the patients who were listed but did not receive transplants were removed from the transplant group. Several other centers have performed similar comparisons, but most have not included an intent-to-transplant group, nor have they excluded incidentally found HCCs in explanted livers as this study has. The authors recommend that in these times of limited donor organs, that resection of HCC should be favored in those patients eligible for transplantation (meeting Milan or UCSF criteria) who have preserved liver function (MELD < 10) (Fig 4). This question will not be resolved until a randomized trial is conducted, but this article gives perspective on practice patterns in major centers and their resulting outcomes.

J. Howe, MD

Melanoma

Sentinel Lymph Node Biopsy for Melanoma: American Society of Clinical Oncology and Society of Surgical Oncology Joint Clinical Practice Guideline
Wong SL, Balch CM, Hurley P, et al (Univ of Michigan, Ann Arbor; Univ of Texas Southwestern, Dallas; American Society of Clinical Oncology, Alexandria, VA; et al)
J Clin Oncol 30:2912-2918, 2012

Purpose.—The American Society of Clinical Oncology (ASCO) and Society of Surgical Oncology (SSO) sought to provide an evidence-based guideline on the use of lymphatic mapping and sentinel lymph node (SLN) biopsy in staging patients with newly diagnosed melanoma.

TABLE 1.—Summary of Clinical Practice Guideline Recommendations

Clinical Question	Recommendation
What are the indications for SLN biopsy?	
Intermediate-thickness melanomas	SLN biopsy is recommended for patients with intermediate-thickness cutaneous melanomas (Breslow thickness, 1 to 4 mm) of any anatomic site. Routine use of SLN biopsy in this population provides accurate staging, with high estimates for PSM and acceptable estimates for FNR, PTPN, and PVP
Thick melanomas	Although there are few studies focusing specifically on patients with thick melanomas (T4; Breslow thickness, > 4 mm), use of SLN biopsy in this population may be recommended for staging purposes and to facilitate regional disease control
Thin melanomas	There is insufficient evidence to support routine SLN biopsy for patients with thin melanomas (T1; Breslow thickness, < 1 mm), although it may be considered in selected patients with high-risk features when the benefits of pathologic staging may outweigh the potential risks of the procedure. Such risk factors may include ulceration or mitotic rate ≥ $1/mm^2$, especially in the subgroup of patients with melanomas 0.75 to 0.99 mm in Breslow thickness
What is the role of CLND?	CLND is recommended for all patients with positive SLN biopsy. CLND achieves regional disease control, although whether CLND after a positive SLN biopsy improves survival is the subject of the ongoing MSLT II

Abbreviations: CLND, completion lymph node dissection; FNR, false-negative rate; MSLT II, Multicenter Selective Lymphadenectomy Trial II; PSM, proportion successfully mapped; PTPN, post-test probability negative; PVP, positive predictive value; SLN, sentinel lymph node.

Methods.—A comprehensive systematic review of the literature published from January 1990 through August 2011 was completed using MEDLINE and EMBASE. Abstracts from ASCO and SSO annual meetings were included in the evidence review. An Expert Panel was convened to review the evidence and develop guideline recommendations.

Results.—Seventy-three studies met full eligibility criteria. The evidence review demonstrated that SLN biopsy is an acceptable method for lymph node staging of most patients with newly diagnosed melanoma.

Recommendations.—SLN biopsy is recommended for patients with intermediate-thickness melanomas (Breslow thickness, 1 to 4 mm) of any anatomic site; use of SLN biopsy in this population provides accurate staging. Although there are few studies focusing on patients with thick melanomas (T4; Breslow thickness, > 4 mm), SLN biopsy may be recommended for staging purposes and to facilitate regional disease control. There is insufficient evidence to support routine SLN biopsy for patients with thin melanomas (T1; Breslow thickness, < 1 mm), although it may be considered in selected patients with high-risk features when staging benefits outweigh risks of the procedure. Completion lymph node dissection (CLND) is recommended for all patients with a positive SLN biopsy and achieves good regional disease control. Whether CLND after a positive SLN biopsy improves survival is the subject of the ongoing Multicenter Selective Lymphadenectomy Trial II (Table 1).

▶ Sentinel lymph node biopsy in melanoma was popularized by Donald Morton in 1992. Large randomized trials, such as the Sunbelt Melanoma Trial and the Multicenter Selective Lymphadenectomy Trial I (MSLT-I), found that the sentinel node biopsy is an excellent staging procedure for intermediate-thickness melanoma; however, whether a survival advantage is provided by this procedure has not yet been determined and is the subject of the MSLT-II trial. A general recommendation has been that after a positive sentinel lymph node biopsy finding, completion lymph node dissection (CLND) should be performed. In this article from the Society of Surgical Oncology and American Society of Clinical Oncology, a meta-analysis was performed to examine 2 specific questions: (1) the indications for sentinel lymph node biopsy in melanoma and (2) the role of CLND after a positive sentinel lymph node biopsy result. This report gives recommendations based on review of the literature (Table 1) and summarizes the current indications. For the first question, it includes all intermediate-thickness melanomas, can be considered in thick melanomas, and its role continues to be controversial in thin melanomas. In the latter, it is generally not recommended; however, it may benefit patients with either ulceration or mitotic rate ≥1 mm^2 in those with 0.75- to 0.99-mm-thick melanomas. With respect to the second question, CLND should be done in cases in which there is a sentinel lymph node that is positive. However, there is morbidity from this, and the Sunbelt Melanoma and MSLT-I trials have found that the rate of additional nonsentinel lymph nodes being positive is only in the 15% to 20% range. But, the risk of nodal recurrence is that it may negatively impact survival, and this is the basis of the recommendation. This article is an excellent resource for the current state of thinking on sentinel lymph node biopsy for melanoma, and we will await the results from the MSLT-II trial to determine its impact on patient survival.

J. Howe, MD

---

1 or 2 cm Margins of Excision for T2 Melanomas: Do They Impact Recurrence or Survival?

Hudson LE, Maithel SK, Carlson GW, et al (Emory Univ School of Medicine & The Winship Cancer Inst, Atlanta, GA)
Ann Surg Oncol 20:346-351, 2013

Background.—NCCN guidelines recommend 1 or 2 cm margins for melanomas 1–2 mm (T2 melanomas) in depth; however, no head-to-head comparison has been performed. We hypothesized 1- or 2-cm margins would have similar local recurrence (LR) and overall survival (OS).

Methods.—An institutional database was queried for patients with 1.0–2.0 mm melanomas treated from July 1995 to January 2011. All had wide excision and sentinel lymph node biopsy. Patients without documented surgical margins or follow-up were excluded. Clinicopathologic and recurrence data were reviewed. Univariate and multivariate analyses were performed.

Results.—Of 2,118 patients, 1,225 met study criteria. Of these, 576 had complete data: 224 (38.9%) had 1 cm margins and 352 (61.1%), 2 cm margins. Median follow-up was 38 months. Mean age was 52.6 years (range 11.3—86.7). Mean thickness was 1.27 and 1.48 mm (1 and 2 cm, respectively, $p < 0.001$) with ulceration more common in the 2 cm group (12.3 and 21.3%, respectively; $p = 0.009$). LR was 3.6 and 0.9% in the 1 cm versus 2 cm group, respectively ($p = 0.044$). OS was 29.1 months with 1 cm and 43.7 months in the 2 cm group. On multivariate analysis, only head and neck location and nodal status were associated with overall survival.

Conclusions.—In this series, 1 cm margins were associated with a small increase in LR that did not impact OS. This is concordant with the NCCN recommendations; however, a prospective, randomized trial would be optimal.

▶ The current recommendations from the National Comprehensive Cancer Network (NCCN) for margins of excision in 1- to 2-mm Breslow depth melanoma is 1 to 2 cm. There has never been a randomized, controlled trial that has looked at 1- vs 2-cm margins for T2 (depth 1.01-2.0 mm) melanoma. However, a previous study by the World Health Organization showed that 1- vs 3-cm excision margins for melanomas < 2 mm in Breslow depth were equivalent, and the Intergroup trial found that there was little difference between 2- or 4-cm margins for melanomas < 4 mm in thickness. This study sought to address the differences in local recurrence and overall survival in a single institutional study that was nonrandomized. They looked at 576 patients with T2 melanomas, of whom 39% had 1-cm margins while 61% had 2-cm margins. The overall recurrence rate was low at 1.9%, but it was 3.6% in the 1-cm group vs 0.9% in the 2-cm group, which was statistically significant. There was no difference in regional or distant recurrence rates in the 2 groups. With respect to overall survival at a mean follow-up of 38 months, there were no differences in the 2 groups. To summarize, there was no difference in overall survival between 1- and 2-cm excision margins, but there was a slightly higher local recurrence rate in the 1-cm group. This validates the NCCN guidelines, but it makes the point that a randomized trial is necessary to fully answer the question as to whether 1-cm margins are justified in T2 melanoma. Therefore, the current practices of using 1-cm margins in difficult sites, such as the head, neck, hands, and feet, appear reasonable.

J. Howe, MD

Long-Term Results of the Randomized Phase III Trial EORTC 18991 of Adjuvant Therapy With Pegylated Interferon Alfa-2b Versus Observation in Resected Stage III Melanoma

Eggermont AMM, Suciu S, Testori A, et al (Institute de Cancérologie Gustave Roussy, Villejuif, Paris-Sud, France; European Organisation for Res and Treatment of Cancer Headquarters, Brussels, Belgium; Istituto Europeo di Oncologia, Milan, Italy; et al)

J Clin Oncol 30:3810-3818, 2012

Purpose.—Adjuvant pegylated interferon alfa-2b (PEG-IFN-α-2b) was approved for treatment of resected stage III melanoma in 2011. Here, we present long-term follow-up results of this pivotal trial.

Patients and Methods.—In all, 1,256 patients with resected stage III melanoma were randomly assigned to observation (n = 629) or PEG-IFN-α-2b (n = 627) for an intended duration of 5 years. Stratification factors were microscopic (N1) versus macroscopic (N2) nodal involvement, number of positive nodes, ulceration and tumor thickness, sex, and center. Recurrence-free survival (RFS; primary end point), distant metastasis-free survival (DMFS), and overall survival (OS) were analyzed for the intent-to-treat population.

Results.—At 7.6 years median follow-up, 384 recurrences or deaths had occurred with PEG-IFN-α-2b versus 406 in the observation group (hazard ratio [HR], 0.87; 95% CI, 0.76 to 1.00; $P = .055$); 7-year RFS rate was 39.1% versus 34.6%. There was no difference in OS ($P = .57$). In stage III-N1 ulcerated melanoma, RFS (HR, 0.72; 99% CI, 0.46 to 1.13; $P = .06$), DMFS (HR, 0.65; 99% CI, 0.41 to 1.04; $P = .02$), and OS (HR, 0.59; 99% CI, 0.35 to 0.97; $P = .006$) were prolonged with PEG-IFN-α-2b. PEG-IFN-α-2b was discontinued for toxicity in 37% of patients.

Conclusion.—Adjuvant PEG-IFN-α-2b for stage III melanoma had a positive impact on RFS, which was marginally significant and slightly diminished versus the benefit seen at prior follow-up (median, 3.8 years). No significant increase in DMFS or OS was noted in the overall population. Patients with ulcerated melanoma and lower disease burden had the greatest benefit.

▶ Adjuvant interferon treatment of node positive melanomas has been an area of controversy ever since the publication of the Eastern Cooperative Oncology Group (ECOG) 1684 trial in 1996, but improved survival did not hold up in the ECOG 1690 trial. The current study, European Organisation for Research and Treatment of Cancer (EORTC) 18991, was designed to randomize patients to receive pegylated interferon alpha-2b vs observation in patients with stage III melanoma. This is an excellent randomized, clinical trial with 7.6 years of median follow-up, which involved 1256 patients. The bottom line is that 37% of patients had significant complications from the therapy, which required discontinuation of treatment. Treatment was given on a weekly basis and was intended to be given for 5 years. Examination of overall survival rates showed that there was no significant difference in patients who received interferon vs not receiving interferon with approximate 7-year overall survival rates of 46% to 48%. In evaluation of specific subgroups, however, there were some differences seen. In those patients who had microscopic disease in their lymph nodes, there was no difference in overall survival; however, there was an 18% reduction in risk of recurrence or death, which approached significance, and a similar finding was seen when patients had disease in just 1 lymph node. When there was microscopic involvement of more than 1 node or palpable nodes, then there was no difference in survival. The study was not intended to look at the subgroup of microscopically positive patients who had ulcerated melanomas, but this subgroup did have a significant difference in overall survival. This particular study did not mention whether there were differences in those patients who just had ulcerated melanomas overall or with microscopic disease in ulcerated melanomas. Over the course of the study, there were similar numbers of deaths in each group and there was a very similar incidence of death from disease in both groups. The conclusions were that the patients most likely to benefit from interferon were those with a low disease burden, such as those patients with only a single positive sentinel lymph node, and possibly those with low disease burden and ulceration. Therefore, the benefits of interferon based on this large, well-conducted, randomized trial for patients with nodal disease in melanomas still remain questionable. There is a significant incidence of toxicity requiring cessation of treatment, and the overall survival differences are not significant. The EORTC plans to follow up with a randomized trial in patients with stage II melanoma with ulceration, which may help to answer the question of whether interferon will show benefit in these patients.

J. Howe, MD

Sentinel Lymph Nodes Containing Very Small (<0.1 mm) Deposits of Metastatic Melanoma Cannot Be Safely Regarded as Tumor-Negative

Murali R, DeSilva C, McCarthy SW, et al (Royal Prince Alfred Hosp, Sydney, New South Wales, Australia; Melanoma Inst Australia, Sydney, New South Wales; et al)
Ann Surg Oncol 19:1089-1099, 2012

Background.—Some authors have suggested that patients with very small (< 0.1 mm) deposits of metastatic melanoma in sentinel lymph nodes (SLNs) should be considered SLN-negative, whereas others have reported that such patients can have adverse long-term outcomes. The aims of the present study were to determine whether extensive sectioning of SLNs resulted in more accurate categorization of histologic features of tumor deposits and to assess prognostic associations of histologic parameters obtained using more intensive sectioning protocols.

Methods.—From patients with a single primary cutaneous melanoma who underwent SLN biopsy between 1991 and 2008, those in which the maximum size of the largest tumor deposit (MaxSize) in SLNs was < 0.1 mm in the original sections were identified. Five batches of additional sections were cut from the SLN tissue blocks at intervals of 250 μm. The 1st batch was cut from the blocks without any trimming; these sections were therefore immediately adjacent to the original sections. Each batch included 5 sequential sections, the 1st and 5th stained with hematoxylin-eosin, and the 2nd, 3rd, and 4th stained immunohistochemically with S-100, HMB-45, and Melan-A, respectively. In each batch of sections, the following histologic features of tumor deposit(s) in the SLNs were evaluated: MaxSize; tumor penetrative depth (TPD) (defined as the maximum depth of tumor deposit(s) from the inner margin of the lymph node capsule), and intranodal location (classified as subcapsular if the tumor deposit(s) were confined to the subcapsular zone or parenchymal if there was any involvement of the nodal parenchyma beyond the subcapsular zone). The measured histologic parameters were compared in each batch of sections. The association of histologic parameters with overall survival was assessed for the parameters measured in each batch of sections.

Results.—There were 20 eligible patients (15 females, 5 males, median age 60 years). After a median follow-up duration of 40 months, 4 patients had died from melanoma and 2 patients of unknown causes. Completion lymph node dissection (CLND) was performed in 13 cases (65%) and was negative in all cases. Relative to the measured values on the original sections, all 3 parameters were upstaged in subsequent batches of sections, but no further upstaging of MaxSize, TPD, or location was seen beyond batch 3, batch 4, and batch 2, respectively. Increasing MaxSize was associated with significantly poorer overall survival in batches 1, 2, and 3. Parenchymal involvement was significantly associated with poorer survival in batches 2–5. TPD was not significantly associated with overall survival.

Conclusions.—The results of this study indicate that very small (< 0.1 mm) deposits of melanoma in SLNs may be associated with adverse clinical outcomes and that this is due, at least in part, to the underestimation of SLN tumor burden in the initial sections. Our evidence does not support clinical decision-making on the assumption that patients with very small melanoma deposits in SLNs have the same outcome as those who are SLN-negative.

▶ Sentinel lymph node biopsy for melanoma has become a very popular and widespread technique for improving the staging of this disease. It is generally recommended that patients with positive sentinel lymph nodes undergo completion lymphadenectomy; however, a subset of patients, specifically those with just microscopically positive sentinel lymph node biopsies, are less straightforward. This study looked at patients from the Sydney Melanoma Unit who had sentinel lymph node metastases less than 1 mm in size. The question of this study was whether these patients should be considered as sentinel lymph node negative with respect to their clinical behavior or whether they should be treated the same as others with positive sentinel lymph nodes. To do this, they retrieved paraffin blocks from patients who had sentinel lymph nodes with deposits less than 0.1 mm and cut 5 additional sections at 250-μm intervals, which were then stained with hematoxylin and eosin as well as by immunohistochemistry. They found 20 such patients from a group of more than 400 patients with positive sentinel lymph nodes; in 13 cases patients had completion lymph node dissection, and in all cases there were no additional positive lymph nodes found, raising the question of whether these patients needed to have nodal dissection. When they did cut the extra sections they found that in 8 cases the maximum size increased with the additional sections. In those patients with the increase in maximum size, one died of unknown causes. Two patients with maximum size greater than 1 mm on repeat section died, one of melanoma and one of unknown cause. Of the other 12 patients in whom the tumor remained less than 0.1 mm on repeat sections, 1 had recurrence and 3 died of melanoma. The authors conclude that patients with very small deposits of melanoma should not be considered sentinel lymph node negative. It is clear from this study that even in this subgroup, several patients died; therefore, it is not justified to treat them differently and omit regional node dissection as conjectured by some.

J. Howe, MD

Pancreatic

Neoadjuvant/Preoperative Gemcitabine for Patients with Localized Pancreatic Cancer: A Meta-analysis of Prospective Studies
Andriulli A, Festa V, Botteri E, et al ("Casa Sollievo Della Sofferenza" Hosp, San Giovanni Rotondo, Italy; "San Filippo Neri" Hosp, Rome, Italy; European Inst of Oncology, Milan, Italy; et al)
Ann Surg Oncol 19:1644-1662, 2012

Background.—Long-term prognosis for localized pancreatic cancer remains poor. We sought to assess the benefit of neoadjuvant/preoperative chemotherapy with or without radiotherapy.

Methods.—Prospective studies where gemcitabine with or without radiotherapy was provided before surgery in patients with initially resectable or unresectable disease were reviewed by meta-analysis. Primary outcome was survival, and secondary outcomes were tumor response after therapy, toxicity, surgical exploration, and resection rates.

Results.—Twenty independent studies with 707 participants were included, 366 with resectable lesions and 341 with unresectable lesions. Seven studies were phase I/II trials, 10 phase II, and 3 prospective cohort studies. Estimated 1- and 2-year survival probabilities after resection were 91.7% (95% confidence interval [CI] 75—100) and 67.2% (95% CI 38—87) for initially resectable patients, and 86.3% (95% CI 78—100) and 54.2% (95% CI 25—100) for initially unresectable patients. The complete/partial response rate was 12% (95% CI 4—23) and 27% (95% CI 18—38) in resectable and unresectable lesions, respectively. The rate of treatment-related grade 3—4 toxicity was 31% (95% CI 21—42). Of resectable patients evaluable after restaging, 91% (95% CI 83—97) underwent surgery, and 82% (95% CI 65—95) of explored patients underwent resection. R0 resections amounted to 89% (95% CI 83—94). Of unresectable patients evaluable after restaging, 39% (95% CI 28—50) underwent surgery, and 68% (95% CI 53–82) of explored patients were resected, with 60% (95% CI 50–71) R0 resections.

Conclusions.—Current analysis provides marginal support to the assumed benefits of neoadjuvant therapies for patients with resectable cancer, and indicates a potential advantage only for a minority of those with unresectable lesions.

▶ Patients with pancreatic cancer continue to have dismal long-term survival, even after resection. Therefore, many have advocated preoperative chemotherapy and/or radiation to potentially improve survival, identify those who will progress under therapy (and, as a result, may not benefit from surgery), and increase the number of patients with margin-negative resections. In this study by Andriulli et al, a meta-analysis of prospective studies was performed in which patients received gemcitabine with or without radiation before attempted resection. They were fairly stringent on selection of trials to include only those that were prospective, used gemcitabine, and had both resectable tumors and borderline resectable tumors. The most significant findings from this meta-analysis were that nearly one-quarter of patients had complete or partial responses, whereas 50% had stable disease and approximately 25% had tumor progression. Furthermore, significant toxicity was seen in 32% of patients receiving gemcitabine alone vs 38% when gemcitabine was administered with radiation. Ninety percent of patients with potentially resectable lesions were explored, and 82% were resected. Of the patients deemed borderline resectable or unresectable, 46% were explored, and 68% of these had resections. After resection, median survival was 28 months; it was 31 months in those having resection and initially deemed resectable vs 18 months for those initially thought to be unresectable. The bottom line of this study was that there was marginal benefit for neoadjuvant treatment with gemcitabine in those patients thought to be resectable and minimal downstaging in patients thought to be unresectable. It is difficult to make clear conclusions from this meta-analysis because of the heterogeneity of the studies included, although the authors did a good job of trying to only include prospective and well-performed trials. Without randomization to neoadjuvant treatment vs no treatment, it will always be difficult to fully assess the potential benefits of such therapy.

J. Howe, MD

Laparoscopic Distal Pancreatectomy: Trends and Lessons Learned Through an 11-Year Experience
Kneuertz PJ, Patel SH, Chu CK, et al (Emory Univ School of Medicine, Atlanta, GA; et al)
J Am Coll Surg 215:167-176, 2012

Background.—As compared with open distal pancreatectomy, laparoscopic distal pancreatectomy (LDP) is associated with lower morbidity and shorter hospital stays. Existing reports do not elucidate trends in patient selection, technique, and outcomes over time. We aimed to determine outcomes after LDP at a specialized center, analyze trends of patient selection and operative technique, and validate a complication risk score (CRS).

Study Design.—Patients undergoing LDP between January 2000 and January 2011 were identified and divided into 2 equal groups to represent our early and recent experiences. Demographics, tumor characteristics, operative technique, and perioperative outcomes were examined and compared between groups. A CRS was calculated for the entire cohort and examined against observed outcomes.

Results.—A total of 132 LDPs were attempted, of which 8 (6.1%) were converted to open procedures. Thirty-day overall and major complication rates were 43.2% and 12.9%, respectively, with mortality < 1%. Pancreatic fistulas occurred in 28 (21%) patients, of which 14 (11%) were clinically significant. Recent LDPs (n = 66) included patients with increasingly severe comorbidities (Charlson scores > 2, 40.9% vs 16.7%, $p = 0.003$), more proximal tumors (74.2% vs 26.2%, $p < 0.001$), more extended resections (10.6 vs 8.3 cm, $p < 0.001$), shorter operative times (141 vs 172 minutes, $p = 0.007$), and less frequent use of a hand port (25.8% vs 66.6%, $p < 0.001$). No significant differences were found in perioperative outcomes between the groups. As compared with the hand access technique, the total laparoscopic approach was associated with shorter hospital stays (5.3 vs 6.8 days, $p = 0.032$). Increasing CRS was associated with longer operative time, significant fistulas, wound infections, blood transfusions, major complications, ICU readmissions, and rehospitalizations.

Conclusions.—This large, single-institution series demonstrates that despite a shift in patient selection to sicker patients with more proximal tumors, similar perioperative outcomes can be achieved with laparoscopic distal pancreatectomy. The CRS appears to be a reliable preoperative assessment tool for assessing other adverse perioperative outcomes in addition to predicting overall complications and fistulas as originally published.

▶ Over the past decade, there has been increasing use of laparoscopic pancreatectomy, and this series reviews one institution's earlier vs later experience with this procedure. The value of this study is that the authors determined which techniques and outcomes were used more frequently. Initially, hand ports were used in nearly two-thirds of cases, whereas only one-quarter of cases used them in the more recent experience, and, interestingly, splenic vessel preservation was performed less and less with time. The authors favored the medial to lateral approach, as they believed it was more oncologic and showed a trend toward decreasing operative times with no change of pancreatic fistula rate or complication rates over the series. Another interesting trend was an increasing use of vascular loads for the stapler in 50% of the more recent cases vs only one-third of the earlier cases, and no significant change in reinforcement along the staple line with approximately 40% of cases early and late. This study allows us to look into the experience gained at a high-volume center and the modifications and procedures that they came up with over time.

J. Howe, MD

Grafts for Mesenterico-Portal Vein Resections Can Be Avoided during Pancreatoduodenectomy

Wang F, Arianayagam R, Gill A, et al (Royal North Shore Hosp and North Shore Private Hosp, St Leonards, New South Wales, Australia)
J Am Coll Surg 215:569-579, 2012

Background.—The aim of this study was to assess whether pancreatoduodenectomy (PD) and en bloc mesenterico-portal resection (PD+VR) could be performed with primary venous reconstruction, avoiding a vascular graft. In addition, the short-term surgical outcomes of this approach were compared with a standard PD (PD-VR).

Study Design.—Two hundred twelve patients underwent PD between January 2004 and June 2011. Clinical data, operative results, pathologic findings, and postoperative outcomes were collected prospectively and analyzed.

Results.—One hundred fifty patients (71%) had PD-VR and 62 patients underwent PD+VR. The majority (82%) of the venous reconstructions were performed with primary end-to-end anastomosis. Only 1 patient had synthetic interposition graft repair. The volume of intraoperative blood loss and the perioperative blood transfusion requirements were significantly greater, and the duration of the operation was significantly longer in the PD+VR group compared with the PD-VR group. There were no significant differences in the length of hospitalization, postoperative morbidity, or grades of complications between the 2 groups. Multivariate logistic regression identified American Society of Anesthesiologists score as the only predictor of postoperative morbidity. Fifty percent of patients with pancreatic adenocarcinoma (n = 101) required VR. A significantly higher rate of positive resection margins ($p < 0.001$) was noted in the PD+VR subgroup compared with PD-VR subgroup. Furthermore, high intraoperative blood loss and neural invasion were predictive of a positive resection margin.

Conclusions.—Pancreatoduodenectomy with VR and primary venous anastomosis avoids the need for a graft and has comparable postoperative morbidity with PD-VR. However, it is associated with an increased operative time, higher intraoperative blood loss, and, for pancreatic ductal adenocarcinoma, a higher rate of positive resection margins compared with PD-VR.

▶ In the past few decades, it has been demonstrated that portal or superior mesenteric vein resection can be done safely in patients undergoing pancreaticoduodenectomy, with similar survival as compared to patients not having vein resection. Typically, a vein resection will require an interposition of prosthetic graft or vein, although primary anastomosis is also feasible, as is repair with a vein patch. This study from Australia looked at the authors' experience with 212 pancreaticoduodenectomies, in which a venous resection was performed in 62. In only 1 patient did they place a synthetic graft, and the remainder had primary venous reconstruction, with more than 80% having end-to-end anastomosis. The advantage of an end-to-end anastomosis is that there is only 1 suture line, which reduces the risk of thrombosis and shortens mesenteric clamp time. Other reasons given for not using prosthetic grafts are increased risk of thrombosis as well as the opportunity for infection because of pancreatic fistula formation.

The authors showed that they could do this without significant morbidity with complication and mortality rates similar to patients who did not have vein resection. There were differences among the 2 groups in terms of increased blood loss, need for blood transfusion, and increase in tumor size in the subset undergoing vein resection. On histologic analysis, three-quarters of the patients who underwent vein resection had histologic evidence of invasion, whereas 25% did not. The authors also noted that the mean length of vein resection was 20 mm and suggested that lengths up to 4 cm can be taken with primary anastomosis. The article gives interesting technical details on how to facilitate this, including division of the splenic vein and closing any lateral wall defects with a transverse suture line. This study did not look at survival analysis as this was not the intent of the study.

J. Howe, MD

Retroperitoneal Dissection in Patients with Borderline Resectable Pancreatic Cancer: Operative Principles and Techniques
Katz MHG, Lee JE, Pisters PWT, et al (The Univ of Texas MD Anderson Cancer Ctr, Houston)
J Am Coll Surg 215:e11-e18, 2012

Pancreatectomy with aggressive vascular resection is increasingly being recognized as an appropriate treatment strategy for patients with borderline resectable PDAC after administration of chemotherapy and/or chemoradiation. Because tumor downstaging is an uncommon event, both venous and hepatic arterial resection and reconstruction might be necessary to achieve negative surgical margins and the favorable short-term and long-term outcomes we have reported previously. The technical approaches we have described here can be used as a basic foundation for operative safety and efficiency during these challenging operations.

▶ Aggressive surgical resection of pancreatic adenocarcinoma has been performed with increasing frequency over the past decade, including on patients with borderline resectable tumors. This is defined as radiographic abutment or encasement greater than 180° of the superior mesenteric vein or portal vein, common hepatic artery, or limited abutment to the superior mesenteric artery (SMA) or celiac trunk. This article from M.D. Anderson gives several helpful pointers to performing these advanced resections. Most of these patients will have received neoadjuvant chemotherapy with or without radiation, which often does not shrink the primary tumor radiographically but may improve surgical margins. A strategy discussed in this article is retroperitoneal dissection of the right side of the SMA with the tissue adjacent being swept toward the right. Careful note is made to not circumferentially dissect the SMA because this can lead to sympathectomy and intractable diarrhea. In cases in which there is encroachment on the superior mesenteric vein (SMV) or significant abutment of the SMV, it may be necessary to divide and ligate the first jejunal branch, the inferior mesenteric vein if it enters the SMV directly, and/or the splenic vein. Sometimes when the splenic vein is divided, the stomach will show signs of impaired venous drainage and one should then consider performing a splenorenal shunt. The author has described that when the SMA itself is encroached that heparinization and proximal and distal control of the SMA may be necessary to divide the inferior pancreaticoduodenal arteries from the side of the SMA so they can be sutured primarily. They also described cases of hepatic artery encasement or replaced right hepatic artery encasement that can be treated by resection of the artery and interposition graft. This article contains nice illustrations to show how these techniques are done. Not everyone would agree that vascular resection, especially arterial resection, is indicated in many cases, but this article does describe several technical details that would be helpful in these instances.

J. Howe, MD

Genetic Basis of Pancreas Cancer Development and Progression: Insights from Whole-Exome and Whole-Genome Sequencing
Iacobuzio-Donahue CA, Velculescu VE, Wolfgang CL, et al (Johns Hopkins Univ School of Medicine, Baltimore, MD)
Clin Cancer Res 18:4257-4265, 2012

Pancreatic cancer is caused by inherited and acquired mutations in specific cancer-associated genes. The discovery of the most common genetic alterations in pancreatic cancer has provided insight into the fundamental pathways that drive the progression from a normal cell to noninvasive precursor lesions and finally to widely metastatic disease. In addition, recent genetic discoveries have created new opportunities to develop gene-based approaches for early detection, personalized treatment, and molecular classification of pancreatic neoplasms (Tables 2 and 4).

▶ Knowledge of the human genome and application of next-generation sequencing methodologies are nicely reviewed in this report with respect to their application to pancreatic cancers. Sequencing the exomes or coding sequences of all the known genes is an excellent way to determine the fundamental genetic basis of these diseases, both in sporadic pancreatic cancer (Table 2) and in cases in which patients are born with a predisposition and strong family history of

TABLE 2.—Common Somatic Changes in Ductal Adenocarcinoma of the Pancreas

Gene	Chromosome	Cancers with a Mutation (%)
KRAS	12p	95
P16/CDKN2A	9p	>90
TP53	17p	75
SMAD4	18q	55

TABLE 4.—Familial Pancreatic Cancer Genes

Gene[a]	Chromosome	Syndrome Name	Other Tumor Types
BRCA2	13q	Familial breast cancer 2	Breast, ovary, and prostate
P16/CDKN2A	9p	Familial atypical multiple mole melanoma	Melanoma
PRSS1	7q	Familial pancreatitis	None
PALB2	16p		Breast
ATM	11q	Ataxia telangiectasia	Leukemia and lymphoma (homozygotes), breast (heterozygotes)
STK11	19p	Peutz-Jeghers	Gastrointestinal tract, breast, gynecologic, testis, and lung

[a]The BRCA2, p16/CDKN2A, STK11, ATM, PALB2, and PRSS1 genes account for less than 20% of the familial aggregation of pancreatic cancer.

pancreatic cancer (Table 4). This report reviews studies that include invasive ductal adenocarcinoma, pancreatic intraepithelial neoplasia, intraductal papillary mucinous neoplasm, familial pancreatic cancers, pancreatic neuroendocrine tumors, and rarer pancreatic cancers. Knowledge of the fundamental genetic basis of these conditions allows for identification of gene carriers in those with a familial predisposition and screening for other components of these syndromes. It also allows one to understand the progression of cancer and, therefore, has therapeutic implications as well. Knowledge of the genetic perturbations in an individual tumor can also help in the classification of this tumor into a specific subtype if this is not clear. Overall, it is an exciting time that we live in, to be able to understand the fundamental DNA changes that lead to this highly lethal disease. Hopefully, new and effective therapies will follow from this knowledge.

J. Howe, MD

Rectal

Postoperative Adjuvant Chemotherapy Use in Patients With Stage II/III Rectal Cancer Treated With Neoadjuvant Therapy: A National Comprehensive Cancer Network Analysis

Khrizman P, Niland JC, ter Veer A, et al (Lurie Comprehensive Cancer Ctr of Northwestern Univ, Chicago, IL; City of Hope Comprehensive Cancer Ctr, Los Angeles, CA; et al)
J Clin Oncol 31:30-38, 2013

Purpose.—Practice guidelines recommend that patients who receive neoadjuvant chemotherapy and radiation for locally advanced rectal cancer complete postoperative adjuvant systemic chemotherapy, irrespective of tumor downstaging.

Patients and Methods.—The National Comprehensive Cancer Network (NCCN) Colorectal Cancer Database tracks longitudinal care for patients treated at eight specialty cancer centers across the United States and was used to evaluate how frequently patients with rectal cancer who were treated with neoadjuvant chemotherapy also received postoperative systemic chemotherapy. Patient and tumor characteristics were examined in a multivariable logistic regression model.

Results.—Between September 2005 and December 2010, 2,073 patients with stage II/III rectal cancer were enrolled in the database. Of these, 1,193 patients receiving neoadjuvant chemoradiotherapy were in the analysis, including 203 patients not receiving any adjuvant chemotherapy. For those seen by a medical oncologist, the most frequent reason chemotherapy was not recommended was comorbid illness (25 of 50, 50%); the most frequent reason chemotherapy was not received even though it was recommended or discussed was patient refusal (54 of 74, 73%). After controlling for NCCN Cancer Center and clinical TNM stage in a multivariable logistic model, factors significantly associated with not receiving adjuvant chemotherapy were age, Eastern Cooperative Oncology Group performance status ≥ 1, on Medicaid or indigent compared with private insurance, complete pathologic response, presence of re-operation/wound infection, and no closure of ileostomy/colostomy.

Conclusion.—Even at specialty cancer centers, a sizeable minority of patients with rectal cancer treated with curative-intent neoadjuvant chemoradiotherapy do not complete postoperative chemotherapy. Strategies to facilitate the ability to complete this third and final component of curative intent treatment are necessary.

▶ Neoadjuvant chemotherapy and radiation for rectal cancer has been shown to decrease local recurrence rates, but it generally does not improve overall survival. An important issue in these patients is that current recommendations are for 6 months of postoperative adjuvant chemotherapy, but many patients will not receive this follow-up chemotherapy. This study looked at patients from the National Comprehensive Cancer Network (NCCN) with rectal cancer to determine the number of patients who did not receive adjuvant therapy after neoadjuvant treatment of rectal cancer. This was done in an effort to determine potential reasons why these patients did not receive postsurgical adjuvant treatment. They focused on patients with stage II and stage III rectal cancer, and of 1193 patients who received neoadjuvant therapy (72% of the total number of patients with rectal cancer), 83% received adjuvant therapy and 17% did not. It was determined that 20% of the latter patients were not seen by a medical oncologist, and in 13% of cases it was unknown whether or not they saw a medical oncologist. In the two-thirds of these patients who did see a medical oncologist, chemotherapy was not recommended in 37%, was recommended in 54%, and in 13% of cases it was not clear. The most common reasons for not recommending chemotherapy were comorbidity, that the therapy was not indicated, a combination of comorbidity and older age, and disease recurrence or death. In those patients in whom it was recommended but who did not get adjuvant treatment, the majority of the cases were because the patients declined treatment (54 of 74 cases), followed by recurrence prior to treatment, patient deaths, or unknown reasons. In multivariate analysis, the study found that the factors most likely to be associated with not receiving adjuvant therapy included older age, Eastern Cooperative Oncology

Group status performance > 1, Medicaid or indigent patients, patients who had complete response, or those patients who had reoperation for wound infection or had not had closure of their ileostomy or colostomy. This study does have the limitation that the patients included were seen at academic medical centers and may not reflect the US population as a whole. However, it does provide a good estimate of why as many as one-fifth of patients do not receive postoperative adjuvant therapy for rectal cancer, as currently recommended by the NCCN.

J. Howe, MD

Robot-Assisted Versus Conventional Laparoscopic Surgery for Colorectal Disease, Focusing on Rectal Cancer: A Meta-Analysis
Yang Y, Wang F, Zhang P, et al (Shanghai Tenth People's Hosp Affiliated to Tongji Univ, People's Republic of China; et al)
Ann Surg Oncol 19:3727-3736, 2012

Background.—Robotic colorectal surgery may solve some of the problems inherent to conventional laparoscopic surgery (CLS). We sought to evaluate the advantages of robot-assisted laparoscopic surgery (RALS) using the da Vinci Surgical System over CLS in patients with benign and malignant colorectal diseases.

Methods.—PubMed and Embase databases were searched for relevant studies published before July 2011. Studies clearly documenting a comparison of RALS with CLS for benign and malignant colorectal diseases were selected. Operative and postoperative measures, resection margins, complications, and related outcomes were evaluated. Weighted mean differences, relative risks, and hazard ratios were calculated using a random-effects model.

Results.—The meta-analysis included 16 studies comparing RALS and CLS in patients with colorectal diseases and 7 studies in rectal cancer. RALS was associated with lower estimated blood loss in colorectal diseases ($P = 0.04$) and rectal cancer ($P < 0.001$) and lower rates of intraoperative conversion in colorectal diseases ($P = 0.03$) and rectal cancer ($P < 0.001$) than CLS. In patients with colorectal diseases, however, operating time ($P < 0.001$) and total hospitalization cost ($P = 0.06$) were higher for RALS than CLS.

Conclusions.—RALS was associated with reduced estimated blood loss and a lower intraoperative conversion rate than CLS, with no differences in complication rates and surrogate markers of successful surgery. Robotic colorectal surgery is a promising tool, especially for patients with rectal cancer.

▶ Laparoscopic colorectal surgery has been shown to be safe and results for colon cancer have revealed it to have similar oncologic outcomes as conventional open surgery. Robot-assisted laparoscopic surgery for colorectal procedures has been performed since 2002, and this study set out to determine the safety, feasibility, and efficacy of performing robot-assisted laparoscopic colectomy vs conventional laparoscopic colectomy. To do this they performed a meta-analysis and ultimately had 16 studies to compare, most of which were nonrandomized, case-control studies; however, 2 were randomized. The findings of this study were that the cost and operative times were slightly longer for the robot-assisted procedures; however, there were no differences in intraoperative blood loss, postoperative complications, and distal resection margins, and there was only a minimal difference in length of stay. The intraoperative conversion rate was also similar between the 2 methods. This study reveals that there are not significant differences in most parameters for laparoscopic vs robot-assisted colectomy, and the costs were higher for the robot-assisted colectomy, which did not include the cost of buying the device in this analysis. The operative time for benign and malignant disease of the colorectum was longer for robot-assisted procedures; however, it was the same in patients undergoing these procedures for rectal cancer. These results suggest that robot-assisted colorectal resection is equivalent to standard laparoscopic resection, but it remains to be determined whether the increases in costs will be justified with this equivalency of results.

J. Howe, MD

Is the 1-cm Rule of Distal Bowel Resection Margin in Rectal Cancer Based on Clinical Evidence? A Systematic Review
Bujko K, Rutkowski A, Chang GJ, et al (Maria Sklodowska-Curie Memorial Cancer Centre, Warsaw, Poland; Univ of Texas MD Anderson Cancer Ctr, Houston, TX)
Ann Surg Oncol 19:801-808, 2012

Background.—Distal intramural spread is present within 1 cm from visible tumor in a substantial proportion of patients. Therefore, ≥ 1 cm of distal bowel clearance is recommended as minimally acceptable. However, clinical results are contradictory in answering the question of whether this rule is valid. The aim of this review was to evaluate whether in patients undergoing anterior resection, a distal bowel gross margin of < 1 cm jeopardizes oncologic safety.

Methods.—A systematic review of the literature identified 17 studies showing results in relation to margins of approximately < 1 cm (948 patients) versus > 1 cm (4626 patients); five studies in relation to a margin of ≤ 5 mm (173 patients) versus > 5 mm (1277 patients), and five studies showing results in a margin of ≤ 2 mm (73 patients). In most studies, pre- or postoperative radiation was provided.

Results.—A multifactorial process was identified resulting in selection of favorable tumors for anterior resection with the short bowel margin and unfavorable tumors for abdominoperineal resection or for anterior resection with the long margin. In total, the local recurrence rate was 1.0% higher in the < 1-cm margin group compared to the > 1-cm margin group (95% confidence interval [CI] −0.6 to 2.7; $P = 0.175$). The corresponding figures for ≤ 5 mm cutoff point were 1.7% (95% CI −1.9 to 5.3; $P = 0.375$). The pooled local recurrence rate in patients having ≤ 2 mm margin was 2.7% (95% CI 0 to 6.4).

Conclusions.—In the selected group of patients, <1 cm margin did not jeopardize oncologic safety.

▶ A National Cancer Institute consensus panel recommended in 2001 that a 1-cm margin of tumor clearance is important in the treatment of rectal cancer. Over time, with increased use of preoperative and postoperative radiation and chemotherapy, surgeons have questioned the need for a 1-cm margin. Furthermore, with the use of total mesorectal excision it may also be less important. The current study looked at several thousand patients from 17 studies using a meta-analysis approach. The findings from this study were surprising. There was only a 1% increase in local recurrence in those patients with <1-cm vs >1-cm margins and, therefore, the authors conclude that current clinical data do not support the rule that a 1-cm margin is necessary. It should be noted that there was some inherent bias associated with this study. This is underlined by the fact that it included only patients undergoing lower anterior resection and, therefore, patients who are deemed to have larger tumors and higher risk tumors who underwent abdominal perineal resection may not have been included. Also, surgeons might be more likely to accept a closer margin if they feel there has been a good response to preoperative chemotherapy and radiation. However, these potential biases not withstanding, the need to adhere to a 1-cm margin may not be as important as previously thought.

J. Howe, MD

Carcinoid Tumors of the Rectum: A Multi-institutional International Collaboration

Shields CJ, the International Rectal Carcinoid Study Group (Mater Misericordiae Univ Hosp and Dublin Academic Med Centre, Ireland; et al)
Ann Surg 252:750-755, 2010

Objective.—This study aims to describe recent experience with rectal carcinoids in European and North American centers.

Background.—While considered indolent, the propensity of carcinoids to metastasize can be significant.

Methods.—Rectal carcinoid patients were identified from prospective databases maintained at 9 institutions between 1999 and 2008. Demographic, clinical, and histologic data were collated. Median follow-up was 5 years (range, 0.5—10 years).

Results.—Two hundred two patients were identified. The median age was 55 years (range, 31—81 years). The majority of tumors were an incidental finding (n = 115, 56.9%). The median tumor size was 10 mm (range, 2—120 mm). Overall, 93 (49%) tumors were limited to the mucosa or submucosa, 45 (24%) involved the muscularis propria, 29 (15%) extended into the perirectal fat, and 6 (3%) reached the visceral peritoneum. The primary treatment modalities were endoscopic resection (n = 86, 43%)

TABLE 3.—Multiple Variable Logistic Regression Analysis of Risk Factors for Lymph Node Metastases*

Variables	Odds Ratio	95% CI	P
Tumor size >10 mm	32.7	14.8–72.3	0.006
Lymphovascular invasion	19.6	12.3–146.0	< 0.001

*Risk factors for nodal involvement calculated in patients who underwent formal surgical resection (n = 100).

TABLE 4.—Multiple Variable Logistic Regression Analysis of Risk Factors for Distant Metastases*

Variables	Odds Ratio	95% CI	P
Lymph node metastases	12.3	1.8-84.7	0.033
Lymphovascular invasion	74.4	4.6-120.2	0.022

*Risk factors for distant metastases calculated in patients who underwent formal surgical resection (n = 100).

and surgical extirpation (n = 102, 50%). Forty-one patients (40%) underwent a high anterior resection, whereas 45 (44%) underwent anterior resection with total mesorectal excision. Seven patients (7%) underwent Hartman's procedure, 7 (7%) underwent abdomino-perineal resection, and 6 (6%) had transanal endoscopic microsurgery, whereas 4 (4%) patients underwent a transanal excision. Multiple variable logistic regression analysis demonstrated that tumor size greater than 10 mm and lymphovascular invasion were predictors of nodal involvement ($P = 0.006$ and < 0.001, respectively), whereas the presence of lymph node metastases and lymphovascular invasion was associated with subsequent development of distant metastases ($P = 0.033$ and 0.022, respectively). The presence of nodal metastases has a profound effect upon survival, with a 5-year survival rate of 70%, and 10-year survival of 60% for node positive tumors. Patients with distant metastases have a 4-year survival of 38%.

Conclusion.—Tumor size greater than 10 mm and lymphovascular invasion are significantly associated with the presence of nodal disease, rendering mesorectal excision advisable. Transanal excision is adequate for smaller tumors (Tables 3 and 4).

▶ Carcinoid or neuroendocrine tumors (NETs) of the rectum account for 2% of rectal tumors, and the incidence has increased 10-fold over the past several decades. Local resection has been recommended for those tumors smaller than 20 mm and limited to the submucosa, but even these can metastasize to nodes or distantly. The significance of this study was that 1 American and 8 European centers collected data, including 202 adults with rectal carcinoid tumors; this is the largest collective series outside of national databases, with these retrospective data thought to be more reliable and complete. Of these tumors, 57% were found incidentally, 18% because of rectal bleeding, 10% for change in bowel habits, and 3% from carcinoid syndrome. Patients who had surgical resection (not endoscopic) were evaluated for risk factors for lymph node metastases, and independent predictors were tumor size > 10 mm (odds ratio 32.7) and lymphovascular invasion (OR 19.6; Table 3); for distant metastases, independent predictors were lymph node metastases (OR 12.3) and lymphovascular invasion (OR 74.4; Table 4). Disease-specific 5-year survival rates were 100% for localized disease, 68% with nodal metastases, and < 40% with distant metastases. Rectal carcinoids account for 7% to 27% of all NETs depending on race, and generally have some of the highest overall survival rates (75%–90% 5-year survival). This study demonstrated the features that need to be looked at that increase the risk for nodal and distant metastases, and therefore more aggressive surgery (to include mesorectal excision). These included tumor size > 10 mm, lymphovascular invasion, and possibly T2-4 lesions.

J. Howe, MD

Other

Early- and Long-Term Outcome Data of Patients With Pseudomyxoma Peritonei From Appendiceal Origin Treated by a Strategy of Cytoreductive Surgery and Hyperthermic Intraperitoneal Chemotherapy

Chua TC, Moran BJ, Sugarbaker PH, et al (Univ of New South Wales, Sydney, Australia; Basingstoke and North Hampshire Natl Health Service Foundation Trust, UK; Washington Hosp Ctr, DC; et al)
J Clin Oncol 30:2449-2456, 2012

Purpose.—Pseudomyxoma peritonei (PMP) originating from an appendiceal mucinous neoplasm remains a biologically heterogeneous disease. The purpose of our study was to evaluate outcome and long-term survival after cytoreductive surgery (CRS) and hyperthermic intraperitoneal chemotherapy (HIPEC) consolidated through an international registry study.

Patients and Methods.—A retrospective multi-institutional registry was established through collaborative efforts of participating units affiliated with the Peritoneal Surface Oncology Group International.

Results.—Two thousand two hundred ninety-eight patients from 16 specialized units underwent CRS for PMP. Treatment-related mortality was 2% and major operative complications occurred in 24% of patients. The median survival rate was 196 months (16.3 years) and the median progression-free survival rate was 98 months (8.2 years), with 10- and 15-year survival rates of 63% and 59%, respectively. Multivariate analysis identified prior chemotherapy treatment ($P < .001$), peritoneal mucinous carcinomatosis (PMCA) histopathologic subtype ($P < .001$), major postoperative complications ($P = .008$), high peritoneal cancer index ($P = .013$), debulking surgery (completeness of cytoreduction [CCR], 2 or 3; $P < .001$), and not using HIPEC ($P = .030$) as independent predictors for a poorer progression-free survival. Older age ($P = .006$), major postoperative complications ($P < .001$), debulking surgery (CCR 2 or 3; $P < .001$), prior chemotherapy treatment ($P < .001$), and PMCA histopathologic subtype ($P < .001$) were independent predictors of a poorer overall survival.

Conclusion.—The combined modality strategy for PMP may be performed safely with acceptable morbidity and mortality in a specialized unit setting with 63% of patients surviving beyond 10 years. Minimizing nondefinitive operative and systemic chemotherapy treatments before definitive cytoreduction may facilitate the feasibility and improve the outcome of this therapy to achieve long-term survival. Optimal cytoreduction achieves the best outcomes.

▶ Although appendiceal cancers are rare, as they grow in this relatively enclosed diverticulum, they may frequently spread through the wall, leading to seeding of the peritoneal cavity that results in pseudomyxoma peritonei. This is a big problem, and early studies looking at debulking surgery alone revealed a high incidence of recurrence and low long-term survival rates. Significant progress has been made over the past several decades in this disease, however, thanks to the efforts of those surgeons who have dedicated themselves to dealing with this difficult problem. The current state of the art begins with removal of the peritoneal lining and all visible disease, followed by heated intraperitoneal chemotherapy (HIPEC), most recently with mitomycin C and oxaliplatin. Using this strategy, impressive 10- and 15-year survivals have been described, and this report represents the largest series of appendiceal peritoneal mucinous carcinomatosis and diffuse peritoneal adenomucinosis. This study retrospectively reviewed 2298 patients from 16 institutions between 1993 and 2011. Interesting findings of this study were that optimal cytoreduction could be achieved in 83% of patients (ie, no visible disease or disease less than 2.5 mm in size for any single nodule), with a median operative time of 9 hours. Clearly, these are labor-intensive procedures. The major complication rate was 24% and mortality rate was 2%. The median survival in these patients was 196 months, and progression-free survival was 98 months; 5-year survival was 74%, 10-year survival was 63%, and 15-year survival was 59%, which has significantly improved over historical controls of debulking surgery alone. This study looked at factors that were associated with increased risk of progression, and that included prior chemotherapy and mucinous adenocarcinoma subtype in addition to those patients having postoperative complication, higher peritoneal cancer index, or suboptimal debulking surgery. The authors could not show that HIPEC itself was an independent significant factor for improved long-term survival, but it was clear that optimal cytoreduction was. The study demonstrated that in specialized centers with expertise in this technique, it is certainly worthwhile for patients to undergo cytoreductive surgery and HIPEC, because the complication rates were not as high as might be expected and there was significant long-term survival benefit.

J. Howe, MD

A Population-Based Comparison of Adenocarcinoma of the Large and Small Intestine: Insights Into a Rare Disease

Overman MJ, Hu C-Y, Kopetz S, et al (Univ of Texas MD Anderson Cancer Ctr, Houston)
Ann Surg Oncol 19:1439-1445, 2012

Background.—Because of its rarity, adenocarcinoma of the small intestine is frequently compared to adenocarcinoma of the colon, although the validity of this comparison is not known.

Methods.—Patients with small and large bowel adenocarcinoma (SBA and LBA) diagnosed between 1988 and 2007 were identified from the Surveillance, Epidemiology, and End Results registry. Age-standardized incidence and mortality rates were determined. Cancer-specific survival (CSS) stratified by stage and by number of assessed lymph nodes was calculated.

Results.—A total of 4518 and 261,521 patients with SBA and LBA, respectively, were identified. In comparison to LBA, patients with SBA were younger and presented with disease of higher stage and histologic grade. The age-standardized incidence rates decreased for LBA (-1.24% per year) but increased for SBA ($+1.47\%$ per year). Although age-standardized mortality rates decreased for both LBA and SBA, the decreases were more pronounced for LBA. Five-year CSS was worse for resected SBA compared with resected LBA, although this difference diminished when comparing cases having eight or more lymph nodes assessed. The relative reduction in CSS when selecting eight or more lymph nodes was much greater for duodenal as opposed to jejunal/ileal subsite of the small bowel. With nodal selection the absolute difference in CSS between LBA and SBA for stages I, II, and III was 13, 15.9, and 18.5%, respectively.

Conclusions.—Adequate nodal assessment is much less common in SBA than LBA; and it appears that SBA, in particular duodenal adenocarcinoma, is understaged. Even after corrections to minimize the effect of stage migration and inadequate lymph node evaluation, SBA demonstrated distinctly worse CSS than LBA.

▶ Small bowel adenocarcinoma (SBA) is a relatively rare disease, and there have been few studies showing the optimal management for this condition. For this reason, and because it shares origin within the intestine, surgical procedures (resection with lymphadenectomy), as well as adjuvant treatment for stage III and IV disease have generally been similar as that in colon cancer. This study evaluated patients in the Surveillance, Epidemiology, and End Results database between 1988 and 2007 to look for differences between patients diagnosed with SBA and large bowel adenocarcinoma (LBA) during this period. There were 4518 cases of SBA, approximately 1.7% of the incidence of LBA. Interesting findings included a higher incidence of SBA in male patients, black race, poorly differentiated tumors, and stage IV tumors. Over the study period, there was an increase in incidence of SBA but a decrease in LBA. Stage for stage, survival was better in LBA relative to SBA. In this study, a correction was performed to include resections which included 8 or more lymph nodes, and with this there continued to be stage-for-stage improvement in survival for LBA. However, the degree of difference was not as great for stage I and stage II SBA, suggesting stage migration. The difference was greatest for patients with duodenal adenocarcinoma with respect to the improvement of survival when 8 or more lymph nodes were harvested in stage I and II. The authors conclude that there may be differences in biology between the SBA and LBA to explain these differences in survival and stage; however, an other option would be the impact of screening colonoscopy and earlier detection of colon cancer, although there have been improvements in SBA diagnosis with capsule endoscopy and improved computed tomography imaging. Improvements in mortality for SBA were seen over the study period, which may reflect the increasing use of adjuvant chemotherapy as well as an increasing fraction of stage I and stage II SBA over the study period. Another interesting aspect of this study was that a significant percentage of patients with SBA died of colorectal cancer (22%) and pancreatic cancer (10%) versus SBA itself (68%). This study adds some new twists to the previously reported studies of SBA, which have focused on clinicopathologic features and survival through comparison with its similar counterpart, LBA.

J. Howe, MD

Effect of Adjuvant Chemotherapy With Fluorouracil Plus Folinic Acid or Gemcitabine vs Observation on Survival in Patients With Resected Periampullary Adenocarcinoma: The ESPAC-3 Periampullary Cancer Randomized Trial

Neoptolemos JP, for the European Study Group for Pancreatic Cancer (Univ of Liverpool, UK; et al)
JAMA 308:147-156, 2012

Context.—Patients with periampullary adenocarcinomas undergo the same resectional surgery as that of patients with pancreatic ductal adenocarcinoma. Although adjuvant chemotherapy has been shown to have a survival benefit for pancreatic cancer, there have been no randomized trials for periampullary adenocarcinomas.

Objective.—To determine whether adjuvant chemotherapy (fluorouracil or gemcitabine) provides improved overall survival following resection.

Design, Setting, and Patients.—The European Study Group for Pancreatic Cancer (ESPAC)-3 periampullary trial, an open-label, phase 3, randomized controlled trial (July 2000-May 2008) in 100 centers in Europe, Australia, Japan, and Canada. Of the 428 patients included in the primary analysis, 297 had ampullary, 96 had bile duct, and 35 had other cancers.

Interventions.—One hundred forty-four patients were assigned to the observation group, 143 patients to receive 20 mg/m^2 of folinic acid via intravenous bolus injection followed by 425 mg/m^2 of fluorouracil via intravenous bolus injection administered 1 to 5 days every 28 days, and 141 patients to receive 1000 mg/m^2 of intravenous infusion of gemcitabine once a week for 3 of every 4 weeks for 6 months.

Main Outcome Measures.—The primary outcome measure was overall survival with chemotherapy vs no chemotherapy; secondary measures were chemotherapy type, toxic effects, progression-free survival, and quality of life.

Results.—Eighty-eight patients (61%) in the observation group, 83 (58%) in the fluorouracil plus folinic acid group, and 73 (52%) in the gemcitabine group died. In the observation group, the median survival was 35.2 months (95%% CI, 27.2-43.0 months) and was 43.1 (95%, CI, 34.0-56.0) in the 2 chemotherapy groups (hazard ratio, 0.86; (95% CI, 0.66-1.11; $\chi^2 = 1.33$; $P = .25$). After adjusting for independent prognostic variables of age, bile duct cancer, poor tumor differentiation, and positive lymph nodes and after conducting multiple regression analysis, the hazard ratio for chemotherapy compared with observation was 0.75 (95% CI, 0.57-0.98; Wald $\chi^2 = 4.53$, $P = .03$).

Conclusions.—Among patients with resected periampullary adenocarcinoma, adjuvant chemotherapy, compared with observation, was not associated with a significant survival benefit in the primary analysis; however, multivariable analysis adjusting for prognostic variables demonstrated a statistically significant survival benefit associated with adjuvant chemotherapy.

Trial Registration.—clinicaltrials.gov Identifier: NCT00058201.

▶ There have been no randomized trials looking at adjuvant chemotherapy for periampullary tumors, in contrast to pancreatic adenocarcinomas. This trial, the European Study Group for Pancreatic Cancer 3, randomized patients to receive fluorouracil (5-FU)/leucovorin, gemcitabine, or observation to determine whether there was survival benefit for adjuvant treatment at these sites. Only about half of the patients received the total doses of chemotherapy and 10%–20% never received chemotherapy, presumably because of complications from the procedure. The primary subtypes of periampullary tumors were ampullary, bile duct and others, including duodenal and other periampullary carcinomas. Overall, there was improved median survival with chemotherapy vs observation, which held up for both the 5-FU and the gemcitabine groups. The overall hazard ratio was 0.86 for those receiving chemotherapy vs observation, but the price of this was a serious adverse event incidence of 30%–50% in the chemotherapy group. There was a statistically significant benefit to chemotherapy, and especially with gemcitabine vs 5-FU, and a better safety profile with gemcitabine. Because these periampullary tumors are not very common, the authors had to lump ampullary and bile duct tumors together as well as duodenal. It would be of significant interest to know whether bile duct tumors responded better to chemotherapy because of their more aggressive tumor biology and whether differences were seen in ampullary cancers, which generally have improved survival rates. Unfortunately, this trial does not answer the question, but it shows that, overall, there may be a survival benefit when patients with these tumors are grouped together.

J. Howe, MD

Minimally invasive versus open oesophagectomy for patients with oesophageal cancer: a multicentre, open-label, randomised controlled trial
Biere SSAY, van Berge Henegouwen MI, Maas KW, et al (VU Univ Med Centre, Amsterdam, Netherlands; Academic Med Centre, Amsterdam, Netherlands; et al)
Lancet 379:1887-1892, 2012

Background.—Surgical resection is regarded as the only curative option for resectable oesophageal cancer, but pulmonary complications occurring in more than half of patients after open oesophagectomy are a great concern. We assessed whether minimally invasive oesophagectomy reduces morbidity compared with open oesophagectomy.

Methods.—We did a multicentre, open-label, randomised controlled trial at five study centres in three countries between June 1, 2009, and March 31, 2011. Patients aged 18—75 years with resectable cancer of the oesophagus or gastro-oesophageal junction were randomly assigned via a computer-generated randomisation sequence to receive either open transthoracic or minimally invasive transthoracic oesophagectomy. Randomisation was stratified by centre. Patients, and investigators undertaking interventions, assessing outcomes, and analysing data, were not masked to group assignment. The primary outcome was pulmonary infection within the first 2 weeks after surgery and during the whole stay in hospital. Analysis was by intention to treat. This trial is registered with the Netherlands Trial Register, NTR TC 2452.

Findings.—We randomly assigned 56 patients to the open oesophagectomy group and 59 to the minimally invasive oesophagectomy group. 16 (29%) patients in the open oesophagectomy group had pulmonary infection in the first 2 weeks compared with five (9%) in the minimally invasive group (relative risk [RR] $0 \cdot 30$, 95% CI $0 \cdot 12 - 0 \cdot 76$; $p = 0 \cdot 005$). 19 (34%) patients in the open oesophagectomy group had pulmonary infection in-hospital compared with seven (12%) in the minimally invasive group ($0 \cdot 35$, $0 \cdot 16 - 0 \cdot 78$; $p = 0 \cdot 005$). For in-hospital mortality, one patient in the open oesophagectomy group died from anastomotic leakage and two in the minimally invasive group from aspiration and mediastinitis after anastomotic leakage.

Interpretation.—These findings provide evidence for the short-term benefits of minimally invasive oesophagectomy for patients with resectable oesophageal cancer.

▶ The popularity of minimally invasive esophagectomy has increased significantly over the past decade due to shorter hospital stays and potentially reduced complication rates without compromise of oncological results. This study proposed to undertake a randomized controlled trial to evaluate whether the incidence of pulmonary infections was higher in open esophagectomy vs minimally invasive esophagectomy. A total of 115 patients were randomized at 5 different European hospitals to these 2 treatment groups, all of whom received neoadjuvant chemotherapy with or without radiation. Not surprisingly, there was a shorter length of stay in the minimally invasive esophagectomy group vs the open group and the incidence rate of pulmonary infections was significantly reduced in the minimally invasive group. The adequacy of resection in terms of lymph nodes and margins was similar between groups, as was the need for reoperation. The mortality was higher in the minimally invasive group. This study demonstrates that patients undergoing minimally invasive esophagectomy benefit from lower pulmonary infections as well as shorter length of stay, as was presumed previously, but is now shown conclusively in a randomized controlled trial.

J. Howe, MD

Reoperative Lymph Node Dissection for Recurrent Papillary Thyroid Cancer and Effect on Serum Thyroglobulin
Hughes DT, Laird AM, Miller BS, et al (Montefiore Med Ctr/Albert Einstein College of Medicine, Bronx, NY; Univ of Michigan, Ann Arbor; et al)
Ann Surg Oncol 19:2951-2957, 2012

Background.—Papillary thyroid cancer (PTC) has an excellent prognosis with current treatment methods. However, the rates of locoregional recurrence after initial surgical management remain significant. This study evaluates the effect of reoperative neck dissection for locoregional recurrence of PTC after initial total thyroidectomy and radioiodine therapy on the incidence of cervical recurrence and postoperative serum thyroglobulin (Tg) levels.

Methods.—This is a retrospective cohort study conducted in a single academic medical center of patients with recurrent or persistent PTC isolated to the neck after previous total thyroidectomy with or without lymph node dissection and adjuvant I^{131} therapy who were treated with reoperative lymph node dissection. Outcomes including operative complications, pathologic findings, and effect of surgery on Tg levels and rates of recurrent disease were analyzed.

Results.—From 2001 to 2010, a total of 61 patients had reoperative neck dissections for recurrent cervical PTC with a complication rate of 5%. Seventy-two percent of patients were clinically free of detectable disease, and 28% of patients had recurrent, persistent, or newly metastatic disease detected during the follow-up period. All patients had significant decreases in Tg levels, with a median 98% reduction in preoperative levels. However, only 21% of patients had an undetectable stimulated Tg (< 0.5 ng/mL) during the follow-up period of 15.5 months.

Conclusions.—Reoperative treatment of recurrent or persistent PTC can be performed with low complication rates, and Tg levels greatly decrease in most patients; however, few achieve undetectable stimulated Tg.

▶ Papillary thyroid cancer is a disease in which approximately 30% of patients will have locoregional recurrences. Fortunately, many of these recurrences do not affect patient survival, but they can lead to morbidity due to local invasion. Therefore, it has been recommended that patients have surveillance with stimulated or unstimulated thyroglobulin levels after total thyroidectomy and radioactive iodine ablation as well as physical examination and cervical ultrasound scan. This study evaluated patients who had locoregional recurrence after thyroidectomy and radioiodine therapy and sought to determine the rates of complication of reoperation, biochemical cure rates, and rates of control of disease. This was a well-conducted study done in a retrospective fashion, which agrees with the findings of others; it was limited by having small numbers of patients and a short median follow-up of 15.5 months. There were 61 patients who were ultimately evaluated and underwent reoperation. Of this group, 72% were rendered free of clinically detectable disease; however, there were only 21% who had undetectable stimulated thyroglobulin levels, signifying residual disease in the majority. The morbidity of these explorations was low, and the authors showed that they could be performed safely; the procedures included lateral neck dissections, central neck dissections, and combinations of central and lateral neck dissections. Lessons learned from this study were that because not all patients had biochemical cure, exploration should be directed at reducing complications of locoregional recurrence, which might mean watchful waiting in certain patients rather than surgery, especially in those with small foci of disease. A subset of patients presumed to have recurrent thyroid cancer had negative surgical explorations, suggesting the importance of cytologic confirmation of recurrence before exploration.

J. Howe, MD

12 Vascular Surgery

Introduction

There were three seminal publications included in the 2013 YEAR BOOK OF SURGERY that should be read in their entirety. The long-term results of the Open versus Endovascular Repair (OVER) trial confirmed the initial findings and failed to demonstrate a survival benefit for endovascular aneurysm repair (EVAR). Somewhat surprisingly, there was survival advantage for younger patients with EVAR. Importantly, there were several deaths in the EVAR group from aneurysm rupture, thereby underscoring the importance of long-term surveillance. The long-term follow-up of the Multicenter Aneurysm Screening Study demonstrated that aneurysm screening for men 65–74 years of age reduced mortality although the number needed to treat was 216. There were a few aneurysm ruptures in patients with initial aortic diameters between 2.5 – 2.9 cm, suggesting that this cohort of patients with enlarged but non-aneurysmal aortas should undergo repeat screening. Lastly, the CaVenT trial compared catheter-directed lysis and endovascular treatment with medical management alone for patients with iliofemoral deep venous thrombosis and found a benefit in the interventional group. Notably, there was a lower incidence of post-thrombotic syndrome and a higher iliofemoral patency rate in the interventional group, although there was a 9% incidence of clinically significant bleeding.

Aortic diseases and their treatment continue to be a focus of our discipline. There were two nice reports using the Medicare database included among this year's article looking at the treatment of abdominal aortic aneurysms. Jackson et al reported that there was a long-term survival benefit for EVAR among Medicare beneficiaries, unlike the multiple randomized trials that have failed to show a survival benefit for EVAR despite significantly lower perioperative mortality. Greenblatt et al reported comparable hospital readmission rates after the open and EVAR approach, demonstrating that readmission was associated with increased mortality. Not surprising, readmission correlated with perioperative complications and patient comorbidities. Duran et al described their experience with iliac artery rupture during endovascular aneurysm repair, including a nice description of their remedial approach. This is particularly relevant given the dissemination of the percutaneous valve therapies and their large delivery systems. Donas et al compared open juxtarenal aneurysm repair with the alternative endovascular approaches, including fenestrated grafts and the chimney technique. In their relatively large series, the endovascular approaches were associated

345

with lower mortality, shorter length of stay, and fewer transfusions. These findings largely parallel the experience with the endovascular approach for infrarenal aneurysms and are particularly noteworthy since the better-risk patients underwent open repair. A report from the International Registry of Acute Aortic Dissection has attempted to define the natural history of acute aortic intramural hematomas, emphasizing that there is no role for medical management of the acute type A variant. Kuzmik et al have performed an evidence-based summary of the literature to define the treatment threshold for thoracic aneurysms. They recommended a diameter threshold of 5.5 cm for ascending aneurysms and 6.5 cm for descending aneurysms, although they emphasized that the thresholds should be lower for patients with rapid growth, connective tissue disorders, and those with bicuspid valves. Kasirajan et al called attention to the potential for infolding of thoracic endografts, detailing the potential adverse outcomes including death. This has occurred most frequently in young patients with acute traumatic dissections.

The optimal treatment of lower extremity arterial occlusive disease, both claudication and limb-threatening ischemia, remains one of the larger unanswered questions. The articles included in this year's selection contribute to our overall understanding and address different issues within the continuum of care. Linni et al performed an elegant, randomized trial examining the role of preoperative ultrasound vein mapping prior to infrainguinal revascularization. They reported a benefit in terms of choice of optimal conduit, major infections, and readmission, although there were no differences in terms of long-term bypass patency. Remote endarterectomy appears to be comparable to subintimal angioplasty for patients with TASC II D femoro-popliteal lesions in terms of both primary and secondary patency, although surgical bypass has traditionally been recommended in this setting. The hemodynamic benefit of open and endovascular treatment for diabetics with critical limb ischemia appears to be comparable. Although this potentially dispels a myth about the hemodynamic superiority of the open approach, the report included among the articles does not provide sufficient data about the long-term outcomes. McPhee et al have reported that the patency rates for alternative conduits (ie, other than saphenous vein) in the femoro-below knee popliteal position are comparable. Monaco et al reported that the patency rates for femoro-popliteal bypass were improved with the combination of warfarin/clopidogrel when compared with aspirin/clopidogrel. Although this combination seems quite potent, it was associated with only a small increase in minor bleeding complications. Lastly, Bui et al examined the role of duplex ultrasound surveillance after infrainguinal endovascular treatment and reported that the natural history was distinctly different than lower extremity bypasses. Notably, the duplex criteria for a failing graft are not applicable after endovascular treatment.

The management of cerebrovascular occlusive disease continues to be a major component of most vascular surgical practices. Thapar et al performed a decision analysis to examine the role of carotid endarterectomy for asymptomatic patients using data from the Asymptomatic Carotid

Surgery Trial and concluded that it was beneficial for patients <75 years of age. Notably, these findings were similar to an early-decision analysis based on the Asymptomatic Carotid Atherosclerosis Study. Schechter et al used the American College of Surgeons National Surgical Quality Improvement Program database to examine the age-old question about the choice of regional or general anesthesia for carotid endarterectomy and found no difference in the major endpoints, including death, stroke, and myocardial infarction. Lastly, Mokin et al compared intravenous thrombolysis and endovascular treatment for acute ischemic stroke secondary to internal carotid artery occlusion. They reported no difference in outcome for the two approaches despite an increased rate of intracranial hemorrhage with the endovascular approach.

The balance of the articles included among the selections address a variety of other problems encountered by vascular surgeons. Cull et al described an elegant technique to salvage thrombosed autogenous hemodialysis accesses. Their results were both impressive and noteworthy since thrombosed autogenous accesses, unlike prosthetic accesses, have been traditionally abandoned. An updated report of the Hemodialysis Reliable Outflow (HeRO) graft/catheter was included, documenting impressive patency rates with a low infectious complication. Although it remains to be seen whether these results are reproducible, the HeRO device likely plays a role in the expanding group of patients with complex access problems. An updated version of the Eastern Association for the Surgery of Trauma Guidelines for penetrating lower extremity trauma document the evolution of care with the expanded emphasis on computed tomography (CT) arteriography. They emphasize the role of surgical exploration for the traditional hard signs (eg, pulse deficit, expanding hematoma) and soft signs with an ABI <.9 while detailing that a patient with palpable pulses and an ABI >.9 can likely be discharged without further evaluation, provided they have adequate follow-up. Farber et al used a national trauma database to examine the role of fasciotomy and reported that early fasciotomy was associated with a lower amputation rate and fewer wound complications. Jimenez et al have attempted to perform an evidence-based review of the literature to examine the role of open and endovascular treatment for the median arcuate ligament syndrome, and they report reasonable symptomatic relief with both approaches. Finally, Bruggink et al compared Fluoro-Z-D-glucose position tomography (FDF-PET) FDG-PET and CT scans as diagnostic tools for infected prosthetic grafts, and they reported that FDG-PET was superior, suggesting that it may play a role for equivocal cases.

Thomas S. Huber, MD, PhD

Access

Description and outcomes of a simple surgical technique to treat thrombosed autogenous accesses

Cull DL, Washer JD, Carsten CG, et al (Greenville Hosp System/Univ Med Ctr, SC)
J Vasc Surg 56:861-865, 2012

Objective.—Owing to the difficulty of removing acute and chronic thrombus from autogenous accesses (AA) by standard surgical and endovascular techniques, many surgeons consider efforts to salvage a thrombosed AA as being futile. We describe a simple technique to extract acute and chronic thrombus from a failed AA. This technique involves making an incision adjacent to the anastomosis, directly extracting the arterial plug, and manually milking thrombus from the access. This report details the outcomes of a series of thrombosed AAs treated by surgical thrombectomy/intervention using this technique for manual clot extraction.

Methods.—A total of 146 surgical thrombectomies/interventions were performed in 102 patients to salvage a thrombosed AA. Mean follow-up was 15.6 months. Office, hospital, and dialysis unit records were reviewed to identify patient demographics, define procedure type, and determine functional patency rates. Kaplan-Meier survival analysis was used to estimate primary and secondary functional patency rates.

Results.—Complete extraction of thrombus from the AA was achieved in 140 of 146 cases (95%). The studied procedure itself was technically successful in 127 cases (87%). Reasons for failure were the inability to completely extract thrombus from the AA in six, failed angioplasty due to long segment vein stenosis or sclerosis in seven or vein rupture in two, and central vein occlusion in one. Three failures occurred for unknown causes ≤3 days of successful thrombectomy. No single factor analyzed (age, sex, race, diabetes status, access type or location) was associated with technical failure. The estimated primary and secondary functional patency rates were 27% ± 5% and 61% ± 6% at 12 months.

Conclusions.—The manual clot extraction technique described in this report effectively removed acute and chronic thrombus from failed AAs. Its use, combined with an intervention to treat the underlying cause for AA failure, significantly extended access durability.

▶ The authors describe an effective open surgical technique to salvage thrombosed autogenous accesses (AA) with a technical success rate of 87% and primary and secondary functional patency rates of 27% and 61%, respectively, at 12 months. The report is a follow-up from an early smaller series, but it certainly merits consideration given the large sample size (N = 102) and the total number of surgical procedures (146). The utility of salvaging thrombosed AA has been somewhat unclear, and the traditional dictum has been such that once the AA thrombosed, the patient likely needed another permanent access (either prosthetic or autogenous). Admittedly, this approach is somewhat contradictory to the national initiatives that have emphasized or prioritized the use of AA and the philosophy that each access configuration should be used as long as possible. The inclusion criteria in the current study were quite broad, thereby suggesting that the approach is generally applicable for most thrombosed AA, including those with large aneurysms or pseudoaneurysms. Indeed, the authors reported that the technique was applied in nearly all thrombosed AA that had been usable or functional for dialysis. They did emphasize that salvage was not attempted for nonfunctional or sclerotic AA and those that had been occluded for more than 30 days, stating in the discussion that the technique was no longer attempted in AA that have been occluded more than 14 days. The authors emphasize the importance of several technical points and ascribe the underlying concerns addressed by these points to the mixed results seen with attempted AA thrombectomy historically. First, a transverse incision is made adjacent to the arterial anastomosis, and a transverse incision is made in the access 2 to 3 cm from the actual anastomosis. The arterial anastomosis is thrombectomized with a catheter, but the arterial plug may need to be manually extracted with a pair of forceps. The authors emphasize that the arterial anastomosis and proximal segment of the AA is very compliant and the thromboembolectomy balloon alone may be ineffective. Second, the clot through the length of the AA is manually extracted by milking the access in a retrograde fashion using "vigorous manipulation and firm pressure." They claim that this is very effective, even in the presence of large aneurysms, and that the passage of the thromboembolectomy catheter (although performed) after the completion of the milking process adds little additional benefit in terms of clot extraction. Third, the clot should be extracted at the arterial anastomosis and a clamp applied to the proximal portion of the AA before the retrograde milking to prevent dislodging or pushing clot into the arterial tree. Fourth, a completion fistulagram and definitive treatment of the underlying cause of the AA thrombosis is mandatory because an underlying stenosis was identified in every case. My own experience with the technique has been somewhat limited, and I have attributed my failures to the steep portion of the learning curve. However, the report shows that it is possible to salvage most thrombosed AA, and it has changed my clinical practice.

T. S. Huber, MD, PhD

Multi-center Experience of 164 Consecutive Hemodialysis Reliable Outflow [Hero] Graft Implants for Hemodialysis Treatment

Gage SM, Katzman HE, Ross JR, et al (Duke Univ, Durham, NC; Univ of Miami, FL; Bamberg County Hosp, SC; et al)
Eur J Vasc Endovasc Surg 44:93-99, 2012

Objective.—To report a multi-center experience with the novel Hemo-Dialysis Reliable Outflow (HeRO) vascular access graft.

Materials and Methods.—Four centers conducted a retrospective review of end stage renal disease patients who received the HeRO device from implant to last available follow-up. Data is available on 164 patients with an accumulated 2092.1 HeRO implant months.

Results.—At 6 months, HeRO primary and secondary patency is 60% and 90.8%, respectively and at 12 months, 48.8% and 90.8%, respectively. At 24 months, HeRO had a primary patency of 42.9% and secondary patency was 86.7%. Interventions to maintain or re-establish patency have been required in 71.3% of patients (117/164) resulting in an intervention rate of 1.5/year. Access related infections have been reported in 4.3% patients resulting in a rate of 0.14/1000 implant days.

Conclusions.—In our experience the HeRO device has performed comparably to standard AVGs and has proven superior to TDCs in terms of patency, intervention, and infection rates when compared to the peer-reviewed literature. As an alternative to catheter dependence as a means for hemodialysis access, this graft could reduce the morbidity and mortality associated with TDCs and have a profound impact on the costs associated with catheter related infections and interventions.

▶ The authors report the largest experience of the Hemodialysis Reliable Outflow (HeRO) graft (Hemosphere Inc, Eden Prairie, MN) from the post-market approval of the device. The HeRO Graft is a hybrid "graft-catheter" designed for patients with central vein stenoses or occlusions that preclude the more traditional autogenous or prosthetic arteriovenous accesses. The authors reported impressive 12-month patency rates (primary, 49%; secondary, 91%) and an infectious complication rate of only 4.3% or 0.14/1000 implant days. Notably, both the patency and infections complication rates compared favorably with those historically reported for prosthetic arteriovenous accesses and were far superior to those reported for tunneled dialysis catheters. On first pass, the results seem to suggest that the HeRO device is the "holy grail" for the expanding complex-patient population with central vein problems. However, the results must be interpreted with some caution. First, the study was part of a post-market approval phase for the device and was conducted at 4 institutions with extensive experience with hemodialysis access. Second, the study was conducted in a retrospective fashion and, therefore, was subject to the usual limitations and selection biases. Third, the "control" groups used for comparison for both the patency and infectious complications were obtained from the literature (or historical controls). Fourth, the majority of the authors had a financial interest in the device and the study was funded by the manufacturer. I have been intrigued by the HeRO device and suspect that it has a potential role in the difficult group of patients with central vein occlusions/stenosis. However, we have struggled to define its specific role in our treatment algorithm and have used it almost exclusively for a "terminal" group of patients with limited or no other access options, favoring lower extremity accesses before the HeRO graft. The infectious complication rates for the HeRO Graft in our experience have been significant and have paralleled (or exceeded) those for tunneled dialysis catheters. These infectious complications have further limited our enthusiasm, although we would readily concede that this may be a "center-related" issue and/or reflect our patient selection and use of the device in "terminal" access patients. The impressive secondary patency rates reported likely reflect the authors' commitment to this difficult group of patients as reflected by the requirement of 1.5 interventions/year. The authors stated in the Discussion that the graft failures resulted primarily from intragraft stenoses and/or adherent clot rather than from the graft/catheter coupling mechanism, although this has not been our anecdotal impression and we have favored dissembling (and replacing) the coupling mechanism at the time of thrombectomy. Although not mentioned in the current study, prior reports have suggested that patency may be improved with clopidogrel and that the patency is compromised in the subset of patients with persistent hypotension. Despite my concerns, I remain enthusiastic about the HeRO graft, but I await more rigorous evaluation to help define its role in the collective treatment algorithm for this complex group of patients.

T. S. Huber, MD, PhD

Aneurysm

The role of open and endovascular treatment with fenestrated and chimney endografts for patients with juxtarenal aortic aneurysms

Donas KP, Eisenack M, Panuccio G, et al (Münster Univ Hosp, Germany)
J Vasc Surg 56:285-290, 2012

Objective.—To present endovascular techniques in the treatment of juxtarenal aortic aneurysms (JAAAs) in relation to surgical repair; this is the "gold standard."

Methods.—Between January 2008 and December 2010, 90 consecutive patients were diagnosed with primary degenerative JAAAs ($\geq$5.0 cm) and assigned prospectively to different operative strategies on the basis of morphologic and clinical characteristics. In particular, 59 patients were treated by endovascular means such as fenestrated endovascular abdominal aortic repair (f-EVAR, n = 29) or chimney endovascular abdominal aortic repair (ch-EVAR, n = 30) endografting, and 31 patients underwent open repair (OR, n = 31).

Results.—Early procedure-related and all-cause (30-day) procedure-related mortality was 0% for the endovascular group and 6.4% (n = 2/31) for the OR group, due to systemic inflammatory response syndrome with consecutive multi-organ failure ($P =$.023). Persistent postoperative hemodialysis occurred only after OR (2/31; 6.4%). The overall estimated pre- and postoperative median estimated glomerular filtration rate and creatinine values were similar in the three subgroups. There was one left renal artery occlusion for each endovascular subgroup, which presented as flank pain and was treated by iliaco-renal bypass in both cases. Transfusion requirements and length of hospital stay were significantly less in the endovascular group ($P =$.014 and $P =$.004, respectively).

Conclusions.—Endovascular treatment of JAAA is a safe alternative for the short-term management of JAAA.

▶ The authors report the largest single contemporary experience of patients with juxtarenal abdominal aortic aneurysms treated with either open repair, fenestrated endografts (f-EVAR) or chimney endografts (ch-EVAR). Similar to the randomized trials comparing open and endovascular repair for infrarenal aneurysms, they reported that the endovascular approach was associated with a lower peri-operative mortality rate (0% vs 6%), shorter lengths of hospital stays, and fewer transfusions despite no differences in estimated postoperative glomerular filtration creatinine values. These findings are particularly noteworthy given the authors' treatment algorithm in which low-risk patients were offered open repair, whereas the endovascular approach was reserved for higher risk patients not deemed suitable for open repair. The fenestrated grafts were custom-made Zenith grafts (Cook Medical Inc, Bloomington, IN) and required an obligatory preparation/processing time, thereby precluding their use in the urgent/emergent setting. Notably, these commercially manufactured fenestrated devices are distinctly different from the "off-label," surgeon-modified devices constructed using a standard infrarenal graft and are not currently available outside clinical trials in the United States. The chimney technique represents another off-label use of existing technology in which covered stents are placed in the visceral vessels and configured such that they run parallel to the aortic endograft, thereby creating a parallel conduit. Despite our own group's published experience, I remain incredulous that the chimney technique actually provides an adequate proximal seal, but am reassured by the authors' excellent technical results and the absence of any type I endoleaks. The report suffers from the same limitation of the earlier publications in that the follow-up for the endovascular approaches is still quite short (f-EVAR, mean 13 months; ch-EVAR, mean 15 months). It remains to be determined how well the f-EVAR and ch-EVAR devices will behave in the long term in terms of the proximal seal and whether the early morbidity/mortality advantages will persist. Regardless, the technologies represent the "next frontier" for the aortic endovascular therapies that will hopefully translate into a better, safer alternative to open repair for patients with complex aortic aneurysms.

T. S. Huber, MD, PhD

A Longitudinal View of Improved Management Strategies and Outcomes After Iatrogenic Iliac Artery Rupture During Endovascular Aneurysm Repair
Duran C, Naoum JJ, Smolock CJ, et al (The Methodist Hosp, Houston, TX)
Ann Vasc Surg 27:1-7, 2013

Background.—Intraoperative rupture of the iliac artery is a serious complication of endovascular aneurysm repair (EVAR), the outcomes of which have changed with increasing experience and improved endovascular tools over the past 2 decades. Over the past 15 years, the incidence and management of iliac rupture has changed as devices have improved and experience has grown. This study reviews our longitudinal experience with this complication.

Methods.—All cases of iliac artery rupture during EVAR from 1997 through 2011 were reviewed for presentation, treatment strategies, and outcomes.

Results.—Iliac artery rupture complicated 20 (3%) of 707 EVARs performed. Sixteen (80%) common and four (20%) external iliac arteries were ruptured. Hypotension (systolic blood pressure: < 90 mm Hg) was present in 11 (55%) cases. Five open bypasses were performed (25%), whereas 15 were repaired using an endovascular approach (75%). All open repairs (100%) were associated with postoperative morbidity (one wound infection, four multiorgan system failure), whereas three of the 15 patients (23%) repaired endovascularly experienced postoperative morbidity (cerebrovascular accident, myocardial infarction, line infection). There were no intraoperative deaths. There were four (20%) early deaths in the intensive care unit (< 3 days postoperatively), all of which were associated with resection of bilateral hypogastric arteries and were due to complications of pelvic ischemia and/or multiorgan system failure.

Conclusions.—Iliac artery rupture remains relatively uncommon but can carry a high morbidity and mortality. As device technology, imaging quality for preoperative planning, and experience level have improved, iliac rupture has become less common, and outcomes in the setting of iliac rupture have significantly improved. Endoluminal management has evolved as the primary treatment strategy. Resection of both hypogastric arteries is associated with mortality from pelvic ischemia, a likely indicator of systemic disease.

▶ The authors detail their experience with ruptured iliac arteries during endovascular aneurysm repair (EVAR), although the report is relevant for all endovascular procedures and particularly timely given the proliferation of the percutaneous valve procedures with their requisite large delivery systems. Indeed, there are few complications associated with EVAR that are more serious or anxiety provoking for the attending surgeon than rupture of the iliac artery, as emphasized by the mortality (20%) and complication (open repair, 66%; endovascular repair, 30%) in the current series. Fortunately, the overall incidence of ruptures reported in the authors' series was quite low (3%) and has decreased since 2006 (1%) with their liberal use of endoconduit for patients with severe aortoiliac occlusive disease. The majority of the injuries occurred in the common iliac artery, and it has been our experience that most occur at its bifurcation, likely related to the tethering of the vessel by the internal iliac artery that makes it susceptible to disruption during the forceful delivery of the endovascular device. The authors identified 4 procedural maneuvers that were associated with injury, including device insertion, angioplasty after failed access, angioplasty for type IB endoleak, and device molding (angioplasty) in a noncompliant arterial wall. Additional caution should be exercised during these steps of the procedure. The endovascular approach appears to be the optimal remedial strategy and has largely replaced the open alternative in the authors' experience. Provided that wire access to the vessel has been maintained, the initial step after recognizing the injury is to simply occlude the disrupted vessel with an appropriately sized angioplasty balloon or sheath and allow the anesthesiologists to adequately resuscitate the patient. Definitive treatment can usually be accomplished by simply extending the iliac limb of the device. This may require covering the origin of the internal iliac artery. Unilateral occlusion is usually reasonably welltolerated in terms of the incidence of claudication and sexual dysfunction, but bilateral occlusion can be more problematic, particularly in the acute setting, as underscored by the deaths in the current experience that resulted from multiorgan system failure related to the pelvic ischemia. The best "treatment" for iliac disruptions is appropriate preoperative planning and avoiding the complication altogether with adequate preoperative imaging, use of low-profile delivery systems, angioplasty/dilation of any stenotic iliac vessels, liberal use of alternative delivery conduits (open or endo-), and open repair for patients with prohibitive anatomy.

T. S. Huber, MD, PhD

Causes and Implications of Readmission After Abdominal Aortic Aneurysm Repair
Greenblatt DY, Greenberg CC, Kind AJH, et al (Univ of Wisconsin-Madison; et al)
Ann Surg 256:595-605, 2012

Objective.—To determine the frequency, causes, predictors, and consequences of 30-day readmission after abdominal aortic aneurysm (AAA) repair.

Background Data.—Centers for Medicare & Medicaid Services (CMS) will soon reduce total Medicare reimbursements for hospitals with higher-than-predicted 30-day readmission rates after vascular surgical procedures, including AAA repair. However, causes and factors leading to readmission in this population have never before been systematically analyzed.

Methods.—We analyzed elective AAA repairs over a 2-year period from the CMS Chronic Conditions Warehouse, a 5% national sample of Medicare beneficiaries.

Results.—A total of 2481 patients underwent AAA repair—1502 endovascular aneurysm repair (EVAR) and 979 open aneurysm repair. Thirty-day readmission rates were equivalent for EVAR (13.3%) and open repair (12.8%). Although wound complication was the most common reason for readmission after both procedures, the relative frequency of other causes differed—eg, bowel obstruction was common after open repair, and graft complication after EVAR. In multivariate analyses, preoperative comorbidities had a modest effect on readmission; however, postoperative factors, including serious complications leading to prolonged length of stay and discharge destination other than home, had a profound influence on the probability of readmission. The 1-year mortality in readmitted patients was 23.4% versus 4.5% in those not readmitted ($P < 0.001$).

Conclusions.—Early readmission is common after AAA repair. Adjusting for comorbidities, postoperative events predict readmission, suggesting that proactively preventing, detecting, and managing postoperative complications may provide an approach to decreasing readmissions, with the potential to reduce cost and possibly enhance long-term survival.

▶ The authors have used an administrative database comprising a 5% sample of Medicare beneficiaries from 2004 to 2006 to examine hospital readmissions after open and endovascular aneurysm repair. This analysis is particularly relevant given the 24% readmission rate after all vascular surgical procedures cited by the authors and the anticipated financial penalties (or reduced reimbursements) from the Centers for Medicare and Medicaid Services for these readmissions. The authors reported that the readmission rates for the 2 types of repair were comparable (13.3% vs 12.8%) with wound infections being the leading cause in both groups. Readmission was associated with a mortality rate of 6.5%, exceeding the rate (2.2%) associated with the index hospitalization, and an increased unadjusted mortality rate at one year (23.4% vs 4.5%). Multivariate analysis found several preoperative (congestive heart failure, cancer, age) and postoperative predictors (wound complication, renal/urologic complication, vascular/graft complication, discharge destination other than home) that were associated with readmission, with the postoperative predictors being stronger. The data should be interpreted with some caution given the known limitations of administrative databases, although I suspect that the findings will likely be validated by a prospective study. It is not clear how these data should be used to reduce the risk of readmission and improve the overall quality of patient care. Indeed, it is not particularly surprising to most surgeons that patients who have postoperative complications have increased rates of readmission and lower survival rates. The challenge is clearly to reduce the rate of these postoperative complications. However, the preoperative predictors of readmission (and postoperative complications) are not very helpful and do not provide much guidance in terms of patient selection. This may be because of the limitations of the administrative database, and perhaps the next generation of prospective studies will provide more insight. Inherent in the financial penalties for readmission is the (distasteful) belief that somehow the care provided during the index admission was somehow substandard or inadequate, thereby contributing to the readmission. Indeed, the authors provide a framework for readmission and identify 3 types of complications that potentially contribute: a complication that occurs during the index admission that was inadequately treated, a complication that occurs during the index admission that was not adequately recognized, and a new complication that occurs after discharge from the index admission. Although I would readily concede there is significant room for process improvement in the surgical care of patients with abdominal aortic aneurysms, I am concerned about the punitive actions proposed for readmissions and would contend that there is a finite complication rate associated with every surgical procedure. The challenge remains to optimize patient selection and perioperative management to ensure the best possible outcome, not necessarily withholding care to higher-risk patients for fear of postoperative complications and readmission.

T. S. Huber, MD, PhD

Acute Aortic Intramural Hematoma: An Analysis From the International Registry of Acute Aortic Dissection

Harris KM, Braverman AC, Eagle KA, et al (Abbott-Northwestern Hosp, Minneapolis, MN; Washington Univ School of Medicine, St Louis, MO; Univ of Michigan, Ann Arbor; et al)
Circulation 126,11:S91-S96, 2012

Background.—Acute aortic intramural hematoma (IMH) is an important subgroup of aortic dissection, and controversy surrounds appropriate management.

Methods and Results.—Patients with acute aortic syndromes in the International Registry of Acute Aortic Dissection (1996–2011) were evaluated to examine differences between patients (based on the initial imaging test) with IMH or classic dissection (AD). Of 2830 patients, 178 had IMH (64 type A [42%], 90 type B [58%], and 24 arch). Patients with IMH were older and presented with similar symptoms, such as severe pain. Patients with type A IMH were less likely to present with aortic regurgitation or pulse deficits and were more likely to have periaortic hematoma and pericardial effusion. Although type A IMH and AD were managed medically infrequently, type B IMH were more frequently treated medically. Overall in-hospital mortality was not statistically different for type A IMH compared to AD (26.6% versus 26.5%; $P = 0.998$); type A IMH managed medically had significant mortality (40.0%), although less than classic AD (61.8%; $P = 0.195$). Patients with type B IMH had a hospital mortality that was less but did not differ significantly (4.4% versus 11.1%; $P = 0.062$) from classic AD. One-year mortality was not significantly different between AD and IMH.

Conclusions.—Acute IMH has similar presentation to classic AD but is more frequently complicated with pericardial effusions and periaortic hematoma. Patients with IMH have a mortality that does not differ statistically from those with classic AD. A small subgroup of type A IMH patients are managed medically and have a significant in-hospital mortality.

▶ The report from the International Registry of Acute Aortic Dissection (IRAD) attempts to define the natural history and treatment for patients with acute aortic intramural hematoma (IMH). The IRAD is a registry comprised of unselected, consecutive cases of acute aortic syndromes reported from 30 aortic treatment centers from 10 countries (United States and Europe) that was started in 1996. The report represents the largest published series encompassing 172 patients among the more than 3200 cases of acute aortic syndrome in the database and highlights the relative infrequent nature of the problem (6.3% of all dissections in the IRAD). Strict diagnostic criteria were used to differentiate IMH from the more classic acute aortic dissections (AD) with AD characterized by an intimal flap with 2 lumens, and IMH characterized by a crescentic or circumferential thickening of the aortic wall without evidence of an entry point. The report is particularly noteworthy and timely because there has been an impression in the literature that the natural history and management of IMH are different from those of classic AD. The report documents that the clinical presentation of patients with IMH is indeed somewhat different than those with AD with an older age at presentation, higher incidence of periaortic hematoma, and lower incidence of aortic regurgitation and pulse deficit. However, there were no differences in the in-hospital or 1-year mortality rates, and the treatments (surgical vs medical) provided, as broken down by the type of AD or IMH (A, involvement of the ascending arch; B, no involvement of the arch), were similar. Notably, the in-hospital mortality rate for patients with type A IMH treated medically was 40%, underscoring the emergent nature of the problem. These findings contradict a series of reports from Asia, cited by the authors, suggesting that medical management may be the ideal treatment for type A IMH. The IRAD is a powerful database that has advanced our collective understanding of acute aortic syndromes, although it is still a registry with a tremendous amount of selection bias. Indeed, this report documents how patients with type A and B IMHs were treated, not necessarily the optimal treatment approach. These important questions await appropriate randomized trials. However, the current data would suggest that IMH is likely a variant of classic AD and that the same treatment algorithms are appropriate with emergent surgical repair for patients with type A IMH and medical management for uncomplicated type B IMH.

T. S. Huber, MD, PhD

Natural history of thoracic aortic aneurysms
Kuzmik GA, Sang AX, Elefteriades JA (Aortic Inst at Yale-New Haven Hosp, CT)
J Vasc Surg 56:565-571, 2012

Understanding the natural history of thoracic aortic aneurysms (TAAs) is essential to patient care and surgical decision making. In this evidence summary we discuss some of the most clinically relevant features of the disease. The true incidence of TAAs is likely to be higher than currently reported because of the inherently silent nature of TAAs. However, TAAs can become rapidly lethal once dissection or rupture occurs, highlighting the need for more robust screening. The impressive discovery of familial patterns and novel genetic loci for TAAs challenges the idea that most TAAs are simply sporadic. Although the aorta grows in an indolent manner, its rate of growth and its current diameter both have important clinical implications. Biomechanical studies have supported clinical findings of 6.0 cm as a dangerous threshold. Surgical extirpation of TAAs is currently the mainstay of effective treatment. Although endovascular TAA repair is becoming increasingly common, long-term safety remains unproven. We still need more data to support the concept that any medical therapy is effective (Fig 2).

▶ The article summarizes the evidence for the management of thoracic aortic aneurysms. Although thoracic aneurysms have traditionally been outside the scope of most peripheral vascular surgeons' practices, the advances in endovascular therapies and associated skill sets have affected the treatment of these

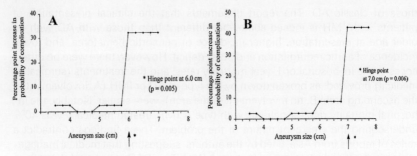

FIGURE 2.—Effects of aortic aneurysm size on risk of complications for the (A) ascending and (B) descending aorta. Reproduced with permission from Coady et al.[13] *Editor's Note*: Please refer to original journal article for full references. (Reprinted from the Journal of Vascular Surgery. Kuzmik GA, Sang AX, Elefteriades JA. Natural history of thoracic aortic aneurysms. *J Vasc Surg*. 2012;56:565-571, Copyright 2012, with permission from The Society for Vascular Surgery.)

aneurysms, particularly those in the descending thoracic aorta. Accordingly, it is incumbent on vascular surgeons to be familiar with their natural history and treatment indications. The "generic" management of thoracic aortic aneurysms is similar to that for infrarenal abdominal aneurysms, and it represents a balance between the risks of expectant management and operative treatment with the risks for expectant management, including both dissection and rupture for the thoracic aneurysms. Similar to infrarenal aneurysms, the diameter of the aorta is the best predictor of adverse outcome with the threshold for adverse outcome or "hinge point" in the curve being 6.0 cm and 7.0 cm for ascending and descending thoracic aneurysms, as shown in Fig 2. Given these risk profiles, treatment is generally recommended at 5.5 cm for ascending aneurysms and 6.5 cm for descending aneurysms, with a lower threshold recommended for symptomatic patients, those with rapid enlargement, those with connective tissue disorders, and those with bicuspid aortic valves. Not surprisingly, the behavior and overall natural history of thoracic aneurysms is very similar to infrarenal aneurysms. They are likely more common than generally appreciated, there appears to be an increase in their overall incidence, most are discovered incidentally, and there is a large familial component (potentially larger than attributed to infrarenal aneurysms). They increase in size over time with an annual growth rate of 0.10 cm/year and 0.29 cm/year for ascending and descending aneurysms, respectively. Furthermore, surgical treatment improves survival with the long-term outcomes approaching the age-matched controls. The optimal treatment in terms of open or endovascular treatment remains unresolved for descending thoracic aneurysms despite the proliferation of the endovascular therapies. The early clinical trials have demonstrated a benefit for the endovascular approach, but concerns have been raised about the long-term durability and survival. There are no effective medical therapies to reduce the risk of rupture and/or dissection, although patients should likely be maintained on antiplatelets, statins, beta blockers, and an angiotensin-converting enzyme inhibitor given their cardiovascular risk profile.

T. S. Huber, MD, PhD

Incidence and outcomes after infolding or collapse of thoracic stent grafts
Kasirajan K, Dake MD, Lumsden A, et al (East Bay Cardiovascular and Thoracic Associates, Concord, CA; Stanford Univ School of Medicine, CA; Methodist Hosp, Houston, TX; et al)
J Vasc Surg 55:652-658, 2012

Objective.—Device-related complications in the thoracic aorta are partly due to the unavoidable proximal angulation and increased flow-related forces. The present study evaluated the incidence, predictors, and outcome of the complication of infolding with the GORE TAG thoracic endoprosthesis (TAG device) to better understand the factors that might help predict these events.

Methods.—We reviewed all complaints reported to W. L. Gore and Associates (Flagstaff, Ariz) related to device infolding after the use of the GORE TAG device on or before December 2008. Events related to device infolding were evaluated. Reporting physicians and local company representatives were contacted, when necessary, to assemble all available imaging, data, and outcomes related to these case reports. When available, computed tomography images were reviewed to confirm aortic landing zone diameters, which were subsequently compared with the implanted device size.

Results.—From 1998 through December 2008, device infolding was reported in 139 patients (mean age, 40 ± 17 years; 73.4% men) from 33,289 device implants (reported incidence, 0.4%). Events were noted in implants for trauma (60%), dissection (19%), aneurysm (10%), and other (9%) and unknown (2%) etiologies. In 77 patients with available imaging, the average minimum aortic diameter was 21.4 ± 4.4 mm. The mean device diameter was 28.5 ± 3.5 mm, with an average oversizing of nearly 33%. Of reported patients, 51% were asymptomatic, with the diagnosis being made on routine chest imaging. Time to diagnosis was 76 ± 222 days (median, 9.5 days). Only 16 patients received no intervention after the diagnosis of device infolding, all of whom were asymptomatic. The other 123 patients underwent 135 interventions. Of these, 30 patients (24%) underwent open surgical conversion and complete or partial endograft removal. The other interventions included a variety of endovascular techniques, such as large balloon-expandable stent(s) in 40%, relining with additional endograft(s) in 31%, and repeat ballooning in seven patients. Ten patients died after device infolding, all after one or more attempts to repair the infolded device: five died of symptoms related to the infolding and five secondary to the intervention undertaken to correct the device infolding.

Conclusions.—TAG device infolding appears to be an infrequent event, primarily occurring in young trauma patients secondary to excessive oversizing and severe proximal aortic angulation. However, there clearly exists a need for devices that treat such patients. As a result, future device designs should consider the compression failure mode when being designed in order to help prevent such events.

▶ The authors call attention to an important complication associated with the deployment of GORE TAG thoracic endoprosthesis (TAG device; W. L. Gore and Associates, Flagstaff, AZ), although the findings are likely relevant to the other thoracic endografts. Specifically, the thoracic endografts can develop compression or invagination at either the proximal or distal fixation sites, collectively referred to as *infolding*. The authors document the event in 139 patients among 33 289 device implantations for an overall incidence of 0.4%, although it must be emphasized that these were reported complaints, and it is likely that the actual number of events and associated rates were both considerably higher. Most of the events (60%) occurred in young trauma patients, and the imputed etiology was related to device oversizing with an overall oversizing rate of 36% in the trauma patients. It is worth emphasizing that the TAG device was approved for the treatment of degenerative aneurysms with the recommendations for 10%–20% oversizing relative to the inner lumen of the native aorta and, thus, the use in the trauma population was off label. The young trauma population presents several anatomic and physiologic challenges for which the TAG device is poorly suited, including the relatively small aortic diameter that contributed to the oversizing because of the limited device sizes (ie, no small diameter devices) and the tight radius of curvature of the aortic arch that can lead to poor device apposition. It is interesting to note that the median time from deployment to recognition of the infolding was only 9.5 days and that only 30% of the patients developed symptoms. However, the 7% mortality rate underscores the significance of the problem and the requirement for early recognition and treatment. Furthermore, it is important that a variety of different health care providers (eg, radiologists, emergency room physicians, primary care physicians, intensivists, trauma surgeons) recognize the potential for this complication, because "symptomatic" patients are more likely to present to these other types of physicians than to their endovascular surgeon, and because the spectrum of symptoms can be somewhat cryptic, including hypertension, chest/back pain, oliguria, claudication, and paraplegia. The authors have developed a classification scheme and thoughtful treatment recommendations that merit review (Table 2 in the original article). The current (and future) generations of thoracic endografts should overcome some of the device limitations outlined above and be more appropriate for expanded indications including trauma patients. However, it is important to keep in mind this complication given the potential for a catastrophic outcome.

T. S. Huber, MD, PhD

Long-Term Comparison of Endovascular and Open Repair of Abdominal Aortic Aneurysm

Lederle FA, for the OVER Veterans Affairs Cooperative Study Group (Veterans Affairs Med Ctrs in Minneapolis, MN; et al)
N Engl J Med 367:1988-1997, 2012

Background.—Whether elective endovascular repair of abdominal aortic aneurysm reduces long-term morbidity and mortality, as compared with traditional open repair, remains uncertain.

Methods.—We randomly assigned 881 patients with asymptomatic abdominal aortic aneurysms who were candidates for both procedures to either endovascular repair (444) or open repair (437) and followed them for up to 9 years (mean, 5.2). Patients were selected from 42 Veterans Affairs medical centers and were 49 years of age or older at the time of registration.

Results.—More than 95% of the patients underwent the assigned repair. For the primary outcome of all-cause mortality, 146 deaths occurred in each group (hazard ratio with endovascular repair versus open repair, 0.97; 95% confidence interval [CI], 0.77 to 1.22; $P = 0.81$). The previously reported reduction in perioperative mortality with endovascular repair was sustained at 2 years (hazard ratio, 0.63; 95% CI, 0.40 to 0.98; $P = 0.04$) and at 3 years (hazard ratio, 0.72; 95% CI, 0.51 to 1.00; $P = 0.05$) but not thereafter. There were 10 aneurysm-related deaths in the endovascular-repair group (2.3%) versus 16 in the open-repair group (3.7%) ($P = 0.22$). Six aneurysm ruptures were confirmed in the endovascular-repair group versus none in the open-repair group ($P = 0.03$). A significant interaction was observed between age and type of treatment ($P = 0.006$); survival was increased among patients under 70 years of age in the endovascular-repair group but tended to be better among those 70 years of age or older in the open-repair group.

Conclusions.—Endovascular repair and open repair resulted in similar long-term survival. The perioperative survival advantage with endovascular repair was sustained for several years, but rupture after repair remained a concern. Endovascular repair led to increased long-term survival among younger patients but not among older patients, for whom a greater benefit from the endovascular approach had been expected. (Funded by the Department of Veterans Affairs Office of Research and Development; OVER ClinicalTrials.gov number, NCT00094575.)

▶ These authors report on the long-term follow-up (mean 5.2 years, maximum 9 years) of the Open versus Endovascular Repair (OVER) trial. Similar to both the DREAM (Dutch Randomised Endovascular Aneurysm Management) and the EVAR-1 (Endovascular Aneurysm Repair) trials, they reported no long-term survival benefit for the endovascular (EVAR) approach (see Fig 1A in the original article). In contrast to the earlier OVER publication, the initial perioperative survival benefit was found to persist until 3 years. The explanation for the convergence of the survival curves seen in all 3 major trials is unclear, but it is likely because of survival of the fittest, with the frailest patients in the open group dying in the perioperative period and those in the EVAR group dying somewhat later.

Analysis of the factors associated with mortality between the treatment groups demonstrated that randomization period after April 15, 2005 (hazard ratio [HR] 0.75; $P = .05$) and age less than 70 years (HR 0.65; $P = .006$) favored the endovascular approach, while the Medtronic AneuRx device (HR 1.49; $P = .06$) and age greater than 70 years (HR 1.31; $P = .006$) favored the open approach. The observation that the younger patients did better with the endovascular approach and vice versa was somewhat counterintuitive because it is the general impression that a major advantage of EVAR is to facilitate aneurysm repair in a cohort of patients not well suited for the open repair. Further analysis of the between-group mortality suggested that there was a higher incidence of cancer-related deaths in the younger patients, which may have accounted for the observed differences. Somewhat surprisingly, there were no differences in the incidence of therapeutic procedures. However, the nature and extent of the interventions varied between the groups, with 100 of 105 procedures in the EVAR group being endovascular procedures and 48 of 78 procedures in the open group being incisional hernia repairs. There were 6 aneurysm ruptures and 9 open conversions among the EVAR group. These results underscore the importance of dedicated surveillance, particularly with the Medtronic AneuRx device. However, the rupture risk in the EVAR group was quite low, at 6 ruptures during 4576 patient-years of follow-up. That statistic may be somewhat misleading because 1 of the rupture patients refused aneurysm repair after randomization, 1 refused to return for follow-up, and 1 refused treatment for his enlarged sac and graft migration. Finally, there were no differences in the health-related quality of life or erectile function between the groups. I would echo the seminal conclusions in the final paragraph of the discussion that EVAR is a safe alternative to open repair, but late rupture remains a concern and there is no difference in long-term survival, particularly among older patients.

T. S. Huber, MD, PhD

Final follow-up of the Multicentre Aneurysm Screening Study (MASS) randomized trial of abdominal aortic aneurysm screening
Thompson SG, on behalf of the Multicentre Aneurysm Screening Study (MASS) Group (Univ of Cambridge, UK; et al)
Br J Surg 99:1649-1656, 2012

Background.—The long-term effects of abdominal aortic aneurysm (AAA) screening were investigated in extended follow-up from the UK Multicentre Aneurysm Screening Study (MASS) randomized trial.

Methods.—A population-based sample of men aged 65–74 years were randomized individually to invitation to ultrasound screening (invited group) or to a control group not offered screening. Patients with an AAA (3·0 cm or larger) detected at screening underwent surveillance and were offered surgery after predefined criteria had been met. Cause-specific mortality data were analysed using Cox regression.

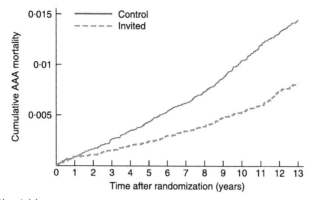

No. at risk

Control	33 887	33 049	32 102	31 055	29 995	28 872	27 674	26 347	25 030	23 841	22 664	21 405	20 185	11 015
Invited	33 883	33 020	32 080	31 127	30 108	29 012	27 873	26 627	25 406	24 155	22 907	21 676	20 497	11 161

FIGURE 1.—Abdominal aortic aneurysm (AAA)-related mortality over 13 years in the Multicentre Aneurysm Screening Study. (Reprinted from Thompson SG, on behalf of the Multicentre Aneurysm Screening Study (MASS) Group. Final follow-up of the Multicentre Aneurysm Screening Study (MASS) randomized trial of abdominal aortic aneurysm screening. *Br J Surg.* 2012;99:1649-1656, © British Journal of Surgery Society Ltd. Reproduced with permission. Permission is granted by John Wiley & Sons Ltd on behalf of the BJSS Ltd.)

Results.—Some 67 770 men were enrolled in the study. Over 13 years, there were 224 AAA-related deaths in the invited group and 381 in the control group, a 42 (95 per cent confidence interval 31 to 51) per cent reduction. There was no evidence of effect on other causes of death, but there was an overall reduction in all-cause mortality of 3 (1 to 5) per cent. The degree of benefit seen in earlier years of follow-up was slightly diminished by the occurrence of AAA ruptures in those with an aorta originally screened normal. About half of these ruptures had a baseline aortic diameter in the range 2·5—2·9 cm. It was estimated that 216 men need to be invited to screening to save one death over the next 13 years.

Conclusion.—Screening resulted in a reduction in all-cause mortality, and the benefit in AAA-related mortality continued to accumulate throughout follow-up. Registration number: ISRCTN37381646 (http://www.controlled-trials.com) (Fig 1).

▶ This report details the long-term follow-up of the United Kingdom Multicenter Aneurysm Screening Study and confirms that an invitation for screening in men 65 to 74 years of age resulted in a 42% (95% CI 31-51) reduction of aneurysm-related mortality, with a number needed to treat of 216. In the study, appropriate-aged men were invited for a screening ultrasound with repeat imaging for aneurysms > 3.0 cm and referral to a vascular surgeon for aneurysm > 5.5 cm or those with an annual expansion rate of > 1.0 cm. Notably, the participation rate for the screening ultrasound was an impressive 80.3% among the 33 883 men invited, with a complete clinic follow-up of 70.6% over the 13-year study period among the 4.9% of the patients detected to have an aneurysm on the original ultrasound. There were roughly twice as many elective aneurysm repairs in the screening group (600 vs 277), but half as many emergent repairs (80 vs 166), with operative mortality rates of 4.2% and 34.1% for the elective and ruptured procedures, respectively. The cumulative aneurysm-related mortality curves are shown (Fig 1), and it is worth emphasizing that the majority of the 273 aneurysm-related deaths in the screening group were patient-related (eg, refusal to participate in screening, failure to complete follow-up, refusal to undergo aneurysm repair). There was a disturbing number (N = 59) of ruptured aneurysms among patients originally detected to be normal (< 3.0 cm). Further analysis of this cohort revealed that the ruptures occurred after 8 years of follow-up in patients with a baseline aortic diameter between 2.5 and 2.9 cm, suggesting that this group should be rescreened at some time. Overall, the results seem to justify aneurysm screening in men 65 to 74 years of age, and the early benefit seems to be maintained over time. Although the number needed to treat to save 1 aneurysm-related death seems high, it is less than for breast cancer screening (roughly 400, according to the authors). Furthermore, the strategy appears to be cost-effective in terms of cost per life-year gained with a value of £7600 at 10 years, which is well below the accepted £20 000 threshold. These results must be interpreted with some caution because the overall compliance and follow-up rates were very excellent. In contrast, the overall participation in the Screening Abdominal Aortic Aneurysms Very Efficiently Act ultrasound screening program in the United States has been modest and has not had a discernable effect on mortality.[1]

T. S. Huber, MD, PhD

Reference

1. Shreibati JB, Baker LC, Hlatky MA, Mell MW. Impact of the Screening Abdominal Aortic Aneurysms Very Efficiently (SAAAVE) Act on abdominal ultrasonography use among Medicare beneficiaries. *Arch Intern Med.* 2012;172:1456-1462.

Comparison of Long-Term Survival After Open vs Endovascular Repair of Intact Abdominal Aortic Aneurysm Among Medicare Beneficiaries
Jackson RS, Chang DC, Freischlag JA (Georgetown Univ Hosp, Washington, DC; Univ of California, San Diego; Johns Hopkins Med Institutions, Baltimore, MD)
JAMA 307:1621-1628, 2012

Context.—Endovascular repair of abdominal aortic aneurysm (AAA) compared with open repair increases perioperative survival, but it is not known if it increases long-term survival.

Objective.—To compare long-term outcomes after open vs endovascular repair of AAA.

Design, Setting, and Patients.—Retrospective analysis of patients 65 years or older in the Medicare Standard Analytic File, 2003-2007, who underwent isolated repair of intact AAA. Cause of death was determined from the National Death Index.

Main Outcome Measures.—The primary outcome was all-cause mortality. Secondary outcomes were AAA-related mortality, hospital length of stay, 1-year readmission, repeat AAA repair, incisional hernia repair, and lower extremity amputation.

Results.—Of 4529 included patients, 703 were classified as having undergone open repair and 3826 as having undergone endovascular repair. Mean and median follow-up times were 2.6 (SD, 1.5) and 2.5 (interquartile range, 2.4) years, respectively. In unadjusted analysis, both all-cause mortality (173 vs 752; 89 vs 76/1000 person-years, $P = .04$) and AAA-specific mortality (22 vs 28; 11.3 vs 2.8/1000 person-years, $P < .001$) were higher after open vs endovascular repair. After adjusting for emergency admission, age, calendar year, sex, race, and comorbidities, there was a higher risk of both all-cause mortality (hazard ratio [HR], 1.24 [95% CI, 1.05-1.47]; $P = .01$) and AAA-related mortality (HR, 4.37 [95% CI, 2.51-7.66]; $P < .001$) after open vs endovascular repair. The adjusted hospital length of stay was, on average, 6.5 days (95% CI, 6.0-7.0 days, $P < .001$) longer after open repair (mean, 10.4 days), compared with endovascular repair (mean, 3.6 days). Incidence of incisional hernia repair was higher after open AAA repair (19 vs 23; 12 vs 3 per 1000 person-years; adjusted HR, 4.45 [95% CI, 2.37-8.34, $P < .001$]), whereas the incidence of 1-year readmission (188 vs 1070; 274 vs 376/1000 person-years; adjusted HR, 0.96 [95% CI, 0.85-1.09, $P = .52$]), repeat AAA repair (15 vs 93; 9.7 vs 12.3/1000 person-years; adjusted HR, 0.80 [95% CI, 0.46-1.38, $P = .42$]), and lower extremity amputation (3 vs 25; 1.9 vs 3.3/1000 person-years; adjusted HR, 0.55 [95% CI, 0.16-1.86, $P = .34$]) did not differ by repair type.

Conclusion.—Among older patients with isolated intact AAA, use of open repair compared with endovascular repair was associated with increased risk of all-cause mortality and AAA-related mortality.

▶ The authors have used the Medicare database to look at perioperative and long-term survival after open and endovascular repair for intact abdominal aortic aneurysms. Similar to the earlier randomized trials, they found that the perioperative mortality rate was higher for the open approach. However, this survival benefit for the endovascular approach persisted in the current study (mean follow-up 2.6 years) unlike the pivotal randomized trials, even after adjusting for several potential confounding factors (Fig 2 in the original article). Interestingly, it was the difference in the perioperative mortality rates that accounted for the observed difference in survival because there was no difference in the unadjusted mortality after the perioperative events were excluded. Although the long-term mortality rates were significantly different, the adjusted hazard ratios associated with open repair (HR 1.24 [95% CI 1.05—1.47]) were relatively modest, and the number needed to treat to save 1 year of life was 77. These findings confirm the original collective bias that the endovascular approach was safer than the open alternative and should be associated with better long-term survival. The baseline characteristics and propensity scores were similar between the open and endovascular groups, suggesting that the endovascular approach was likely selected based on anatomic features of the aneurysm rather than patient comorbidities. The endovascular approach was also associated with a decreased length of hospital stay and a lower incidence of incisional hernia repair as would be predicted based on multiple previous studies. Unfortunately, the authors did not examine health care costs or the incidence of all aneurysm-associated remedial procedures, although these would likely have been higher in the endovascular group. The finding should be interpreted with some caution given the retrospective study design and the database. The Medicare database is an administrative database that suffers from the usual limitations in terms of the accuracy and completeness of documenting comorbidities and clinical outcomes. Furthermore, the mean follow-up is relatively short and may not be sufficiently long to see a separation in the survival curves. The annual breakdown in the number of open and endovascular procedures (Fig 1 in the original article) underscores the fact that the endovascular approach has established itself as the preferred choice, initially based on its less invasive approach and favorable perioperative outcome, but now supported by improved longer-term survival.

T. S. Huber, MD, PhD

Carotid

Regional versus general anesthesia for carotid endarterectomy: The American College of Surgeons National Surgical Quality Improvement Program perspective

Schechter MA, Shortell CK, Scarborough JE (Duke Univ Med Ctr, Durham, NC)
Surgery 152:309-314, 2012

Background.—The ideal anesthetic technique for carotid endarterectomy remains a matter of debate. This study used the American College of Surgeons National Surgical Quality Improvement Program to evaluate the influence of anesthesia modality on outcomes after carotid endarterectomy.

Methods.—Postoperative outcomes were compared for American College of Surgeons National Surgical Quality Improvement Program patients undergoing carotid endarterectomy between 2005 and 2009 with either general or regional anesthesia. A separate analysis was performed on a subset of patients matched on propensity for undergoing carotid endarterectomy with regional anesthesia.

Results.—For the entire sample of 24,716 National Surgical Quality Improvement Program patients undergoing carotid endarterectomy and the propensity-matched cohort of 8,050 patients, there was no difference in the 30-day postoperative composite stroke/myocardial infarction/death rate based on anesthetic type. Within the matched cohort, the rate of other complications did not differ (2.8% regional vs 3.6% general anesthesia; $P = .07$), but patients receiving regional anesthesia had shorter operative (99 ± 36 minutes vs 119 ± 53 minutes; $P < .0001$) and anesthesia times (52 ± 29 minutes vs 64 ± 37 minutes; $P < .0001$) and were more likely to be discharged the next day (77.0% vs 64.4%; $P < .0001$).

Conclusion.—Anesthesia technique does not impact patient outcomes after carotid endarterectomy, but may influence overall cost of care.

▶ The authors have used the American College of Surgeons National Surgical Quality Improvement Program (ACS-NSQIP) database to analyze the choice of anesthesia (regional vs general) for carotid endarterectomy. The question about the optimal choice of anesthesia has lingered for many years, with proponents on either side citing the relative advantages (ie, their inherent biases). The authors found that there were no differences in the important, composite endpoint of 30-day mortality/myocardial infarction/death, although there were significant advantages in the softer endpoints of operating time, anesthesia time, and discharge on the following day that favored the regional technique along with a trend toward a significant difference in the incidence of other complications ($P = .07$). The ACS-NSQIP database, with its prospective data collection, is well suited to answer the study question, although the study is not comparable to a true randomized, controlled trial despite the authors' attempts to reduce the selection bias with their propensity matching analyses. Furthermore, the sample size of 24 716 procedures is by far the largest ever used to examine the question. The composite adverse outcome rates (2.2% regional vs 2.6% general) were low and attest to the safety of the procedure among the 300 participating centers, although it must be recognized that roughly 60% of the procedures were performed for asymptomatic carotid occlusive disease. Unfortunately, the data do not completely resolve the issue about the optimal choice, and the proponents of either choice can use the data to support their biases. It was interesting that only about one-fifth of the procedures were performed with the regional approach, and the patients were somewhat younger and healthier. The study reinforces my own bias in that it doesn't necessarily matter so much which approach you select, as long as your outcomes are acceptable. Indeed, I have always counseled our trainees that you need to identify a consistent approach or series of steps (eg, regional vs general, shunt vs no shunt) for carotid endarterectomy that works and then stick with it, particularly given the small margin of error required for the "prophylactic" carotid endarterectomy to be beneficial for both symptomatic and asymptomatic patients.

T. S. Huber, MD, PhD

Intravenous Thrombolysis and Endovascular Therapy for Acute Ischemic Stroke With Internal Carotid Artery Occlusion: A Systematic Review of Clinical Outcomes
Mokin M, Kass-Hout T, Kass-Hout O, et al (Univ at Buffalo, NY)
Stroke 43:2362-2368, 2012

Background and Purpose.—Strokes secondary to acute internal carotid artery (ICA) occlusion are associated with extremely poor prognosis. The best treatment approach to acute stroke in this setting is unknown. We sought to determine clinical outcomes in patients with acute ischemic stroke attributable to ICA occlusion treated with intravenous (IV) systemic thrombolysis or intra-arterial endovascular therapy.

Methods.—Using the PubMed database, we searched for studies that included patients with acute ischemic stroke attributable to ICA occlusion who received treatment with IV thrombolysis or intra-arterial endovascular interventions. Studies providing data on functional outcomes beyond 30 days and mortality and symptomatic intracerebral hemorrhage (sICH) rates were included in our analysis. We compared the proportions of patients with favorable functional outcomes, sICH, and mortality rates in the 2 treatment groups by calculating χ^2 and confidence intervals for odds ratios.

Results.—We identified 28 studies with 385 patients in the IV thrombolysis group and 584 in the endovascular group. Rates of favorable outcomes and sICH were significantly higher in the endovascular group than the IV thrombolysis-only group (33.6% vs 24.9%, $P = 0.004$ and 11.1% vs 4.9%, $P = 0.001$, respectively). No significant difference in mortality rate was found between the groups (27.3% in the IV thrombolysis group vs 32.0% in the endovascular group; $P = 0.12$).

Conclusions.—According to our systematic review, endovascular treatment of acute ICA occlusion results in improved clinical outcomes. A higher rate of sICH after endovascular treatment does not result in increased overall mortality rate.

▶ The authors performed a systematic review of the literature comparing intravenous thrombolysis with intra-arterial endovascular therapy for acute ischemic stroke secondary to internal carotid artery occlusion. Indeed, this is a relevant question in light of the evolution of the various endovascular therapies and the widespread proliferation of stroke centers. They identified 28 studies encompassing 969 patients that satisfied their search criteria, but unfortunately none were randomized trials comparing the 2 modalities. They reported that both therapies were associated with comparable rates of favorable outcomes (thrombolysis 25% vs endovascular 34%) as defined using standardized scoring systems (ie, Rankin Scale or Barthel Index). The rates of symptomatic intracranial hemorrhage were significant and found to be increased in the endovascular group (34% vs 25%, $P = .0040$), although there were no differences in mortality (27% vs 32%). These rates of symptomatic intracranial hemorrhage must be interpreted with some caution because the endovascular approach was used in several series when or if thrombolysis was ineffective, suggesting that the endovascular therapies were attempted during a period associated with an increased risk of intracranial bleeding. Notably, intravenous thrombolysis is approved within 4.5 hours of an acute stroke, and the risk of intracranial bleeding associated with administration increases beyond 6 hours after the acute event. The associated 30-day mortality and adverse events rates for both treatments were sobering, underscoring the gravity of the underlying problem and highlighting the need for definitive randomized trials, likely including a medical or nontreatment group (ie, no thrombolysis or endovascular treatment). Indeed, the authors emphasize in the discussion that the endovascular approach has been criticized for the lack of direct evidence, the bias among the neurointerventional community for devices/interventions, and the higher associated costs relative to thrombolysis, all justifications for a randomized trial. The treatment modalities are outside the scope of practice for most vascular surgeons, but it is incumbent on us to recognize their respective roles and indications given our central role in treating extracranial carotid disease.

T. S. Huber, MD, PhD

Modelling the cost-effectiveness of carotid endarterectomy for asymptomatic stenosis
Thapar A, Garcia Mochon L, Epstein D, et al (Imperial College London, UK; Andalusian School of Public Health, Granada, Spain; Univ of York, UK)
Br J Surg 100:231-239, 2013

Background.—The aim of this study was to model the cost-effectiveness of carotid endarterectomy for asymptomatic stenosis *versus* medical therapy based on 10-year data from the Asymptomatic Carotid Surgery Trial (ACST).

Methods.—This was a cost-utility analysis based on clinical effectiveness data from the ACST with UK-specific costs and stroke outcomes. A Markov model was used to calculate the incremental cost-effectiveness ratio (ICER, or cost per additional quality-of-life year) for a strategy of early endarterectomy *versus* medical therapy for the average patient and published subgroups. An exploratory analysis considered contemporary event rates.

Results.—The ICER was £7584 per additional quality-adjusted life-year (QALY) for the average patient in the ACST. At thresholds of £20 000 and £30 000 there was a 74 and 84 per cent chance respectively of early endarterectomy being cost-effective. The ICER for men below 75 years of age was £3254, and that for men aged 75 years or above was £71 699. For women aged under 75 years endarterectomy was less costly and more effective than medical therapy; for women aged 75 years or more endarterectomy was less effective and more costly than medical therapy. At contemporary perioperative event rates of 2·7 per cent and background any-territory stroke rates of 1·6 per cent, early endarterectomy remained cost-effective.

Conclusion.—In the ACST, early endarterectomy was predicted to be cost-effective in those below 75 years of age, using a threshold of £20 000 per QALY. If background any-territory stroke rates fell below 1 per cent per annum, early endarterectomy would cease to be cost-effective.

▶ The authors have used the 10-year data from the Asymptomatic Carotid Surgery Trial (ACST) to construct a Markov model examining the cost-effectiveness of carotid endarterectomy or the incremental cost-effectiveness ratio. The ACST was a randomized, controlled European trial comparing medical management and early carotid endarterectomy, encompassing 3120 patients. Notably, the ACST published its 10-year data in 2010 and reported a 4.6% absolute risk reduction for stroke in patients randomized to early carotid endarterectomy, suggesting that it was beneficial for patients < 75 years of age. The current study largely reaches the same conclusions but establishes that early carotid endarterectomy is also cost-effective using the standard £20 000 quality-adjusted life-years threshold. These findings largely echo an earlier publication based on the Asymptomatic Carotid Atherosclerosis Study (ACAS) that in the mid-1970s appeared to be the cost-effective breakpoint.[1] There has been an impression that both the perioperative stroke risk and the stroke risk associated with medical therapy have decreased since the ACAS, particularly because of the introduction of statins, and this has potentially impacted the risk/benefit of the procedure and its cost-effectiveness. The current findings appear to justify carotid endarterectomy for patients < 75 years with the caveat that the event's rates are comparable to the ACST. In our own practice, we have been particularly conservative about recommending carotid endarterectomy for asymptomatic patients and have used this 75-year age cutoff in good-risk patients, based mostly on the analysis from the ACAS.[1] The authors found that carotid endarterectomy would cease to be cost-effective for asymptomatic stenosis if the baseline fell below 1% per year. This suggests that improving the medical therapies and/or patient compliance with these therapies in an attempt to attain this baseline stroke risk of < 1% may have a greater impact on public health than carotid endarterectomy. It was interesting to note that cost-effectiveness of early carotid endarterectomy for asymptomatic patients did not seem to vary by gender, although the absolute values were somewhat different, with young women (< 75 years) deriving more benefit and older women deriving less than their male counterparts. This is somewhat contradictory to the ACAS that failed to identify a significant benefit for women on subgroup analysis, although admittedly the impact of gender was not the study objective.

T. S. Huber, MD, PhD

Reference

1. Cronenwett JL, Birkmeyer JD, Nackman GB, et al. Cost-effectiveness of carotid endarterectomy in asymptomatic patients. *J Vasc Surg.* 1997;25:298-309.

Peripheral Arterial Occlusive Disease

The natural history of duplex-detected stenosis after femoropopliteal endovascular therapy suggests questionable clinical utility of routine duplex surveillance

Bui TD, Mills JL Sr, Ihnat DM, et al (Univ of Arizona Health Sciences Ctr, Tucson)
J Vasc Surg 55:346-352, 2012

Objective.—Duplex ultrasound (DU) surveillance (DUS) criteria for vein graft stenosis and thresholds for reintervention are well established. The natural history of DU-detected stenosis and the threshold criteria for reintervention in patients undergoing endovascular therapy (EVT) of the femoropopliteal system have yet to be determined. We report an analysis of routine DUS after infrainguinal EVT.

Methods.—Consecutive patients undergoing EVT of the superficial femoral artery (SFA) or popliteal artery were prospectively enrolled in a DUS protocol (≤ 1 week after intervention, then at 3, 6, and 12 months thereafter). Peak systolic velocity (PSV) and velocity ratio (Vr) were used to categorize the treated artery: normal was PSV < 200 cm/s and Vr < 2, moderate stenosis was PSV = 200-300 cm/s or Vr = 2-3, and severe stenosis was PSV > 300 cm/s or Vr > 3. Reinterventions were generally performed for persistent or recurrent symptoms, allowing us to analyze the natural history of DU-detected lesions and to perform sensitivity and specificity analysis for DUS criteria predictive of failure.

Results.—Ninety-four limbs (85 patients) underwent EVT for SFA-popliteal disease and were prospectively enrolled in a DUS protocol. The initial scans were normal in 61 limbs (65%), and serial DU results remained normal in 38 (62%). In 17 limbs (28%), progressive stenoses were detected during surveillance. The rate of thrombosis in this subgroup was 10%. Moderate stenoses were detected in 28 (30%) limbs at initial scans; of these, 39% resolved or stabilized, 47% progressed to severe, and occlusions developed in 14%. Five (5%) limbs harbored severe stenoses on initial scans, and 80% of lesions resolved or stabilized. Progression to occlusion occurred in one limb (20%). The last DUS showed 25 limbs harbored severe stenoses; of these, 13 (52%) were in symptomatic patients and thus required reintervention regardless of DU findings. Eleven limbs (11%) eventually occluded. Sensitivity and specificity of DUS to predict occlusion were 88% and 60%, respectively.

Conclusions.—DUS does not reliably predict arterial occlusion after EVT. Stenosis after EVT appears to have a different natural history than restenosis after vein graft bypass. EVT patients are more likely to have severe stenosis when they present with recurrent symptoms, in contrast to vein graft patients, who commonly have occluded grafts when they present with recurrent symptoms. The potential impact of routine DU-directed reintervention in patients after EVT is questionable. The natural history of DU-detected stenosis after femoropopliteal endovascular therapy suggests questionable clinical utility of routine DUS.

▶ The authors have attempted to define the role of duplex ultrasound surveillance after endovascular treatment (ie, angioplasty, angioplasty/stenting, and atherectomy) for femoropopliteal lesions. This is an extremely relevant clinical question given the number of peripheral endovascular procedures performed across the country and their high incidence of recurrence, frequently leading to a second or third endovascular procedure at the same site. Patients were prospectively enrolled in a surveillance program, similar to that after infrainguinal bypass, with ultrasound studies performed within a week of the intervention and then at 3 months, 6 months, 12 months, and yearly thereafter. The duplex criteria for the stenoses were also similar to those used after bypass procedures, based on the peak systolic velocities and their ratios. Notably, remedial interventions were generally performed only for recurrent symptoms. The authors reported that the initial duplex studies were normal in 65% of the cases and remained normal in 62% of these at a mean follow-up of 22 months. However, the natural histories of the index, treated lesions, and the postprocedure stenoses were distinctly different after endovascular treatment than would have been predicted based on the bypass graft surveillance experience. First, a higher proportion of the lesions noted to be normal at the initial ultrasound progressed to moderate/severe stenoses or occlusion. Second, a higher percentage of the moderate and severe lesions remained stable or resolved. Third, a larger percentage of the patients presented with severe symptoms and a recurrent stenosis rather than an occlusion. Fourth, only a small percentage of the patients with a thrombosis of the index endovascular lesion had a severe stenosis on the ultrasound preceding the occlusion. Taken together, these findings suggest that the duplex criteria used for lower extremity bypass procedures are not applicable to patients undergoing endovascular treatment of femoropopliteal occlusive disease and that routine surveillance studies are not indicated. I would echo the authors' concerns that the sample size is relatively small and the data were collected retrospectively, but the findings merit consideration. Importantly, a moderate to severe stenosis in the femoropopliteal region in an asymptomatic patient after endovascular treatment may not merit early reintervention.

T. S. Huber, MD, PhD

Randomized controlled trial of remote endarterectomy versus endovascular intervention for TransAtlantic Inter-Society Consensus II D femoropopliteal lesions

Gabrielli R, Rosati MS, Vitale S, et al (Policlinico Casilino, Rome, Italy; Sapienza Univ of Rome, Italy)
J Vasc Surg 56:1598-1605, 2012

Objective.—This study evaluated outcomes of remote endarterectomy (RE) vs endovascular (ENDO) interventions on TransAtlantic Inter-Societal Consensus (TASC)-II D femoropopliteal lesions and identified factors predictive of restenosis.

Methods.—From October 2004 to December 2008, 95 patients with TASC-II D lesions were randomized 1:1 to receive RE of the superficial femoral artery (SFA) with end point stenting (51 patients) or ENDO, consisting of subintimal angioplasty with stenting (44 patients). The groups were balanced for age, sex, atherosclerotic risk factors, and comorbidities. Categoric data were analyzed with χ^2 tests, and time to event provided two-sided P values with a level of significance at .05 and 95% confidence intervals (CIs). Survival curves for primary patency were plotted using the Kaplan-Meier method. Univariate analysis for diabetes, hypertension, dyslipidemia, smoking, and critical ischemia was performed according to the Cox proportional hazards model.

Results.—The mean follow-up was 52.5 months (range, 35-75 months). Five RE patients and four ENDO patients were lost to follow-up (censored). Primary patency was 76.5% (39 of 51) in RE and 56.8% (25 of 44) in ENDO (hazard ratio [HR], 2.6; 95% CI, 0.99-4.2; $P = .05$) at 24 months and was 62.7% (32 of 46) in RE and 47.7% (21 of 40) in ENDO (HR, 1.89; 95% CI, 0.94-3.78; $P = .07$) at 36 months. Assisted primary patency was 70.6% (36 of 51) in RE and 52.3% (23 of 44) in ENDO (HR, 2.45; 95% CI, 1.20-5.02; $P = .01$). Secondary patency overlapped the primary comparison data at 12 and 24 months; at 36 months, there was a slight but significative advantage for RE (HR, 2.26; 95% CI, 1.05-4.86; $P = .03$). Univariate analysis demonstrated that hypercholesterolemia and critical limb ischemia (CLI) were significantly related to patency failure, whereas diabetes was significant only in ENDO. These factors (hypercholesterolemia and CLI) were independent predictors of patency on Cox multivariate analysis.

Conclusions.—RE is a safe, effective, and durable procedure for TASC-II D lesions. Our data demonstrate a significantly higher primary, assisted primary, and secondary patency of RE vs ENDO procedures. Furthermore, overall secondary patency rates remain within the standard limits, although preoperative CLI and dyslipidemia continue to be associated with worse outcomes. Taken together, these data suggest that RE should be considered better than an endovascular procedure in SFA long-segment occlusion treatment.

▶ The authors report the results of a small, but elegant, randomized, controlled trial comparing remote endarterectomy/stenting (RE) with subintimal angioplasty/stenting (ENDO) in patients with TransAtlantic Inter-Societal Consensus (TASC)-II D femoropopliteal lesions. The RE was performed with a Vollmar Stripper (Aesculap, San Jose, CA), and the distal endpoint was tacked down with a self-expanding stent. Notably, these TASC-II D lesions are defined as a chronic total occlusion of the common femoral artery or superficial femoral artery (> 20 cm, involving the popliteal artery) or total chronic occlusion of the popliteal artery and proximal trifurcation vessels. The TASC-II document recommends surgical bypass for these lesions; thus, the current randomized trial reflects the evolution of care or the proverbial "pushing the envelope" for alternative, less-invasive therapies. Overall, the primary and secondary patency rates were quite good for both procedures with the values approaching or achieving significance for RE (3-year primary, 74% vs 51%, $P = .07$; 3-year secondary, 73% vs 55%, $P = .02$), and they serve to define a benchmark for what is feasible in this setting. Not surprisingly, chronic limb ischemia was associated with worse outcome and likely served as a marker for more advanced disease. These results challenge the TASC-II recommendations for surgical bypass in this setting, but I am not certain that they justify a major change in clinical practice until more data have accumulated given the relative small sample size. The optimal treatment for patients with peripheral vascular occlusive disease presenting with both claudication and limb-threatening ischemia remains one of the most important questions in our discipline. However, the question about the optimal treatment is broader than the optimal intervention and also requires defining the role of medical management.

T. S. Huber, MD, PhD

Comparison of initial hemodynamic response after endovascular therapy and open surgical bypass in patients with diabetes mellitus and critical limb ischemia

Zhan LX, Bharara M, White M, et al (Univ of Arizona, Tucson)
J Vasc Surg 56:380-386, 2012

Background.—While endovascular (ENDO) therapy has increasingly become the initial intervention of choice to treat lower extremity peripheral arterial disease, reported outcomes for ENDO in patients with critical limb ischemia (CLI) and diabetes have been reported to be inferior compared to open bypass surgery (OPEN). Objective data assessing the hemodynamic success of ENDO compared to the established benchmark of OPEN are sparse. We therefore evaluated and compared early hemodynamic outcomes of ENDO and OPEN in patients with diabetes with CLI at a single academic center.

Methods.—We studied 85 consecutive patients with diabetes and CLI who underwent 109 interventions, either ENDO (n = 78) or OPEN (n = 31). The mean patient age was 69 years; 62% were men. All patients presented with either rest pain and/or ulcer/gangrene. Per protocol, all were assessed using ankle brachial index (ABI) and toe pressure (TP) determinations before and early postintervention.

Results.—Both ENDO (ΔABI = 0.36 ± 0.24, $P < .0001$; ΔTP = 35.6 ± 24.1, $P < .0001$) and OPEN (ΔABI = 0.39 ± 0.17, $P < .0001$; ΔTP = 34.3 ± 24.0, $P < .0001$) resulted in significant hemodynamic improvement. There was no statistically significant initial difference between the two types of intervention (ABI, $P = .6$; TP, $P = .6$).

Conclusions.—These data suggest that with appropriate patient selection, each intervention is similarly efficacious in initially improving hemodynamics. If the intermediate or long-term results of ENDO for CLI in people with diabetes are inferior, the problem is not one of initial hemodynamic response, but more likely due to differing patient characteristics or durability of the intervention.

▶ The authors compared the initial hemodynamic response after open and endovascular treatment for diabetic patients with critical limb ischemia and found that both therapies resulted in a comparable hemodynamic improvement as measured by ankle brachial index and traumatic brain injuries. There has been a bias among many surgeons, including myself, that the hemodynamic benefits of the endovascular approach were inferior and, thus, open bypass was likely a better choice for patients with critical limb ischemia, particularly those with extensive tissue loss.[1] The current findings seem to dispel this bias for the initial hemodynamic response, but it is important to emphasize that they provide no insight into the longer-term durability of the treatment options. These findings are consistent with the Bypass vs angioplasty in severe ischaemia of the leg (BASIL) Trial 1 that demonstrated that the early amputation-free survival was comparable between patients with severe limb ischemia randomized to an endovascular or open-first approach.[2] Presumably, any differences in the longer-term outcomes for this cohort of diabetics with critical limb ischemia must be due to the durability of the procedures and/or specific patient characteristics, again consistent with the BASIL Trial 2 that suggested patients with a life expectancy of more than 2 years may be better served with open revascularization. The larger question about the choice between endovascular and open revascularization for patients with lower extremity arterial occlusive disease (both claudication and limb-threatening ischemia) has been difficult and remains one of the larger unanswered questions in our discipline. Despite the importance of the question, it has been difficult to design (and fund) the necessary critical studies given the range of presenting symptoms (ie, claudication, rest pain, minor tissue loss, major tissue loss), anatomic location of disease (ie, aortoiliac, femoropopliteal, tibial) extent of occlusive disease (ie, TransAtlantic Inter-Society Consensus A—D), diversity of endovascular treatment options (eg, angioplasty, angioplasty/stent, atherectomy), and differences in outcomes, among other factors. The current findings provide further insight into the complex question regarding the optimal treatment for patients with lower extremity arterial occlusive disease. However, they should be interpreted with some caution given the retrospective nature of the study design, the inherent selection bias, the small sample size, and the clinical expertise of the authors.

T. S. Huber, MD, PhD

References

1. Adam DJ, Beard JD, Cleveland T, et al. Bypass versus angioplasty in severe ischaemia of the leg (BASIL): multicentre, randomised controlled trial. *Lancet.* 2005;366:1925-1934.
2. Bradbury AW, Adam DJ, Bell J, et al. Bypass versus angioplasty in severe ischaemia of the leg (BASIL) trial: an intention-to-treat analysis of amputation-free and overall survival in patients randomized to a bypass surgery-first or a balloon angioplasty-first revascularization strategy. *J Vasc Surg.* 2010;51:5S-17S.

Optimal conduit choice in the absence of single-segment great saphenous vein for below-knee popliteal bypass
McPhee JT, Barshes NR, Ozaki CK, et al (Brigham and Women's Hosp, Boston, MA)
J Vasc Surg 55:1008-1014, 2012

Background.—Single-segment great saphenous vein (SSGSV) remains the conduit of choice for femoral to below-knee popliteal (F—BK) surgical revascularization. The purpose of this study was to determine the optimal conduit in patients with inadequate SSGSV.

Methods.—This was a retrospective review of a prospectively maintained vascular registry. Patients underwent F—BK bypass with alternative vein (AV; arm vein, spliced GSV, or composite vein) or prosthetic conduit (PC).

Results.—From January 1995 to June 2010, 83 patients had unusable SSGSV for F—BK popliteal reconstruction. Thirty-three patients had an AV conduit and 50 had PC. The AV group was a lower median age than the PC group (69 vs 75 years). The two groups were otherwise similar in comorbid conditions of diabetes mellitus (57.6% vs 58.0%; $P > .99$), smoking (15.2% vs 32.0%; $P = .12$), and hemodialysis (3% vs 12%; $P = .23$). The groups were similar in baseline characteristics such as limb salvage as indication (93.9% vs 86.0%; $P = .31$), mean runoff score (5.2 vs 4.6; $P = .39$), and prior ipsilateral bypass attempts (18.2% vs 18.0%; $P > .99$). The AV and PC groups were also similar in 30-day mortality (6.1% vs 4.0%; $P > .99$) and wound infection rates (6.1% vs 6.0%; $P > .99$). PC patients were more likely to be discharged on Coumadin (Bristol-Myers Squibb, Princeton, NJ) than AV patients (62.0% vs 27.3%; $P = .002$). Seventeen of the 50 PC patients (34%) had a distal anastomotic vein cuff. A log-rank test comparison of 5-year outcomes for the AV and PC groups found no significant difference in primary patency (55.3% ± 9.9% vs 51.9% ± 10.8%; $P = .82$), assisted primary patency (68.8% ± 9.6% vs 54.0% ± 11.0%; $P = .45$), secondary patency (68.4% ± 9.6% vs 63.7% ± 10.4% for PC; $P = .82$), or limb salvage rates (96.2% ± 3.8% vs 81.1% ± 8.1%; $P = .19$). Multivariable analysis demonstrated no association between conduit type and loss of patency or limb. The factors most predictive of primary patency loss were limb salvage as the indication for surgery (hazard ratio [HR], 4.23; 95% confidence interval [CI], 1.65-10.9; $P = .003$) and current hemodialysis (HR, 3.51; 95% CI, 1.08-11.4; $P = .037$). The most predictive factor of limb loss was current hemodialysis (HR, 7.02; 95% CI, 1.13-43.4; $P = .036$).

Conclusions.—For patients with inadequate SSGSV, PCs, with varying degrees of medical and surgical adjuncts, appear comparable to AV sources in graft patency for below-knee popliteal bypass targets. This observation is tempered by the small cohort sample size of this single-institutional analysis. Critical limb ischemia as the operative indication and current hemodialysis predict impaired patency, and hemodialysis is associated with limb loss.

▶ The authors address a clinically relevant question about the optimal conduit for femoral, below-knee popliteal bypass in patients without a suitable, single segment of saphenous vein. The authors retrospectively compared their experience with alternative autogenous (ie, arm vein, spliced great saphenous vein, composite) and prosthetic conduits in this location, although the study and title were somewhat misleading because they also included bypasses to the tibioperoneal trunk. Somewhat surprisingly, they reported that the patency and limb salvage rates were comparable, and choice of conduit was not associated with adverse outcome on multivariate analysis. They did find that current hemodialysis and limb salvage indication were associated with adverse outcome, consistent with numerous other reports. These findings are somewhat reassuring to those surgeons who favor prosthetic bypass in this anatomic configuration, although the results must be interpreted with some caution. First, the experience was relatively small (N = 83) considering the overall volume of infrainguinal bypass procedures performed by the authors and the duration of the experience (ie, 1995−2010). Second, there was a tremendous selection bias as would be predicted based on the study design and, thus, the findings may not be widely applicable outside of the authors' practices. Third, the prosthetic conduit group was very heterogeneous in terms of prosthetic conduit type (ie, expanded polytetra-fluoroethylene [ePTFE], heparin-bonded ePTFE, Dacron, flared ePTFE), anastomotic configuration (ie, vein patch versus no vein patch), and long-term anticoagulation (ie, coumadin versus no coumadin). Accordingly, it was difficult to determine the relative contribution of these factors (if any) to the excellent long-term results. In our own practice, we have favored an all autogenous approach for infrainguinal bypass and have reserved prosthetic and cadaveric conduits for patients without sufficient vein. Although I am not quite ready to abandon our approach, the authors' findings merit further critical review of this practice.

T. S. Huber, MD, PhD

Ultrasonic vein mapping prior to infrainguinal autogenous bypass grafting reduces postoperative infections and readmissions
Linni K, Mader N, Aspalter M, et al (Paracelsus Med Univ Salzburg, Austria)
J Vasc Surg 56:126-133, 2012

Objective.—Although duplex vein mapping (DVM) of the great saphenous vein (GSV) is common practice, there is no level I evidence for its application. Our prospective randomized trial studied the effect of preoperative DVM in infrainguinal bypass surgery.

Methods.—Consecutive patients undergoing primary bypass grafting were prospectively randomized for DVM of the GSV (group A) or no DMV of the GSV (group B) before surgery. Society for Vascular Surgery reporting standards were applied.

Results.—From December 2009 to December 2010, 103 patients were enrolled: 51 (group A) underwent DVM of the GSV, and 52 (group B) did not. Group A and group B not differ statistically in age (72.8 vs 71.1 years), sex (women, 29.4% vs 34.6%), cardiovascular risk factors, body mass index (25.9 vs 26.1 kg/m^2), bypass anatomy, and runoff. Group A and B had equal operative time (151.4 vs 151.1 minutes), incisional length (39.4 vs 39.9 cm), and secondary bypass patency at 30 days (96.1% vs 96.2%; $P = .49$). Conduit issues resulted in six intraoperative changes of the operative plan in group B vs none in group A ($P = .014$). Median postoperative length of stay was comparable in both groups ($P = .18$). Surgical site infections (SSIs) were classified (in group A vs B) as minor (23.5% vs 23.1%; $P = 1.0$) and major (1.9% vs 21.2%; $P = .004$). Readmissions due to SSIs were 3.9% in group A vs 19.2% in group B ($P = .028$). Two patients in group B died after complications of SSIs. Multivariate analysis identified preoperative DVM as the only significant factor influencing the development of major SSI ($P = .0038$).

Conclusions.—Routine DVM should be recommended for infrainguinal bypass surgery. The study found that preoperative DVM significantly avoids unnecessary surgical exploration, development of major SSI, and reduces frequency of readmissions for SSI treatment.

▶ The authors have performed an elegant, randomized trial examining the role of ultrasound vein mapping prior to infrainguinal bypass. Although the practice is fairly widespread and generally considered the standard of care, it is somewhat surprising that the supporting evidence is so limited. Preoperative vein mapping theoretically facilitates selection of the optimal vein for use as a conduit (presumably improving bypass graft patency), facilitates vein harvest by minimizing the skin/soft tissue flaps, and reduces both operating time and wound complications. In this study, patients undergoing their first bypass (ie, no redo or reoperative procedure) were randomly assigned to preoperative mapping of the saphenous vein or exploration without imaging with a vein diameter greater than 2.5 mm deemed adequate. The operative plan changed at the time of the procedure in 6 of 51 (12%) patients without preoperative imaging because of conduit-related issues, whereas the major surgical site infection rate (1.9% vs 21.2%) and the readmissions due to surgical site infections (3.9% vs 19.2%) were both significantly higher in this group. Notably, there were 2 deaths related to surgical site infections among the patients that did not undergo preoperative vein mapping, and its use was the only factor identified as a predictor of major surgical site infections in the multivariate analysis. It is somewhat surprising that preoperative vein mapping did not improve graft patency, reduce the operative time, or reduce the length of the incision, given its purported advantages. The overall data provide support for routine preoperative vein mapping in the study cohort, although it is worth emphasizing that these were first-time procedures performed with good-quality saphenous vein and the patients were thin (mean body mass index, 26 kg/m^2). I would contend that it may provide an even greater benefit for obese patients, those undergoing redo procedures, and those with compromised or alternative autogenous conduits (eg, composite arm veins). Indeed, I couldn't imagine performing a complex distal bypass in an obese patient without preoperative imaging to mark the location of the conduit and confirm that it is suitable. The overall wound complication rate for both study groups was a sobering 35% and is largely consistent with those of other reports in the literature. This finding underscores the importance of the various strategies to reduce wound complications, including the use of interval incisions (ie, skip incisions) for the vein harvest as implemented in this study.

T. S. Huber, MD, PhD

Combination therapy with warfarin plus clopidogrel improves outcomes in femoropopliteal bypass surgery patients
Monaco M, Di Tommaso L, Pinna GB, et al (Istituto Clinico Pineta Grande, Castel Volturno, Italy; Univ Federico II, Naples, Italy)
J Vasc Surg 56:96-105, 2012

Background.—Patients having undergone femoropopliteal bypass surgery remain at significant risk of graft failure. Although antithrombotic

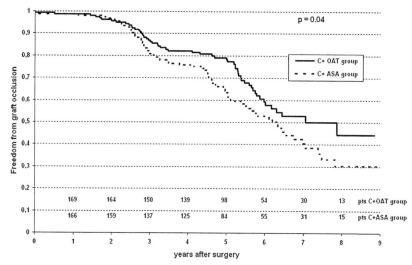

FIGURE 3.—Freedom from major adverse cardiovascular events, including mortality, for the two study groups. C + ASA, Clopidogrel plus acetylsalicylic acid therapy patients; C + OAT, clopidogrel plus oral anticoagulation therapy patients. (Reprinted from the Journal of Vascular Surgery. Monaco M, Di Tommaso L, Pinna GB, et al. Combination therapy with warfarin plus clopidogrel improves outcomes in femoropopliteal bypass surgery patients. *J Vasc Surg.* 2012;56:96-105, Copyright 2012, with permission from The Society for Vascular Surgery.)

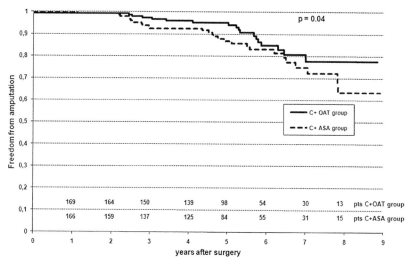

FIGURE 5.—Freedom from amputation for the two study groups. C + ASA, Clopidogrel plus acetylsalicylic acid therapy patients; C + OAT, clopidogrel plus oral anticoagulation therapy patients. (Reprinted from the Journal of Vascular Surgery. Monaco M, Di Tommaso L, Pinna GB, et al. Combination therapy with warfarin plus clopidogrel improves outcomes in femoropopliteal bypass surgery patients. *J Vasc Surg.* 2012;56:96-105, Copyright 2012, with permission from The Society for Vascular Surgery.)

therapy is of paramount importance in these patients, the effect of oral anti-coagulation therapy (OAT) on outcomes remains unresolved. We performed a randomized, prospective study to assess the impact of OAT plus clopidogrel vs dual antiplatelet therapy on peripheral vascular and systemic cardiovascular outcomes in patients who had undergone femoropopliteal bypass surgery.

Methods.—Three hundred forty-one patients who had undergone femoropopliteal surgery were enrolled and randomized: 173 patients received clopidogrel 75 mg/d plus OAT with warfarin (C + OAT), and 168 patients received dual antiplatelet therapy with clopidogrel 75 mg/d plus aspirin 100 mg/d (C + acetylsalicylic acid [ASA]). Study end points were graft patency and the occurrence of severe peripheral arterial ischemia, and the incidence of bleeding episodes.

Results.—Follow-up ranged from 4 to 9 years. The graft patency rate and the freedom from severe peripheral arterial ischemia was significantly higher in C + OAT group than in C + ASA group ($P = .026$ and .044, respectively, Cox-Mantel test). The linearized incidence of minor bleeding complications was significantly higher in C + OAT group than in C + ASA group (2.85% patient-years vs 1.37% patient-years; $P = .03$). The incidence of major adverse cardiovascular events, including mortality, was found to be similar ($P = .34$) for both study groups.

Conclusions.—In patients who have undergone femoropopliteal vascular surgery, combination therapy with clopidogrel plus warfarin is more effective than dual antiplatelet therapy in increasing graft patency and in reducing severe peripheral ischemia. These improvements are obtained at the expenses of an increase in the rate of minor anticoagulation-related complications (Figs 3 and 5).

▶ The optimal anticoagulation and/or antiplatelet regimen after infrainguinal bypass (both prosthetic and autogenous conduits) remains unresolved with the various studies reporting somewhat contradictory results. In the current study, the authors performed a randomized, prospective trial comparing clopidogrel + warfarin (C + OAT) with clopidogrel + aspirin (C + ASA) in patients undergoing femoral above-knee popliteal bypass with prosthetic material and femoral below-knee popliteal bypass with saphenous vein. They reported that the combination of C + OAT was associated with improved graft patency (Fig 3) and fewer ischemic events leading to amputation (Fig 5) with only a small increase in the number of minor bleeding complications. The findings are supported by the relatively large sample size (n = 341) and the duration of the follow-up that ranged from a minimum of 4 years to maximum of 9 years. It is notable that there was no difference in the major adverse cardiac event rates between the groups, similar to the CHARISMA (Clopidogrel for High Atherothrombotic Risk and Ischemic Stabilization, Management, and Avoidance) trial that found no difference in the same endpoint when comparing aspirin alone with aspirin + clopidogrel.[1] The inclusion of both prosthetic above-knee and autogenous below-knee bypasses seems somewhat odd. The authors justified lumping together the different conduits/configurations to "obtain a strong uniformity of population," although it was interesting that the type of bypass (and conduit) did not affect the primary endpoints among multivariate analysis. The combination of C + OAT seems excessive on first pass, although it is likely safe given the findings that the major bleeding risk was < 2% per year and not different between the 2 experimental groups. It was interesting that the largest separation between the graft patency and freedom from amputation curves occurred between 5 and 6 years, suggesting that the optimal benefit of the C + OAT regimen requires long-term therapy. The current findings add another piece of important data to the debate about the most appropriate postoperative regimen after infrainguinal bypass and seem to justify the combination of C + OAT.

T. S. Huber, MD, PhD

Reference

1. CHARISMA Investigators. Clopidogrel and aspirin versus aspirin alone for the prevention of atherothrombotic events. *N Engl J Med*. 2006;354:1706-1717.

Venous

Long-term outcome after additional catheter-directed thrombolysis versus standard treatment for acute iliofemoral deep vein thrombosis (the CaVenT study): A randomised controlled trial

Enden T, on behalf of the CaVenT Study Group (Oslo Univ Hosp, Norway; et al)
Lancet 379:31-38, 2012

Background.—Conventional anticoagulant treatment for acute deep vein thrombosis (DVT) effectively prevents thrombus extension and recurrence, but does not dissolve the clot, and many patients develop post-thrombotic syndrome (PTS). We aimed to examine whether additional treatment with catheter-directed thrombolysis (CDT) using alteplase reduced development of PTS.

Methods.—Participants in this open-label, randomised controlled trial were recruited from 20 hospitals in the Norwegian southeastern health region. Patients aged 18−75 years with a first-time iliofemoral DVT were included within 21 days from symptom onset. Patients were randomly assigned (1:1) by picking lowest number of sealed envelopes to conventional treatment alone or additional CDT. Randomisation was stratified for involvement of the pelvic veins with blocks of six. We assessed two co-primary outcomes: frequency of PTS as assessed by Villalta score at 24 months, and iliofemoral patency after 6 months. Analyses were by intention to treat. This trial is registered at ClinicalTrials. gov, NCT00251771.

Findings.—209 patients were randomly assigned to treatment groups (108 control, 101 CDT). At completion of 24 months' follow-up, data for clinical status were available for 189 patients (90%; 99 control, 90 CDT). At 24 months, 37 (41·1%, 95% CI 31·5−51·4) patients allocated additional CDT presented with PTS compared with 55 (55·6%, 95% CI 45·7−65·0) in the control group ($p = 0·047$). The difference in PTS corresponds to an absolute risk reduction of 14·4% (95% CI 0·2—27·9), and the number needed to treat was 7 (95% CI 4—502). Iliofemoral patency after 6 months was reported in 58 patients (65·9%, 95% CI 55·5—75·0) on CDT versus 45 (47·4%, 37·6—57·3) on control ($p = 0·012$). 20 bleeding complications related to CDT included three major and five clinically relevant bleeds.

Interpretation.—Additional CDT should be considered in patients with a high proximal DVT and low risk of bleeding.

▶ The CaVenT study is among the first randomized controlled trials to examine the role of catheter-directed thrombolysis (CDT) in patients with iliofemoral deep venous thrombosis (DVT). Notably, registry data and a Cochrane review have both suggested a benefit of CDT in this setting, but the strength of the recommendations has been limited by the quality of the underlying studies. In the CaVenT Study, patients with first-time DVT within 21 days of symptoms were randomized to best medical management (anticoagulation + compression) or CDT with adjunct endovascular treatment (eg, angioplasty, stenting) in combination with best medical management, and accordingly, the findings are widely applicable outside the clinical trial setting. The authors reported that CDT resulted in a significant reduction in the incidence of postthrombotic syndrome at 2 years as assessed with the Villalta scale with an absolute risk reduction of 14% (number needed to treat = 7) and a higher incidence of iliofemoral vein patency at 6 months. Although statistically significant, these outcome data are not as compelling as suggested by some of the nonrandomized trials and do not necessarily provide widespread support for the routine use of CDT for all patients with iliofemoral DVT. Fortunately, the incidence of bleeding complications was relatively low with a "clinically relevant" rate of 9% and no permanent bleeding complications attributed to the lysis. These data should be interpreted with some caution because the follow-up period (ie, 2 years) is relatively short and may not be adequate to capture all of the potential adverse sequelae after femoral DVT. Furthermore, the patient compliance in terms of both anticoagulation and use of compression hose was quite good and likely better than anticipated outside a clinical trial. It is noteworthy that the CDT was quite successful from a technical standpoint with only 2 procedural failures (2/93) and a complete lysis rate in roughly half of the patients (43/93), although the mean duration of lysis was 2.4 days and a significant proportion of the patients (39/93) required some type of adjunct procedure. I would echo the authors' generic conclusion that "CDT should be considered in patients with high proximal DVT and low risk of bleeding," but would continue to reserve its use for good-risk patients with a reasonable life expectancy while limiting the overall duration of therapy.

T. S. Huber, MD, PhD

Miscellaneous

Accuracy of FDG-PET–CT in the Diagnostic Work-up of Vascular Prosthetic Graft Infection

Bruggink JLM, Glaudemans AWJM, Saleem BR, et al (Univ Med Ctr Groningen, The Netherlands; et al)

Eur J Vasc Endovasc Surg 40:348-354, 2010

Objectives.—To investigate the diagnostic accuracy of fluoro-2-deoxy-D-glucose positron emission tomography (FDG-PET) compared with computed tomography (CT) scanning and added value of fused FDG-PET–CT in diagnosing vascular prosthetic graft infection.

Design.—Prospective cohort study with retrospective analysis.

Materials.—Twenty five patients with clinically suspected vascular prosthetic infection underwent CT and FDG-PET scanning.

Methods.—Two nuclear medicine physicians assessed the FDG-PET scans; all CT scans were assessed by two radiologists. Fused FDG-PET/CT were judged by the radiologist and the nuclear medicine physician. The concordance between CT and FDG-PET and the inter-observer agreement between the different readers were investigated.

Results.—Fifteen patients had a proven infection by culture. Single FDG-PET had the best results (sensitivity 93%, specificity 70%, positive predictive value 82% and negative predictive value 88%). For CT, these values were 56%, 57%, 60% and 58%, respectively. Fused CT and FDG-PET imaging also showed high sensitivity and specificity rates and high positive and negative values. Inter-observer agreement for FDG-PET analysis was excellent (kappa = 1.00) and moderate for CT and fused FDG-PET–CT analysis (0.63 and 0.66, respectively).

Conclusion.—FDG-PET scanning showed a better diagnostic accuracy than CT for the detection of vascular prosthetic infection. This study suggests that FDG-PET provides a useful tool in the work-up for diagnosis of vascular prosthetic graft infection.

▶ The authors have compared fluoro-2-deoxy-D-glucose positron emission tomography (FDG-PET) and computed tomography (CT) scans as a diagnostic tool for infected prosthetic grafts using a positive graft gram stain as the proverbial "gold standard." They reported that the diagnostic accuracy of FDG-PET was superior to CT in terms of the usual sensitivity, specificity, positive predictive value, and negative predictive value. Although the sample size is relatively small, the report suggests that FDG-PET scanning could play an important role in the diagnostic algorithm of infected grafts, certainly for equivocal cases. The diagnosis is simple for patients with exposed grafts and/or a draining sinus tract that communicate with the graft, although it can be more challenging in patients with nonspecific signs of infection (eg, fever, leukocytosis, generalized malaise) but no overt physical findings. We have used CT as the initial diagnostic imaging setting in these cases and have reserved exploratory laparotomy or graft exploration for scenarios in which the CT findings are equivocal, but our clinical suspicion is high. The CT findings suggestive of a graft infection as detailed by the authors are worth reviewing and include aortoenteric fistula, pseudoaneurysm, intergraft thrombus, hydronephrosis, perigraft fluid/soft tissue/air, focal bowel thickening, and discontinuity of the aneurysm wrap. These largely reflect our own practice, and it has been our clinical impression that hydronephrosis is pathognomonic of an aortic graft infection, even in the absence of more overt signs. The FDG-PET scan may replace graft exploration as a less-invasive, diagnostic study in our treatment algorithm provided that other reports confirm the current report. Indeed, I can imagine extending the application to other clinical scenarios when the suspicion of a prosthetic graft infection is entertained, such as in dialysis patients with persistent fevers and a nonfunctional access. It was somewhat surprising that the diagnostic accuracy of CT was so low in the current report, given its pivotal role in most diagnostic algorithms. The authors attribute this to the fact that many of the patients had already been treated with antibiotics and that they had low-grade infections. I would also add that these may have been caused by low-virulent organisms such as *Staphylococcus epidermidis*.

T. S. Huber, MD, PhD

Open and laparoscopic treatment of median arcuate ligament syndrome
Jimenez JC, Harlander-Locke M, Dutson EP (David Geffen School of Medicine at the Univ of California, Los Angeles)
J Vasc Surg 56:869-873, 2012

Background.—Median arcuate ligament syndrome (MALS) is a syndrome associated with chronic abdominal pain and radiographic evidence of celiac artery compression. We compared the evidence for both open and laparoscopic treatment of patients with MALS.

Methods.—We reviewed the English-language literature between 1963 and 2012. Presenting symptoms, clinical improvement, operative details, and intraoperative and postoperative complications were noted.

Results.—A total of 400 patients underwent surgical (open and laparoscopic) treatment for MALS. Three hundred thirty-nine patients reported immediate postoperative symptom relief (85%). Late recurrence of symptoms was reported in 19 patients in the open group (6.8%) and seven patients in the laparoscopic group (5.7%). Eleven out of 121 patients (9.1%) in the laparoscopic group required open conversion secondary to bleeding.

Conclusions.—The available evidence demonstrates that both laparoscopic and open ligament release, celiac ganglionectomy, and celiac artery revascularization may provide sustained symptom relief in the majority of patients diagnosed with MALS. The role of arterial revascularization following ligament release remains unclear. The rate of open conversion

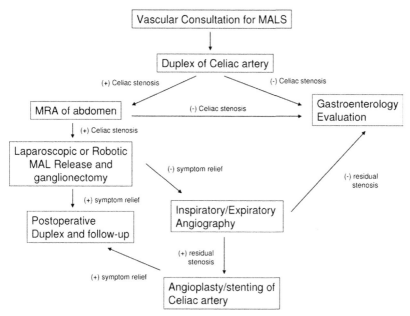

FIGURE.—Current treatment algorithm for median arcuate ligament syndrome (*MALS*) at our institution. *MRA*, Magnetic resonance angiography. (Reprinted from the Journal of Vascular Surgery. Jimenez JC, Harlander-Locke M, Dutson EP. Open and laparoscopic treatment of median arcuate ligament syndrome. *J Vasc Surg*. 2012;56:869-873, Copyright 2012, with permission from The Society for Vascular Surgery.)

with the laparoscopic approach is high, but no perioperative deaths have been reported (Fig).

▶ The authors have attempted to perform an evidence-based review of the literature to compare open and endovascular treatment for median arcuate ligament syndrome. They identified 20 retrospective studies between 1963 and 2012, encompassing a total of 400 patients. Not surprisingly, the majority of the open reports were published before 1991, whereas all of the endovascular reports were published after 2004. Overall, the results were quite impressive, with the overwhelming majority of the patients (85%) reporting early symptomatic relief with a low recurrence rate (< 7%) in both groups. Somewhat surprisingly, the open conversion rate for bleeding was 9% among the laparoscopic group, which was largely attributed to the proverbial learning curve, given the relatively small sample sizes. It is not certain how these data should be used given the retrospective study design and inherent selection bias. Indeed, the diagnosis of median arcuate ligament syndrome itself is among the most controversial in vascular surgery, potentially only rivaled by neurogenic thoracic outlet. Fortunately or unfortunately, patients with the diagnosis of median arcuate ligament syndrome are referred to most busy vascular surgery practices with some frequency. In the usual scenario, the patients have undergone extensive, exhaustive medical evaluations for their chronic abdominal pain and the only abnormality identified on their evaluation is the compression of the celiac axis by the crura of the diaphragm with some poststenotic dilation, a normal anatomic variant seen in approximately 20% of autopsy studies. Unfortunately, there is no definitive diagnostic test with the potential exception of the definitive decompression itself. Gastric tonometry has shown some promise, although the published experience is limited. The etiology of the pain has been attributed to ischemia and neuropathy. Justification for the ischemic etiology is provided in the gastric tonometry series, and the early reports demonstrated that the long-term results were improved when the ligament decompression was combined with celiac revascularization. The neurogenic etiology is supported by the extensive collateral arterial network that is frequently seen and the clinical improvement observed with the dissection/excision of the celiac ganglion performed in combination with the ligament decompression. Like most surgical procedures, the key to good outcome after open or laparoscopic decompression is proper patient selection. The authors have provided a nice, thoughtful algorithm (Fig) that may provide some help in patient selection. It is reassuring that the laparoscopic approach appears to be relatively safe and that no deaths have been reported despite the open conversion rate for bleeding.

T. S. Huber, MD, PhD

Evaluation and management of penetrating lower extremity arterial trauma: An Eastern Association for the Surgery of Trauma practice management guideline
Fox N, Rajani RR, Bokhari F, et al (Cooper Univ Hosp, Camden, NJ; Emory Univ School of Medicine, Atlanta, GA; Hosp of Cook County, Chicago, IL; et al)
J Trauma Acute Care Surg 73:S315-S320, 2012

Background.—Extremity arterial injury after penetrating trauma is common in military conflict or urban trauma centers. Most peripheral arterial injuries occur in the femoral and popliteal vessels of the lower extremity. The Eastern Association for the Surgery of Trauma first published practice management guidelines for the evaluation and treatment of penetrating lower extremity arterial trauma in 2002. Since that time, there have been advancements in the management of penetrating lower extremity arterial trauma. As a result, the Practice Management Guidelines Committee set out to develop updated guidelines.

Methods.—A MEDLINE computer search was performed using PubMed (www.pubmed.gov). The search retrieved English language articles regarding penetrating lower extremity trauma from 1998 to 2011. References of these articles were also used to locate articles not identified through the MEDLINE search. Letters to the editor, case reports, book chapters, and review articles were excluded. The topics investigated were prehospital management, diagnostic evaluation, use of imaging technology, the role of temporary intravascular shunts, use of tourniquets, and the role of endovascular intervention.

Results.—Forty-three articles were identified. From this group, 20 articles were selected to construct the guidelines.

Conclusion.—There have been changes in practice since the publication of the previous guidelines in 2002. Expedited triage of patients is possible with physical examination and/or the measurement of ankle-brachial indices. Computed tomographic angiography has become the diagnostic study of choice when imaging is required. Tourniquets and intravascular shunts have emerged as adjuncts in the treatment of penetrating lower extremity arterial trauma. The role of endovascular intervention warrants further investigation.

▶ This report details the Eastern Association for the Surgery of Trauma Guidelines for penetrating lower extremity trauma and updates the 2002 version. The update was stimulated by several recent changes in clinical practice. Although the authors state that the 2002 guidelines were reviewed and "remain relevant as previously written," there were several notable changes. Computed tomography (CT) arteriography has emerged as the primary diagnostic imaging study and has largely replaced catheter-based arteriography (level 1 recommendation). CT arteriography has been found to have an acceptable sensitivity and specificity in this setting and offers the additional benefits that it is noninvasive, readily available in most centers, cheaper than catheter-based arteriography, and definitive for the evaluation of almost all other traumatic injuries (ie, nonvascular). Indeed, the transition from catheter-based arteriography to CT arteriography has largely paralleled the evolution of diagnostic imaging for most vascular surgery problems over the past decade. Emergent operative exploration without further imaging for the hard signs of peripheral vascular injury is still justified, whereas patients with soft signs and ankle/brachial indices (ABI) less than .9 merit further evaluation, and those with palpable distal pulses and ABI greater than .9 are likely suitable for discharge without further evaluation in the absence of other injuries (all level 2 recommendations). The authors emphasize that 1% to 4% of patients with a normal pulse examination will have a delayed presentation of their vascular injury, thereby underscoring the importance of close follow-up. The remaining recommendations (all level 3) were largely unsupported by evidence in the literature and primarily repeat the 2002 guidelines. The important additions (albeit somewhat lacking in data) addressed the use of tourniquets, temporary intravascular shunts, and endovascular interventions. Tourniquets were deemed acceptable if direct pressure was ineffective, although they should be removed when definitive care is available, and the overall duration of their use should be limited. Intravascular shunts are an important adjunct for damage control surgery when the patient's physiologic status or available surgical expertise preclude definitive repair. Lastly, coil embolization of the branch vessels in the lower extremity (eg, profunda branches, tibial branches) appears to be effective, although the use of stent grafts for the larger vessels remains unresolved.

T. S. Huber, MD, PhD

Early fasciotomy in patients with extremity vascular injury is associated with decreased risk of adverse limb outcomes: A review of the National Trauma Data Bank

Farber A, Tan T-W, Hamburg NM, et al (Boston Univ Med Ctr, MA; et al)
Injury 43:1486-1491, 2012

Introduction and Objectives.—Lower extremity (LE) arterial trauma and its treatment may lead to extremity compartment syndrome (ECS). In that setting, the decision to perform fasciotomies is multifactoral and is not well delineated. We evaluated the outcomes of patients with surgically treated LE arterial injury who underwent early or delayed fasciotomies.

Methods.—The National Trauma Data Bank (NTDB) was retrospectively reviewed for patients who had LE arterial trauma and underwent both open vascular repair and fasciotomies. Exclusion criteria were additional non-LE vascular trauma, head or spinal cord injuries, crush injuries, burn injuries, and declaration of death on arrival. Patients were divided into those who had fasciotomies performed within 8 h (early group) or >8 h after open vascular repair (late group). Comparative analyses of demographics, injury characteristics, complications, and outcomes were performed.

Results.—Of the 1469 patient admissions with lower extremity arterial trauma that met inclusion criteria there were 612 patients (41.7%) who underwent fasciotomies. There were 543 and 69 patients in the early and late fasciotomy groups, respectively. There was no significant difference in age, injury severity, mechanism of injury, associated injuries, and type of vascular repair between the groups. A higher rate of iliac artery injury was observed in the late fasciotomy group (23.2% vs. 5.9%, $P < .001$). Patients in the early fasciotomy group had lower amputation rate (8.5% vs. 24.6%, $P < .001$), lower infection rate (6.6% vs. 14.5%, $P = .028$) and shorter total hospital stay (18.5 ± 20.7 days vs. 24.2 ± 14.7 days, $P = .007$) than those in the late fasciotomy group. On multivariable analysis, early fasciotomy was associated with a 4-fold lower risk of amputation (Odds Ratio 0.26, 95% CI 0.14—0.50, $P < .0001$) and 23% shorter hospital LOS (Means Ratio 0.77, 95% CI 0.64—0.94, $P = .01$).

Conclusion.—Early fasciotomy is associated with improved outcomes in patients with lower extremity vascular trauma treated with surgical intervention. Our findings suggest that appropriate implementation of early fasciotomy may reduce amputation rates in extremity arterial injury.

▶ The authors call attention to the role of fasciotomy (ie, decompression of the fascial compartments) during lower extremity revascularization for trauma. Despite the limitations of a retrospective analysis from a national database, the findings of the study are interesting and show that early fasciotomy (less than 8 hours after injury) is associated with a lower amputation rate, fewer wound complications, and a shorter length of stay with a 4-fold lower amputation rate upon multivariate analysis. The development of a compartment syndrome is multifactorial and includes direct issue injury, hemorrhage/hematoma, ischemia/reperfusion, and venous obstruction, all relevant to the trauma setting. The role for fasciotomy is clear for patients with a true compartment syndrome, although the indications for a prophylactic fasciotomy at the time of arterial trauma are not as well defined. The proponents have suggested that fasciotomy in this setting helps avoid the development of a compartment syndrome, whereas the detractors have suggested that it can lead to wound complications and is often an additional, unnecessary procedure. Notably, our group has been a liberal proponent of extensive (ie, two-thirds the length of the calf) fasciotomies and have espoused the philosophy that "if you think about performing fasciotomies then you should do it." Our bias has been validated by this study, and it is interesting that the early group had fewer wound complications rather than vice versa, as might have been hypothesized. The authors make the point that the higher incidence of wound complications may have been due to muscle necrosis resulting from the delayed recognition of any compartment syndrome. In our own practice, we close the fasciotomy incisions at the bedside using interrupted sutures if there is no significant swelling and have been impressed with how well the wounds heal, although this is not particularly surprising given that the usual trauma victims are young, healthy men without peripheral vascular disease. It is interesting to note that there was a higher incidence of iliac vascular injuries in the late fasciotomy group. This finding suggests that the potential for a compartment syndrome was not well recognized in this subset of patients and should heighten our collective awareness. I would certainly echo the authors' conclusions that "early amputation may reduce amputation rates in extremity arterial injury" and restate our own philosophy that if you "think about it, do it."

T. S. Huber, MD, PhD

13 General Thoracic Surgery

Miscellaneous

A new classification scheme for treating blunt aortic injury
Starnes BW, Lundgren RS, Gunn M, et al (Univ of Washington, Seattle)
J Vasc Surg 55:47-54, 2012

Background.—There are numerous questions about the treatment of blunt aortic injury (BAI), including the management of small intimal tears, what injury characteristics are predictive of death from rupture, and which patients actually need intervention. We used our experience in treating BAI during the past decade to create a classification scheme based on radiographic and clinical data and to provide clear treatment guidelines.

Methods.—The records of patients admitted with BAI from 1999 to 2008 were retrospectively reviewed. Patients with a radiographically or operatively confirmed diagnosis (echocardiogram, computed tomography, or angiography) of BAI were included. We created a classification system based on the presence or absence of an aortic external contour abnormality, defined as an alteration in the symmetric, round shape of the aorta: (1) intimal tear (IT)—absence of aortic external contour abnormality and intimal defect and/or thrombus of <10 mm in length or width; (2) large intimal flap (LIF)—absence of aortic external contour abnormality and intimal defect and/or thrombus of ≥10 mm in length or width; (3) pseudoaneurysm—presence of aortic external contour abnormality and contained rupture; (4) rupture—presence of aortic external contour abnormality and free contrast extravasation or hemothorax at thoracotomy.

Results.—We identified 140 patients with BAI. Most injuries were pseudoaneurysm (71%) at the isthmus (70%), 16.4% had an IT, 5.7% had a LIF, and 6.4% had a rupture. Survival rates by classification were IT, 87%; LIF, 100%; pseudoaneurysm, 76%; and rupture, 11% (one patient). Of the ITs, LIFs, and pseudoaneurysms treated nonoperatively, none worsened, and 65% completely healed. No patient with an IT or LIF died. Most patients with ruptures lost vital signs before presentation or in the emergency department and did not survive. Hypotension before or at hospital presentation and size of the periaortic hematoma at the level of the aortic arch predicted likelihood of death from BAI.

Conclusions.—As a result of this new classification scheme, no patient without an external aortic contour abnormality died of their BAI. ITs can be managed nonoperatively. BAI patients with rupture will die, and resources could be prioritized elsewhere. Those with LIFs do well, and currently, most at our institution are treated with a stent graft. If a pseudoaneurysm is going to rupture, it does so early. Hematoma at the arch on computed tomography scan and hypotension before or at arrival help to predict which pseudoaneurysms need urgent repair.

▶ The management of blunt aortic injury (BAI) has evolved over time and now demonstrates reduced mortality and paraplegia rates with endovascular repair, along with an increase in device-related complications.

The new classification must consider the presence or absence of external contour abnormality. The classification ranges in severity from intimal tear alone, to large intimal flap, to pseudoaneurysm and, finally, rupture. The 2 most severe forms are noted to have external contour abnormality.

The authors arbitrarily selected 10 mm as the size at which an intimal tear becomes a large intimal flap based on institutional experience. In patients with intimal tear (or minimal aortic injury) less than 10 mm, the treatment was medical with anti-impulse therapy and follow-up computed tomography (CT) scanning until resolution.

Patients with large intimal flaps may or may not require operative therapy. Interestingly, in this series, no patient with normal aortic external contour died of BAI.

Conversely, of patients with the worst injuries, including external contour disruption and suspected rupture, 90% died within 24 hours. The authors note that patients who present in extremis after blunt thoracic trauma and do not respond to resuscitative measures typically fare poorly, with the eventual result being death. It may be appropriate to prioritize scarce resources for other patients with a better chance of survival.

The salient points of this study are sobering. Patients with minimal aortic injury can probably be safely managed expectantly. Patients with large intimal flaps may require endovascular repair. Pseudoaneurysms should be repaired with an endovascular approach whenever feasible. Sadly, those with rupture and in extremis are likely to do very poorly and it may be appropriate to prioritize efforts elsewhere.

There remains some controversy on the endovascular-first approach. However, it must be carefully considered that even in patients who develop device-related complications and require open surgery, it is likely that the patients will be much better candidates at a later time when the acute traumatic injuries have resolved.

This article serves as a reminder that the BAI classification and treatment in contemporary times is changing, and we must carefully consider the historical dogma we bring forward from the historical experiences of angiography-based diagnosis and open surgical correction. The CT scan and endovascular repair era allows an evolving approach and treatment to BAI that more clearly defines expectations and allows for potentially superior results.

C. T. Klodell, Jr, MD

Initial Suction Evacuation of Traumatic Hemothoraces: A Novel Approach to Decreasing Chest Tube Duration and Complications
Ramanathan R, Wolfe LG, Duane TM (Virginia Commonwealth Univ Health Systems, Richmond)
Am Surg 78:883-887, 2012

Between 2 and 4.4 per cent of all patients with trauma chest tubes develop retained hemothoraces. Retained hemothoraces prolong chest tube duration and hospital length of stay, and increase infectious complications like empyema. Early surgical drainage of retained hemothoraces has been shown to decrease complications and reduce hospital length of stay. However, the high resource and expertise requirement may limit the widespread applicability of surgical drainage. We present the results of a relatively simple and novel intervention for traumatic hemothoraces undertaken by our faculty to shorten chest tube duration and prevent empyema formation. At our Level I trauma center, 10 trauma patients underwent initial suction evacuation of their traumatic hemothoraces using a sterile suction catheter before chest tube placement. Compared with propensity matched controls, patients that underwent initial suction evacuation experienced significantly shorter chest tube duration (4.2 ± 1.9 *vs* 5.8 ± 2.3 days, $P = 0.04$). Also, in this population, there was an 8.2 per cent decrease in the number of patients that developed empyema or required additional drainage. Our study suggests that initial suction evacuation of traumatic hemothoraces is an effective and relatively easy intervention that reduces the duration of chest tube therapy, empyema formation, and the need for additional surgical intervention.

▶ About 60% of all polytrauma in some way involves the chest, leading to more than 300 000 chest tubes being placed annually in the United States. Chest tube complications increase with the duration and number of chest tubes required. Retained hemothoraces are problematic for myriad reasons in this same patient population. The retained blood serves as a culture medium, leading to development of empyema. Loculations and adhesions may form in response to the inflammation and lead to trapped lung. The authors trialed direct suction evacuation of the hemothoraces at the time of chest tube insertion and compared it with a propensity-matched control group from their institution. The technique involved insertion of a sterile Yankauer suction catheter at the bedside before insertion of either a 28F or 32F chest tube. Measured endpoints included chest tube duration, empyema formation, the need for a second chest tube, and the need for surgical exploration either by video-assisted thoracoscopy or thoracotomy. This technique resulted in 26.5% greater removal of hemothorax in the first 24 hours when compared with controls. Additionally, more of the control patients experienced the other endpoints.

Hemothorax is second only to rib fractures in frequency of occurrence after chest trauma. Retained hemothorax and subsequent empyema are two of the most troublesome complications. The authors are to be congratulated for studying this technique. Many of us have been trained to use a sterile Yankauer at the time of chest tube insertion for hemothorax to accelerate the removal of the clot. We had relied on the training dogma that it was more effective than placing the chest tube and allowing it to fully drain at a slower rate. The authors have now investigated and reinforced our belief that the addition of this technique to bedside thoracostomy for hemothorax not only allows for more effective removal of the hemothorax but reduces the rate of empyema, likely because of reduction in the retained clot. The only caveat to this technique is that it remains essential to explore the pleural space digitally and ensure it is free from adhesions before passing the suction catheter to avoid iatrogenic injury to the lung tissue.

C. T. Klodell, Jr, MD

Development of posttraumatic empyema in patients with retained hemothorax: Results of a prospective, observational AAST study
DuBose J, the AAST Retained Hemothorax Study Group (Univ of Maryland Med Ctr, Baltimore)
J Trauma Acute Care Surg 73:752-757, 2012

Background.—The natural history of retained hemothorax (RH), in particular factors contributing to the subsequent development of empyema, is not well known. The intent of our study was to establish the modern incidence of empyema among patients with trauma and RH and identify the independent predictors for development of this complication.

Methods.—An American Association for the Surgery of Trauma multicenter prospective observational trial was conducted, enrolling patients with placement of a thoracostomy tube within 24 hours of trauma admission, and subsequent development of RH was confirmed on computed tomography of the chest. Demographics, interventions, and outcomes were analyzed. Logistic regression analysis was used to identify the independent predictors for the development of empyema.

Results.—Among 328 patients with posttraumatic RH from the 20 participating centers, overall incidence of empyema was 26.8% (n = 88). On regression analysis, the presence of rib fractures (adjusted odds ratio [OR], 2.3; 95% confidence interval [CI], 1.3–4.1; $p = 0.006$), Injury Severity Score of 25 or higher (adjusted OR, 2.4; 95% CI, 1.3–4.4; $p = 0.005$), and the need for any additional therapeutic intervention (adjusted OR, 28.8; 95% CI, 6.6–125.5; $p < 0.001$) were found to be independent predictors for the development of empyema for patients with posttraumatic RH. Patients with empyema also had a significantly longer adjusted intensive care unit stay (adjusted mean difference, 4.1; 95% CI, 1.3–6.9; $p = 0.008$) and hospital stay (adjusted mean difference, −7.9; 95% CI, −12.7 to −3.2; $p = 0.01$).

Conclusion.—Among patients with trauma and posttraumatic RH, the incidence of empyema was 26.8%. Independent predictors of empyema development after posttraumatic RH included the presence of rib fractures, Injury Severity Score of 25 or higher, and the need for additional interventions to evacuate retained blood from the thorax. Our findings highlight

the need to minimize the risk associated with subsequent thoracic procedures among patients with critical illness and RH, through selection of the most optimal procedure for initial evacuation.
Level of Evidence.—Prognostic study, level III.

▶ This prospective, observational, multicenter study analyzed patients between 2009 and 2011 with a thoracostomy tube placed within 24 hours of admission for the evacuation of hemothorax or pneumothorax and later found to have retained hemothorax. Patients suspected of retained hemothorax underwent a repeat computed tomography (CT) scan within 14 days of chest tube placement. The retained hemothorax was classified as small or large based on quantification using a radiographic formula.

This study noted that 26.8% of the 328 patients with retained hemothorax subsequently developed empyema. Of the patients with empyema, 82.2% were managed without further therapeutic intervention, whereas 33.5% required thoracoscopy and 22.2% underwent thoracotomy either initially or ultimately.

The empyema patients were more likely to have required bilateral chest tubes and had larger retained hemothorax volumes. Additionally, more than 62% of these patients were noted to have initial thoracostomy tube placement in the emergency department.

It has long been understood that retained blood within the thoracic cavity represents a hazardous situation for the patient with many possible deleterious consequences. Liquefied hemothorax may drain freely through a chest tube, but more often clotted or loculated collections require more aggressive therapy to eliminate this fertile culture medium from the chest. This observational study certainly confirms our long-held belief that allowing clotted blood to remain in the pleural cavity poses a hazardous situation. It further highlights the need for aggressive evacuation of any significant retained hemothorax. My personal practice has been for early CT scanning in any patient who has a persistently abnormal chest x-ray after chest tube placement for hemothorax. Early thoracoscopy can be accomplished with minimal morbidity and frequently allows for complete evacuation of the hemothorax. It allows the added benefit of removal of suspect chest tubes, irrigation of the pleural space, and replacement of chest tube(s) in perfect position under videoscopic visualization.

C. T. Klodell, Jr, MD

Predicting outcome of patients with chest wall injury
Pressley CM, Fry WR, Philp AS, et al (Virginia Tech Carilion School of Medicine, Roanoke; West Penn Allegheny Health System, Pittsburgh, PA; et al)
Am J Surg 204:910-914, 2012

Background.—Rib fractures occur in 10% of injured patients, are associated with morbidity and mortality, and frequently necessitate intensive care unit (ICU) care. A scoring system that identifies the risk for respiratory failure early in the evaluation process may allow early intervention to improve outcomes. The aim of this study was to test the hypothesis that a scoring system based on initial clinical findings can identify patients with rib fractures at greatest risk for morbidity and mortality.

Methods.—A simple scoring system to stratify risk was developed and applied to patients through a retrospective trauma registry review. Points were assigned as follows: age < 45 years = 1 point, age 45 to 65 years = 2 points, age > 65 years = 3 points; < 3 fractures = 1 point, 3 to 5 fractures = 2 points, > 5 fractures = 3 points; no pulmonary contusion = 0 points, mild pulmonary contusion = 1 point, severe pulmonary contusion = 2 points, bilateral pulmonary contusion = 3 points; and bilateral rib fracture absent = 0 points, bilateral rib fracture absent present = 2 points. A review of trauma registry patients with rib fractures (June 2008 to February 2010) at a state-designated level 1 trauma center was performed. Data reviewed included age, number of fractures, bilateral injury, presence of pulmonary contusion, classification of the contusion, length of hospital stay, mechanical ventilation, ICU admission, and length of stay. The scoring system was retrospectively applied to 649 patients to determine validity.

Results.—A score ≤ 7 indicated lower mortality (24 of 579 [4.2%]) compared with patients with scores > 7 (10 of 70 [14.3%]) (Fisher's 2-sided $P = .0018$). Patients with scores ≤ 6 were less likely to be admitted to an ICU (29.7%) compared with those with scores ≥ 7 (56.7%) ($P < .0001$). Patients with total scores < 7 were less likely to require intubation (20.6%) compared with those with scores ≥ 7 (40.0%) ($P < .0001$). Patients with scores ≤ 4 had shorter lengths of stay (36.0% < 5 days) compared with those who had scores > 4 (59.7%) ($P < .0001$).

Conclusions.—A simple scoring system predicts the likelihood that patients will require mechanical ventilation and prolonged courses of care. A score of 7 or 8 predicted increased risk for mortality, admission to the ICU, and intubation. A score > 5 predicted a longer length of stay and a longer period of ventilation. This scoring system may assist in the earlier implementation of treatment strategies such epidural anesthesia, ventilation, and operative fixation of fractures.

▶ Rib fractures occur in greater than 10% of patients with traumatic injuries and are associated with significant morbidity and mortality. Rib fractures may lead to respiratory failure secondary to altered chest wall mechanics or respiratory distress from fracture-associated pain. Additionally, there may be underlying pulmonary contusion that contributes to hypoxia.

Treatments include intercostal nerve blocks, patient-controlled analgesia pumps, and epidural anesthesia to assist with pain control. Other interventions may include initiation of mechanical ventilation and positive end-expiratory pressure or operative intervention with open reduction and internal fixation.

The authors retrospectively reviewed a large volume of experience with chest wall injury in hopes of creating a novel scoring system to help better predict outcomes and potentially allow for future prediction of optimal therapy. The scoring system evaluated age, pulmonary contusion, number of rib fractures, and presence or absence of bilateral rib fractures. The scoring system was able to predict which patients were more likely to require mechanical ventilation and prolonged courses of care as well as those with high mortality risk. The scoring system may also allow for earlier development of treatment strategies, which may include epidural anesthesia, mechanical ventilation, or operative fixation of fractures.

Most importantly, this report should lead to a prospective trial of this scoring system with planned interventions based on the scoring. Rib fractures are too often treated as minor injuries and are just an expected part of trauma care. The authors have shown the ability to predict which patients will have more difficult courses and even a higher mortality based on the magnitude of chest wall injury. It would seem logical to proceed with a randomized trial of the patients with moderate- to high-risk scores and targeted interventions, such as operative fixation of the rib fractures, in hopes of showing reductions in morbidity and mortality.

C. T. Klodell, Jr, MD

Surgical Fixation vs Nonoperative Management of Flail Chest: A Meta-Analysis
Slobogean GP, Macpherson CA, Sun T, et al (Univ of British Columbia, Vancouver, Canada)
J Am Coll Surg 216:302-311.e1, 2013

Background.—Flail chest is a life-threatening injury typically treated with supportive ventilation and analgesia. Several small studies have suggested large improvements in critical care outcomes after surgical fixation of multiple rib fractures. The purpose of this study was to compare the results of surgical fixation and nonoperative management for flail chest injuries.

Study Design.—A systematic review of previously published comparative studies using operative and nonoperative management of flail chest was performed. Medline, Embase, and the Cochrane databases were searched for relevant studies with no language or date restrictions. Quantitative pooling was performed using a random effects model for relevant critical care outcomes. Sensitivity analysis was performed for all outcomes.

Results.—Eleven manuscripts with 753 patients met inclusion criteria. Only 2 studies were randomized controlled designs. Surgical fixation resulted in better outcomes for all pooled analyses including substantial decreases in ventilator days (mean 8 days, 95% CI 5 to 10 days) and the odds of developing pneumonia (odds ratio [OR] 0.2, 95% CI 0.11 to 0.32). Additional benefits included decreased ICU days (mean 5 days, 95% CI 2 to 8 days), mortality (OR 0.31, 95% CI 0.20 to 0.48), septicemia (OR 0.36, 95% CI 0.19 to 0.71), tracheostomy (OR 0.06, 95% CI 0.02 to 0.20), and chest deformity (OR 0.11, 95% CI 0.02 to 0.60). All results were stable to basic sensitivity analysis.

Conclusions.—The results of this meta-analysis suggest surgical fixation of flail chest injuries may have substantial critical care benefits; however, the analyses are based on the pooling of primarily small retrospective studies. Additional prospective randomized trials are still necessary.

▶ Although the treatment of chest wall injuries has evolved significantly over the past several decades, there remains much that is unknown. Many centers still rely on mechanical ventilation and positive end-expiratory pressure as a first-line treatment. However, several investigators have reported excellent results using operative techniques to manage these injuries. Despite the potential benefits for surgical fixation, operative management has been described as an underused treatment.

The authors sought to compare the critical care outcomes of surgical fixation with those of nonoperative management in patients with flail chest injuries using pooled data from previously published studies. Although a large volume of studies were reviewed, ultimately only 11 published studies were found appropriate for inclusion in comparing surgical intervention to nonoperative management for the treatment of flail chest injuries.

The pooled results suggest substantial benefits to surgical intervention, including decreases in the number of mean ventilator days, intensive care unit days, and hospital days, as well as decreased odds for tracheostomy, pneumonia, chest deformity, mortality, and septicemia.

However, even with the overwhelming positive results observed, this must be interpreted with caution. This meta-analysis included only 11 total studies, and only 2 included greater than 100 patients. Additionally, the only 2 randomized trials included 37 and 40 patients, respectively. With that caveat, the study does show a significant advantage to surgical fixation. These benefits were observed across multiple critical care outcomes and with relatively narrow confidence intervals. While it is premature to dramatically change clinical practice based on this study in isolation, certainly it is reasonable to consider surgical fixation of flail chest as an option in daily practice. Our institutional experience with this technique has been very favorable both in the acute and chronic flail chest.

C. T. Klodell, Jr, MD

Aggressive Surgical Treatment of Acute Pulmonary Embolism With Circulatory Collapse
Takahashi H, Okada K, Matsumori M, et al (Kobe Univ Graduate School of Medicine, Japan)
Ann Thorac Surg 94:785-791, 2012

Background.—Acute high-risk pulmonary embolism is a life-threatening condition with high early mortality rates resulting from acute right ventricular failure and cardiogenic shock. We retrospectively analyzed the outcomes of surgical embolectomy among patients with circulatory collapse.

Methods.—Between July 2000 and September 2011, 24 consecutive patients (17 women and 7 men; mean age, 59.9 ± 17.2 years) underwent emergency surgical embolectomy to treat acute pulmonary embolism with circulatory collapse. Nineteen (79.2%) patients were in cardiogenic shock, and 16 (66.7%) patients received preoperative percutaneous cardio-pulmonary support. Eleven (45.8%) patients were in cardiac arrest. The preoperative pulmonary artery obstruction index was 76.9% ± 16.4% (median, 88.9%; range, 44.4%–88.9%). The indications for surgical intervention were cardiogenic shock (n = 16 [66.7%]), failed medical therapy or catheter embolectomy (n = 4 [16.7%]), or contraindication for thrombolysis (n = 4 [16.7%]). Follow-up was 100% complete with a mean of 6.8 ± 3.9 years (median, 5.6 years).

Results.—The in-hospital mortality rate was 12.5% (n = 3). One patient underwent a repeated embolectomy on postoperative day 6. The postoperative course was complicated by cerebral infarction and by mediastinitis in 1 patient each. The 5-year cumulative survival rate was 87.5% ± 6.8%. Mean right ventricular pressure significantly decreased from 66.9 to 28.5 mm Hg among the survivors.

Conclusions.—Surgical pulmonary embolectomy is an excellent approach to treating acute pulmonary embolism with circulatory collapse. Providing immediate percutaneous cardiopulmonary support to patients with cardiogenic shock could help to resuscitate and stabilize cardiopulmonary function and allow for a good outcome of pulmonary embolectomy.

▶ The mortality of acute high-risk pulmonary embolism is high despite advances in diagnosis and therapy. Surgical pulmonary embolectomy is usually indicated for patients with high-risk pulmonary embolism and circulatory collapse. The authors review the outcomes at their center occurring between 2000 and 2011, during which time they treated 24 patients surgically. Their strategy for patients with high-risk pulmonary embolism and cardiogenic shock is to immediately start percutaneous cardiopulmonary support and to achieve prompt and effective hemodynamic stabilization. This retrospective study analyzes the outcomes of surgical embolectomy for patients with circulatory collapse secondary to acute pulmonary embolism.

The authors used percutaneous cardiopulmonary support to restore vital organ perfusion before surgical intervention in 67% of the patients. The femoral artery and vein were cannulated either percutaneously or via cutdown. They then proceeded with standard surgical technique, including median sternotomy and cannulation centrally for cardiopulmonary bypass. Under mild hypothermia, they opened the main pulmonary artery and extended into the left pulmonary artery as needed. In some cases, a separate incision into the right pulmonary artery between the aorta and superior vena cava was also used. In all cases, an interventional radiologist positioned an inferior vena cava filter during the first postoperative week.

Although the mortality rate in the series is high (12.5%), it does compare favorably with much of the published literature for this pathology. Interestingly, they noted a 100% survival rate in patients if preoperative cardiac arrest could be avoided.

The key to the success in this devastating condition is the ability to rapidly provide circulatory support. Although the authors do not mention it in their report, many centers with an interest in this area have a pulmonary embolism rapid response team with a special circuit prepared for circulatory support. Once the hemodynamics are well supported, there are many reasonable options for surgical treatment. We have historically performed surgical embolectomy exactly as the authors describe. However, recently we have had success with the Angiovac device (Vortex Inc.) for removal of clot either in the iliac veins, vena cava, right atrium, or pulmonary arteries. Although the Angiovac can be performed in a more minimally invasive manner, it certainly does require more resources and is best performed in a hybrid operating room. Currently, its use is likely limited to larger centers with more extensive resources.

C. T. Klodell, Jr, MD

A Comparative Study of Thoracoscopic Sympathicotomy Versus Local Surgical Treatment for Axillary Hyperhidrosis

Heidemann E, Licht PB (Odense Univ Hosp, Denmark)
Ann Thorac Surg 95:264-268, 2013

Background.—Axillary hyperhidrosis affects approximately 1.4% of the population. Medical management is often frustrating, and the response generally transient. Surgical methods include thoracoscopic sympathectomy or sympathicotomy and local axillary surgery such as suction-curettage or en-bloc skin resection. Many case series with retrospective follow-up are available in the literature, but no comparative studies between surgical techniques have been published.

Methods.—During a 9-year period, two groups of consecutive patients with isolated axillary hyperhidrosis underwent thoracoscopic sympathicotomy (n = 49) or local axillary surgery (n = 47) at the same university hospital, depending on referral or preference. Patients received identical questionnaires to investigate local effect and side effects after surgery.

Results.—Questionnaires were returned by 92% after a median of 26 months, with no significant difference between the two groups. Local effect was significantly better after axillary surgery compared with sympathicotomy ($p < 0.001$), but mild recurrent axillary symptoms were significantly more frequent after axillary surgery (51% versus 5%, $p < 0.001$). Compensatory and gustatory sweating were significantly more frequent after sympathicotomy (84% versus 25%, $p < 0.001$; and 54% versus 26%, $p = 0.01$, respectively).

Conclusions.—Outcome after surgery for isolated axillary hyperhidrosis was significantly better after local surgical treatment compared with sympathicotomy. Local effect was better and side effects fewer, but milder recurrent symptoms were more frequent. Compensatory sweating also occurs after local axillary surgery and has not been reported before. Our results suggest that local axillary surgery is preferable for isolated axillary hyperhidrosis and that R2-R3 or R2-R4 sympathicotomy should be discouraged.

Sympathicotomy should only be considered for patients who have additional palmar hyperhidrosis.

▶ The authors performed a retrospective comparative study encompassing a 9-year period at their institution. During this period, 96 patients were treated surgically for axillary hyperhidrosis. Almost equal numbers underwent thoracic sympathecotomy (n = 49) and local axillary surgery (n = 47). It is unknown how many patients were treated with topical agents, pharmacotherapy, or botulinum toxin during the same interval.

They report improved local effect with axillary surgery when compared with sympathecotomy. As expected, the compensatory and gustatory sweating were significantly more frequent after sympathecotomy. No mention is made of other known complications, such as Horner's syndrome or regional pain syndrome.

Although the authors' volume of sympathecotomy surgery is relatively low, the local axillary surgery rate is higher than that of most centers, allowing for an interesting study with meaningful conclusions. We have enjoyed a relatively moderate- to high-volume sympathecotomy experience for hyperhidrosis but, similar to the authors, have tried to avoid those patients with isolated axillary hyperhidrosis. The higher incidence of compensatory sweating and seemingly worsened intensity of this complication make the patient satisfaction after the procedure lower. Furthermore, patients with only axillary symptoms are often well managed with local axillary surgery (including suction curettage) and topical methods. One challenge that the authors have clearly overcome is the difficulty in finding surgeons interested in performing the local axillary surgery. At our center, we have been fortunate to have good collaboration with the plastic surgery division for the management of patients with isolated axillary hyperhidrosis. While the surgical treatment of choice for palmar hyperhidrosis clearly should remain endoscopic thoracic sympathecotomy, an initial approach of local axillary surgery for patients with isolated axillary hyperhidrosis seems prudent.

C. T. Klodell, Jr, MD

Tumor Biology and Prognostic Variables

Thoracoscopic Versus Open Pulmonary Metastasectomy: A Prospective, Sequentially Controlled Study
Eckardt J, Licht PB (Odense Univ Hosp, Denmark)
Chest 142:1598-1602, 2012

Background.—Patients with limited metastatic disease in the lung may benefit from metastasectomy. Thoracotomy is considered the gold standard, and video-assisted thoracoscopic surgery (VATS) is controversial because nonimaged nodules may be missed when bimanual palpation is restricted. Against guideline recommendations, metastasectomy with therapeutic intent is now performed by VATS by 40% of thoracic surgeons surveyed. The evidence base for optimal surgical approach is limited to case series and registries, and no comparative surgical studies were observer blinded.

Methods.—Patients considered eligible for pulmonary metastasectomy by VATS prospectively underwent high-definition VATS by one surgical team, followed by immediate thoracotomy with bimanual palpation and resection of all palpable nodules by a second surgical team during the same anesthesia. Both surgical teams were blinded during preoperative evaluation of CT scans and during surgery. Primary end points were number and histology of nodules detected.

Results.—During a 12-month period, 37 patients were included. Both surgical teams observed exactly 55 nodules suspicious of metastases on CT scans. Of these, 51 nodules were palpable during VATS (92%), and during subsequent thoracotomy 29 additional nodules were resected: Six (21%) were metastases, 19 (66%) were benign lesions, three (10%) were subpleural lymph nodes and one was a primary lung cancer.

Conclusions.—Modern VATS technology is increasingly used for pulmonary metastasectomy with therapeutic intent, but several nonimaged, and therefore unexpected, nodules are frequently found during subsequent observer-blinded thoracotomy. A substantial proportion of these nodules are malignant, and, despite modern imaging and surgical technology, they would have been missed if VATS was used exclusively for metastasectomy with therapeutic intent.

▶ There remains much controversy surrounding the treatment of pulmonary metastasis. No randomized trials currently exist to guide us, and the available level of evidence is lacking. The different surgical approaches to pulmonary metastasectomy remain a source of controversy as well. Although the traditional open thoracotomy is still recommended because of the ability to use direct bimanual palpation, a recent survey confirmed that up to 40% of surgeons routinely use thoracoscopy to treat metastatic lesions in some cases. The obvious concern of those who advocate open thoracotomy is the possibility of missing lesions that were below the threshold for imaging but may be palpated directly. Bimanual palpation during thoracoscopy can be limited by the size and location of the port sites.

The authors sought greater clarity on this controversy, citing the improved technology of thoracoscopy, including high-definition cameras and the increasing routine use of thoracoscopy for this therapy. They designed their study to allow the first operating team, the thoracoscopy team, to proceed with the full operation. At the conclusion, a second team, the thoracotomy team, converted the procedure to an open one and sought additional lesions. They studied 37 patients with this method. Both teams agreed on the number of lesions identified on imaging. However, the open team identified 29 additional nodules after the thoracoscopy team completed their procedure. Twenty-one percent of the lesions were unrecognized metastases, and one was found to be a primary lung cancer.

Surgeons in favor of thoracoscopy may argue that resecting all the disease via thoracoscopy and then following up with the patient closely is an equally viable strategy. Certainly, there are no current data to dispute this belief, but it does carry the caveat that some patients will require a second procedure.

Additionally, some may suggest that thoracoscopy minimizes pain and trauma and may maximize compliance and speed initiation of subsequent adjuvant therapy. Conversely, one may consider a muscle-sparing thoracotomy approach, which may offer the best compromise of the 2 approaches. We have often used this approach through a relatively small vertical incision with excellent results, especially in the sarcoma patients in whom multiple smaller nonimaged nodules may be detected.

C. T. Klodell, Jr, MD

Is Lymph Node Dissection Required in Pulmonary Metastasectomy for Colorectal Adenocarcinoma?
Hamaji M, Cassivi SD, Shen KR, et al (Mayo Clinic, Rochester, MN)
Ann Thorac Surg 94:1796-1800, 2012

Background.—The aim of this study was to clarify the clinical outcome and significance of mediastinal lymph node dissection (LND) during pulmonary resection of metastases from colorectal adenocarcinoma.

Methods.—A retrospective chart review was performed. Between April 1985 and December 2009, 518 patients underwent 720 pulmonary metastasectomies for metastatic colorectal adenocarcinoma. Relevant factors were analyzed with the χ^2 or Fisher exact test and the Mann-Whitney test. Survival and lymph node (LN) recurrence-free period after pulmonary metastasectomy were analyzed with Kaplan-Meier and Cox proportional hazards methods.

Results.—The overall 5-year and 10-year survival rate after pulmonary metastasectomy were 47.1% and 27.7%, respectively. The only significant prognostic factor for survival after pulmonary metastasectomy was mediastinal LN metastasis ($p = 0.047$ in univariate and 0.0028 in multivariate analysis); 199 patients did not undergo LND, 279 patients underwent LND that were negative, and 40 patients underwent LND that contained 1 or more positive mediastinal LN for metastases. The sensitivity of positron emission tomographic scan for detecting mediastinal LN metastases was only 35%. Although long-term survivors were present, systematic LND was not a significant factor for prolonged survival ($p = 0.26$) in the positive LND group.

Conclusions.—Mediastinal LN metastases are a significant negative prognostic factor for survival after pulmonary metastasectomy for metastatic colorectal cancer. Computed tomography and positron emission tomography based imaging, as well as preoperative carcinoembryonic antigen levels have poor sensitivity for detecting malignant mediastinal LN in this setting. Systematic mediastinal LND should be performed for prognostic purposes during pulmonary metastasectomy for colorectal metastases.

▶ Colorectal cancer remains one of the leading causes of cancer death and one of the more common referrals for consideration of resection of pulmonary metastasis.

Selected patients can undergo surgical resection of pulmonary metastasis as a curative option. Pulmonary metastasis with or without hepatic metastasis from colorectal cancer is an indication for surgical resection if complete removal of disease is achievable. Previous studies have identified lymph node metastasis, high carcinoembryonic antigen value, number and size of lesions, central location, and short disease-free interval as poor prognostic indicators.

The authors sought to examine the surgical management of lymph node dissection at the time of pulmonary resection of colorectal adenocarcinoma. In the complete report, the authors detail their lymph node dissection, which is quite thorough, including levels 2, 4, 7, 8, 9, 10R, and 11R on the right and 4L, 5, 6, 7, 8, 9, and 10 or 11L on the left. They report an overall survival rate of 47% at 5 years and 27.8% at 10 years. When stratified by those with negative lymph nodes at the time of dissection and compared with those with positive nodes, the involved nodes were a strong predictor of poorer survival.

Although many previous reports have examined the prognosis and outcome of pulmonary resection for colorectal metastasis, few have considered the issue of mediastinal lymph node involvement.

Other interesting findings in this study included no observed survival differences between N1- and N2-level nodal metastasis or between single-level and multiple-level involvement. There were noted to be several long-term survivors in the positive lymph node group, and the authors suggest that patients with N2 disease or multistation disease noted preoperatively need not be excluded from resection for colorectal metastasis. Additionally, it is important to note that the potential therapeutic effects of thoracic and mediastinal lymph node dissection at the time of colorectal metastasis resection are unknown.

C. T. Klodell, Jr, MD

Adjuvant chemotherapy for surgically resected non—small cell lung cancer
Heon S, Johnson BE (Dana-Farber Cancer Inst, Boston, MA; Harvard Med School, Boston, MA)
J Thorac Cardiovasc Surg 144:S39-S42, 2012

Despite surgical resection, patients with early-stage (I to IIIA) non—small cell lung cancer (NSCLC) are at considerable risk of recurrence and death from their lung cancer. In recent years, multiple, large, randomized trials assessing the efficacy of adjuvant chemotherapy for resected NSCLC have been reported. Three of 6 trials with 300 or more patients with early-stage NSCLC have demonstrated that adjuvant cisplatin-based chemotherapy can significantly improve 5-year survival in carefully selected patients with resected NSCLC. These benefits have been confirmed in a meta-analysis of modern cisplatin-based adjuvant trials. The most consistent benefit has been reported in patients with resected stage II and IIIA NSCLC. The benefit of adjuvant chemotherapy in patients with resected stage IB NSCLC is less concrete. Herein, we review the results of the major adjuvant chemotherapy trials and their implications for the treatment of patients with completely resected NSCLC. A future challenge will be to identify the subsets of patients who will derive the greatest benefit from adjuvant chemotherapy. Current trials are also underway to define the role of novel targeted therapies, such as inhibitors of the epidermal growth factor receptor and monoclonal antibodies, in adjuvant treatment strategies.

▶ The number of chemotherapy trials over the past 30 years that relate to lung cancer is significant. The authors attempt to summarize these trials and help us better understand which of our postresection lung cancer patients may benefit from subsequent adjuvant therapy. Three trials have demonstrated a statistically significant survival advantage for the patients treated with chemotherapy after resection. The International Adjuvant Lung Trial enrolled patients with stage I to IIIA non–small-cell lung cancer (NSCLC) and following complete resection randomized to observation or a cisplatin base combination chemotherapy for 3 to 4 cycles. The National Cancer Institute of Canada reported a similar trial that enrolled patients who were stage IB or II NSCLC. A third trial demonstrating survival benefit is the Adjuvant Navelbine International Trialists Association, which enrolled stage IB-IIIA NSCLC patients.

From these trials, it is reasonable to conclude that patients with completely resected stage II and IIIA NSCLC who receive subsequent adjuvant chemotherapy may enjoy a survival advantage. Additionally, when considering T3 lesions with separate tumor nodules in the same lobe (this used to be T4 but has been reclassified), it may be reasonable to consider for cisplatin-based adjuvant chemotherapy.

Patients with resected oligometastatic NSCLC (usually brain or adrenal) may be treated adequately by resection of all disease. No randomized trials have investigated the value of chemotherapy in this situation. However, it would seem reasonable to include chemotherapy in their curative intent treatment plan.

Future directions will focus on better delineation of those likely to derive the greatest benefit by using pharmacogenomics approaches and gene expression profiling. Several current trials should help us better understand the role of these agents, and additional data in the near future may better clarify the best treatment algorithm for patients with stage IB disease.

C. T. Klodell, Jr, MD

Staging of Non-small Cell Lung Cancer

Complete Thoracic Mediastinal Lymphadenectomy Leads to a Higher Rate of Pathologically Proven N2 Disease in Patients With Non-Small Cell Lung Cancer

Cerfolio RJ, Bryant AS, Minnich DJ (Univ of Alabama at Birmingham)
Ann Thorac Surg 94:902-906, 2012

Background.—The American College of Surgery Oncology Group Z0030 study was a prospective randomized study that showed that mediastinal lymph node sampling (MLNS) offered similar results to mediastinal lymph node dissection (MLND) in patients with non-small cell lung cancer (NSCLC). However, that study only randomized patients after thorough samplings that were negative on frozen section in several N2 and N1 nodal stations. The purpose of this study was to evaluate the effect of MLND to the more common practice of ruling out N2 disease preoperatively and then resection without sending lymph nodes for frozen section.

Methods.—This is a retrospective study of patients clinically staged as N0 with NSCLC. The incidence of pathologic N2 disease reported by the Society of Thoracic Surgeons (STS) database was considered to represent MLNS and it was compared with our patients who underwent complete MLND.

Results.—Between January 2002 and December 2009, 1,358 patients clinically staged as N0 underwent lobectomy or segmentectomy and MLND (not MLNS). Our incidence of pathologic N2 disease in 1,107 patients who underwent lobectomy was 10.6% compared with 9.4% in the 24,896 STS lobectomy patients ($p = 0.196$). Our incidence of pathologic N2 disease in 251 patients who underwent segmentectomy was 13.0% compared with 5.3% in the 2,150 STS segmentectomy patients ($p < 0.001$).

Conclusions.—When complete MLND is performed in patients during pulmonary resection who are clinically node negative (have benign N2 nodes after selective endobronchial or esophageal ultrasound or mediastinoscopy) without using intraoperative frozen section of N2 or N1, more patients are pathologically staged with N2 disease; thus, more are considered for adjuvant chemotherapy. The impact on survival in these patients is unproven.

▶ In the current study, suspicious nodes were sampled preoperatively by either endobronchial ultrasound, esophageal ultrasound, or mediastinoscopy. During definitive resection, the authors perform a complete lymph node dissection. They compare their incidence of N2 disease with that of the Society of Thoracic Surgeons (STS) database, thereby assuming that most of the patients in the database had lymph node sampling rather than dissection. The authors' incidence of N2 disease missed by clinical staging was 10.6% compared to 9.4% in the STS database.

Although there continues to be controversy over mediastinal lymph node dissection vs sampling at the time of resection, these data suggest that patients may be more accurately staged and treated by complete lymph node dissection at the time of resection. This argument is further strengthened by the fact that many of us who enroll patients in the STS dataset do perform a full lymph node dissection, further supporting the importance of the findings in this study because that disparity may partially mask an even greater difference in the presence of N2 disease between the 2 approaches.

Many have argued that the complete lymph nodes dissection is more difficult than sampling with various minimally invasive techniques. The authors have not found that to be true, especially with the use of robotic technology. I agree that the enhanced visualization and magnification of the robotic approach greatly facilitates complete lymph node dissection. Although it is unknown if demonstrating more N2 disease will lead to better outcomes, it does allow for patients to be appropriately staged and treated. Furthermore, it allows for greater clarity in the expected prognosis by stage of disease.

C. T. Klodell, Jr, MD

Value of flexible bronchoscopy in the pre-operative work-up of solitary pulmonary nodules
Schwarz C, Schönfeld N, Bittner RC, et al (HELIOS Klinikum Emil von Behring, Berlin, Germany)
Eur Respir J 41:177-182, 2013

The diagnostic value of flexible bronchoscopy in the pre-operative work-up of solitary pulmonary nodules (SPN) is still under debate among pneumologists, radiologists and thoracic surgeons.

In a prospective observational manner, flexible bronchoscopy was routinely performed in 225 patients with SPN of unknown origin.

Of the 225 patients, 80.5% had lung cancer, 7.6% had metastasis of an extrapulmonary primary tumour and 12% had benign aetiology. Unsuspected endobronchial involvement was found in 4.4% of all 225 patients (or in 5.5% of patients with lung cancer). In addition, flexible bronchoscopy clarified the underlying aetiology in 41% of the cases. The bronchoscopic biopsy results from the SPN were positive in 84 (46.5%) patients with lung cancer. Surgery was cancelled due to the results of flexible bronchoscopy in four cases (involvement of the right main bronchus (impaired pulmonary function did not allow pneumonectomy) n = 1, small cell lung cancer n = 1, bacterial pneumonia n = 2), and the surgical strategy had to be modified to bilobectomy in one patient.

Flexible bronchoscopy changed the planned surgical approach in five cases substantially. These results suggest that routine flexible bronchoscopy should be included in the regular preoperative work-up of patients with SPN.

▶ The diagnostic value of flexible bronchoscopy in the preoperative workup of solitary pulmonary nodules is still a subject of much debate. Recent guidelines recommend a very limited use of bronchoscopy, especially for biopsy of nodules in patients who are reasonable candidates for potentially curative surgical resection. These recommendations are based on the fact that bronchoscopy has rarely been shown to change the tumor stage or contraindicate surgery.

The authors performed a prospective study in 225 patients. Macroscopically, in 4.4% of all cases and 5.5% of known lung cancer cases there was found to be unsuspected malignant involvement of the central bronchial tree. Interestingly, the findings changed the surgical plan in 2 patients, forcing a bilobectomy in one patient and a decision to not operate in another.

In contemporary practice, many of our referrals will come already comprehensively evaluated from our pulmonary medicine colleagues. The evaluation often will include not only bronchoscopy, but the use of endobronchial ultrasound scan to better delineate the N2 nodal status. However, some pulmonary nodules will be referred directly from primary care or even present directly to the surgeon. In these patients, it would seem prudent to include diagnostic bronchoscopy as part of the evaluation. As a final point of evaluation, strong consideration should be given to intraoperative flexible bronchoscopy before proceeding to the operative procedure in any patient who has not had bronchoscopy as part of the evaluation.

C. T. Klodell, Jr, MD

Esophageal Cancer

Minimally Invasive Transhiatal Esophagectomy After Thoracotomy
Carter YM, Bond CD, Benjamin S, et al (Georgetown Univ Med Ctr, Washington, DC)
Ann Thorac Surg 95:e41-e43, 2013

Patients with end-stage achalasia may not be candidates for a transhiatal minimally invasive esophageal resection because of anatomic challenges and adhesions from previous interventions, namely, thoracotomy. Given the tactile feedback provided through a GelPort laparoscopic system (Applied Medical, Rancho Margarita, CA) we proposed that a minimally invasive transhiatal esophagectomy would be feasible in this patient cohort. The procedure was successful in 4 patients; seven complications occurred in 3 of the patients. At follow-up all patients demonstrated that they were meeting their nutritional needs with an oral diet.

▶ Minimally invasive esophageal surgery has progressively expanded to encompass for complex and technically challenging procedures in contemporary times. At many centers, the minimally invasive approach has now become the standard first-line approach to many esophageal problems. Esophagectomy is the definitive treatment for end-stage achalasia. However, significant scarring of the hiatus and mediastinum may prohibit a transhiatal minimally invasive approach.

The hand port has been successfully used in laparoscopic surgery to facilitate challenging tasks and speed the course of the operation. The authors adapted the use of the hand port to minimally invasive esophagectomy in a small series of patients with end-stage achalasia.

In contemporary times, the mortality from esophageal resection has been minimized in higher volume centers. However, the associated morbidity remains high. The transhiatal approach may be favored in achalasia secondary to a lower incidence of respiratory complications compared with other approaches that involve a thoracic incision. Additionally, a minimally invasive transhiatal approach may be ideal in that there are no oncologic concerns. Intrathoracic adhesions from previous failed treatments may be formidable. The authors noted that the enhanced tactile feedback and manual retraction associated with the hand port enhanced the safety and speed with which the procedure could be accomplished. The hand port was also removed to hasten the draining of the pylorus, resecting the specimen, and the feeding jejunostomy. The authors noted no anastomotic leaks, nerve injuries, or deaths in their small series.

Although it is unclear the role this technique plays in the spectrum of mini-mally invasive options available today, including the use of robotic technology, it seems prudent to keep this technique in the armamentarium of the esophageal surgeon for complex achalasia cases with a history of previous thoracic interventions.

C. T. Klodell, Jr, MD

Intra-Operative Concerns

The Use of Vacuum-Assisted Wound Closure Therapy in Thoracic Operations
Begum SSS, Papagiannopoulos K (St James's Univ Hosp, Leeds, UK)
Ann Thorac Surg 94:1835-1840, 2012

Background.—Conventional treatment of complex, nonresolving empy-emas after an episode of pneumonia or a chest operation often requires an open-window thoracostomy. This necessitates frequent, often painful dressing changes and is associated with prolonged hospitalization. The wound is often malodorous, causing significant social distress to patients and unquestionably affects their quality of life. We assessed the value of using vacuum-assisted closure (VAC) therapy in managing patients with a persistent infected pleural space.

Methods.—The study included 10 patients. All patients signed an informed consent and were debriefed before the procedure. An empyema developed in 1 patient after an episode of pneumonia. The other 9 had recently undergone a thoracic surgical procedure. All patients underwent initial open drainage of the pleural cavity and debridement. A VAC therapy system was then inserted intraoperatively or on the first postoperative day. The patients were discharged home with a portable VAC therapy system in situ. Subsequent dressing changes were managed by tissue-viability nurses in the community, without the need for further anesthesia or analgesia. Over a period of time, the cavity was sterilized and eventually obliterated spontaneously.

Results.—All patients were mobilized early and fast-tracked through the hospital. This prevented the need for daily dressing changes; hence, mini-mizing the disruption of normal activities and reducing the need for nursing care. Overall, the length of hospitalization was shorter, and the VAC therapy facilitated closure of the infected wound cavity. The use of the VAC therapy system negated the need for a second surgical procedure to close the wound cavity. None of the patients reported pain, odor, or inconvenience associated with the VAC therapy system.

Conclusions.—Our observations suggest that the use of VAC therapy to treat such patients is safe, facilitates early discharge and recovery, and offers a "civilized," cost-effective treatment in a community setting.

▶ Parapneumonic collections develop in 20% to 40% of patients hospitalized for pneumonia, and 5% to 20% of these patients will subsequently have empyema. Early empyema may be adequately treated with a thoracoscopic procedure.

However, longer duration and complexity requires thoracotomy and decortications. The ability of the lung to expand and fill the residual space is paramount in determining the postoperative course. Often in chronic collections, some space-filling procedure is required.

The authors describe the use of vacuum-assisted closure (VAC) therapy as having advantages of promoting the closure while eliminating the social inconvenience of an open Eloesser procedure and perhaps eliminating the need for repeat procedures. They stress the use of a silicone membrane on the lung and mediastinal tissues before application of the VAC, but otherwise the VAC is used in fairly traditional fashion. In their series, they used a negative pressure of −100 mm Hg for the VAC and changed the dressing every 3 to 4 days. Dressing changes were performed by nurses in the community without the need for further anesthesia or analgesia. Over time, the cavity was sterilized and eventually obliterated spontaneously.

The authors report impressive success with this technique and have even used it to obliterate large postpneumonectomy spaces that were measured at 750 mL before initiation of therapy. They have not noted any association between the therapy and development of bronchopleural fistula. This novel use of the VAC is quite interesting and may offer significant advantages to the more traditional methods of treating empyema. Further study will more fully elucidate the benefits, but this report is certainly quite encouraging.

C. T. Klodell, Jr, MD

Thoracoscopic maneuvers for chest wall resection and reconstruction
Demmy TL, Yendamuri S, Hennon MW, et al (Roswell Park Cancer Inst, Buffalo, NY)
J Thorac Cardiovasc Surg 144:S52-S57, 2012

Objective.—The aim of this report is to describe technical maneuvers used to complete minimally invasive resections of the chest wall successfully.

Methods.—Case videos of advanced thoracoscopic chest wall resections performed at a comprehensive cancer center were reviewed, as were published reports. These were analyzed for similarities and also categorized to summarize alternative approaches.

Results.—Limited chest wall resections en bloc with lobectomy can be accomplished with port placement similar to that used for typical thoracoscopic anatomic resections, particularly when the utility incision is close to the region of excision. Generally, chest wall resection precedes lobectomy. Ribs can be transected with Gigli saws, endoscopic shears, or high-speed drills. Division of bone and overlying soft tissue can be planned precisely using thoracoscopic guidance. Isolated primary chest wall masses may require different port position and selective reconstruction using synthetic materials. Patch anchoring can be accomplished by devices that facilitate laparoscopic port site fascial closure.

Conclusions.—Thoracoscopic chest wall resections have been accomplished safely using tools and maneuvers summarized here. Further outcomes research is necessary to identify the benefits of thoracoscopic chest wall resection over an open approach.

▶ The unusual nature of this report merits inclusion for the thoracic section. Similar to the evolution of open abdominal approaches to laparoscopic, there has been steady progression of open thoracic procedures to thoracoscopic. This evolution has been driven by many factors, including patient demand, perception of reduced perioperative pain, early return to function or subsequent treatment, and improved cosmetic result. The evolving technology and techniques now enable surgeons to reproduce the open operations using minimally invasive techniques.

Although the use of thoracoscopic techniques for chest wall resection has not yet become widespread, many similar techniques have become commonplace in other disciplines. The authors reviewed literature on other similar procedures and compiled a list of steps and effective techniques that facilitate the thoracoscopic resection of chest wall lesions. These maneuvers provide the tools necessary to facilitate many of the difficult tasks, such as dividing the ribs, mobilizing the specimen, and reconstructing the chest wall with a patch if required.

Although there are no reports yet available comparing these techniques with open approaches, there is certainly hope that there may be a faster recovery and a more rapid return to full function or progression to subsequent therapy. For those involved in chest wall resections and with some interest in minimally invasive techniques, I strongly encourage review of this complete article. The tips and tricks contained within are a valuable addition to the knowledge of the minimally invasive surgeon.

C. T. Klodell, Jr, MD

Surgical management of pulmonary carcinoid tumors: sublobar resection versus lobectomy
Fox M, Van Berkel V, Bousamra M II, et al (Univ of Louisville, KY)
Am J Surg 205:200-208, 2013

Background.—Surgical resection of bronchopulmonary carcinoid tumors can be curative and remains the primary treatment modality. There are limited data to delineate the optimal extent of resection for this disease.

Methods.—A retrospective review of the 3,270 patients diagnosed with typical and atypical carcinoid tumors between 2000 and 2007 in the Surveillance Epidemiology and End Results registry was performed.

Results.—The mean follow-up period was 46 months (range, 1—95 mo). Overall survival (OS) and disease-specific survival at 5 years was 80% and 90%, respectively. The mean OS was slightly better in the lobectomy group compared with those undergoing sublobar resection (86 vs 83 mo; $P = .008$). After adjusting for age, this finding was no longer present ($P = .513$). By using multivariate analysis, sublobar resection was noninferior to lobectomy with regard to disease-specific survival and OS ($P < .05$).

Conclusions.—Compared with lobectomy, sublobar resection is associated with noninferior survival in patients with typical carcinoid of the lung.

▶ Carcinoid tumors are relatively uncommon and account for 3% or less of all resected lung cancers. Typical carcinoids account for the majority of these tumors and have a very favorable prognosis. Atypical carcinoid tumors have a worse prognosis and more aggressive behavior including regional lymph node metastasis, but they account for only 16% of all carcinoid tumors. Very few large series exist to guide the optimal extent of resection, which led the authors to draw upon a large multicenter database and compare the disease-specific and overall survival in patients undergoing lobar and sublobar resection for carcinoid tumors.

Interestingly, this large dataset suggests that when compared with lobectomy, sublobar resection was statistically noninferior. Lobectomy patients did have a better overall survival, but that finding was eliminated when controlled for age of the patient at the time of resection.

It is challenging to translate this study into changes in current clinical practice. It is a retrospective study and should be interpreted with an appropriate level of caution. The overall survival data may be confounded by selection bias of which patients were selected for larger resections based on presence or absence of significant comorbidities.

Additionally, this study contained an unusually low incidence of atypical carcinoid (5%), which may be an inherent limitation of the dataset. It would suggest that at least some of the atypical carcinoid tumors were misclassified as typical carcinoid tumors. Finally, no data are available about the extent of lymph node dissection at the time of resection.

It is important to remember that 80% to 90% of carcinoid tumors are central tumors and likely require either lobectomy or bronchoplastic resection for extirpation. Additionally, peripheral carcinoids are more likely to be atypical subtype. However, this study does suggest some meaningful clinical considerations. Limited resection may be performed for typical carcinoid tumors when technically feasible. If a wedge resection is performed for excisional biopsy of an unknown nodule and frozen section returns carcinoid results with negative margins, mediastinal lymph nodes should be sampled. In those with negative nodes it may be reasonable to not proceed with lobectomy. Patients with atypical features or with lymph node involvement should have lobectomy until the optimal treatment of this subset of disease is more fully elucidated.

C. T. Klodell, Jr, MD

Minimally Invasive Thymectomy and Open Thymectomy: Outcome Analysis of 263 Patients
Jurado J, Javidfar J, Newmark A, et al (Columbia Univ Med Ctr, NY)
Ann Thorac Surg 94:974-982, 2012

Background.—An open thymectomy is a morbid procedure. If a minimally invasive thymectomy is performed without compromising the tenets of thymic surgery, it has the potential for decreasing morbidity and may offer similar clinical and oncologic results.

Methods.—This is an institutional review board—approved, retrospective study of a single center's experience with both open (transsternal) and minimally invasive (video-assisted thoracoscopic surgery) thymectomy. Survival estimates and statistical comparisons were calculated using standard software.

Results.—From 2000 to 2011, 263 patients (93 men; median age, 49 years; interquartile range, 37 to 60 years) underwent thymectomy for indications including myasthenia gravis (n = 139) and mediastinal mass (n = 108). Seventy-seven thymectomies were performed by minimally invasive approach. Both groups were equally stratified by sex, body mass index, World Health Organization and Masaoka-Koga staging, incidence of myasthenia gravis, and comorbidities except hyperlipidemia and diabetes. The minimally invasive thymectomy cohort had significantly shorter hospital ($p < 0.01$) and intensive care unit lengths of stay ($p < 0.01$) and a lower estimated blood loss ($p < 0.01$). There was an insignificant difference in postoperative cardiac and respiratory complication rates as well as vocal cord paralysis ($p = 0.60$). There was no difference in terms of operative room times ($p = 0.88$) or volume of blood products transfused ($p = 0.16$) between the two groups. Higher estimated blood loss was associated with higher intensive care unit admission rates ($p < 0.01$). All minimally invasive thymoma resections were complete, with negative margins.

Conclusions.—Minimally invasive thymectomy is safe and achieves a comparable resection and postoperative complication profile when used selectively for all indications, including myasthenia gravis and small thymomas without vascular invasion.

▶ Thymectomy remains a standard treatment for mediastinal masses including thymoma, but it also plays a critical role in the acute and long-term treatment of myasthenia gravis. It has long been argued that, especially in myasthenia gravis, a maximal thymectomy was required and, therefore, mandated a transsternal procedure. With improving technology, including thoracoscopic and robotic visualization, this dogma has been called into question. Many authors have now published series of either unilateral or bilateral thoracoscopy or robotic approaches to thymic and mediastinal masses as well as thymic removal for myasthenia gravis.

The authors sought to evaluate the safety and efficacy of open transsternal thymectomy vs minimally invasive thymectomy at their center in a retrospective review. Their study encompasses 11 years and 263 patients, with almost equal numbers undergoing thymectomy via sternotomy and minimally invasive approaches. Essentially all the minimally invasive patients received bilateral thoracoscopy with 3 ports on each side, which is standard practice at the authors' institution to ensure maximal thymectomy. They used primarily the LigaSure to avoid thermal damage to the phrenic nerve during the dissection.

They noted shorter hospital and intensive care unit (ICU) lengths of stay in the minimally invasive group when compared with the open group. Although there was no difference in the blood products transfused, there was a higher estimated blood loss and ICU admission rate in the open surgical group. The median length of stay was shorted in the minimally invasive group. Unfortunately, the authors were able to report remission rates and long-term outcomes in only 37/139 (27%) patients with myasthenia gravis, making it difficult to draw any meaningful conclusions in comparison of the 2 techniques with respect to remission following thymectomy.

The authors seem to have gone through a similar progression that many centers experience as they slowly transitioned from open to minimally invasive techniques. They first embraced the myasthenia patients, followed by small masses, followed by even larger thymomas. The visualization and technical precision of the operation is actually superior using the minimally invasive approach, in my opinion. At our center, we had favored the thymectomy via thoracoscopy for many years and now have begun to favor the robotic approach. The enhanced visualization and magnification allotted by the robotic technology facilitates a very clean and complete removal of the thymus. Many various techniques may be used from either right- or left-sided approaches. We favor a right-sided approach and place the upper robotic port as cephalad as possible without compromising the motion of the robotic arm secondary to the proximity to the right arm.

C. T. Klodell, Jr, MD

Radiologically Predicting When a Sternotomy May Be Required in the Management of Retrosternal Goiters
Riffat F, Del Pero MM, Fish B, et al (Addenbrooke's Hosp, Cambridge, England)
Ann Otol Rhinol Laryngol 122:15-19, 2013

Objectives.—Surgery remains the most effective treatment for retrosternal goiters. These commonly present as asymptomatic lesions in elderly patients, but may also cause airway and esophageal compression and, less commonly, may also be malignant. Although the majority of these goiters are amenable to transcervical thyroidectomy, in a minority of patients sternotomy is required. The ability to predict the need for sternotomy before operation would allow for safer surgery and operative counseling, as well as improved logistical efficiency if coordination with thoracic surgeons is required. In this report, we assess the radiologic factors that might be predictive of the need for sternotomy.

Methods.—We performed a retrospective review of 97 retrosternal goiters for which thyroidectomy was performed within the otolaryngology department at Addenbrooke's Hospital, Cambridge, between 2001 and 2011. There were a total of 80 cervical excisions and 17 cases in which sternotomy was required. A detailed computed tomographic analysis of these 17 cases was undertaken to assess the predictive factors for the requirement of sternotomy. The factors assessed included posterior mediastinal extension, presence of an ectopic nodule, extension below the carina, extension below the aortic arch, a "conical shape" of the goiter, and tracheal compression. These were compared to the same factors in the control group of 80 patients, and Fisher's exact test was used to determine statistical significance.

Results.—The significant predictive factors for sternotomy were posterior mediastinal extension, extension below the carina, and a "conical" goiter in which the thoracic inlet becomes a ring of constriction (all $p < 0.05$).

Conclusions.—Our results suggest that it is possible to predict on the basis of computed tomographic imaging the need for sternotomy in retrosternal goiters.

▶ Thyroidectomy is a very effective treatment for symptomatic goiters. Worldwide series estimate that retrosternal goiters are found in 3% to 30% of individual series. Retrosternal goiters often demonstrate slow growth and may remain asymptomatic for many years. They ultimately may cause compressive symptoms within the upper aerodigestive tract and superior vena cava. Although the incidence of malignancy is low, many require surgical removal for symptomatic relief. Surgery remains the most effective therapy for this condition.

Most retrosternal goiters may be safely removed from a cervical approach. However, if the thoracic portion cannot be liberated, a sternotomy may be required. The need for sternotomy varies largely across series, as does the exact definition of how much thyroid must extend below the thoracic inlet to be labeled as retrosternal goiter.

The authors retrospectively studied 10 years of experience with retrosternal goiter removal and carefully analyzed the preoperative computed tomography (CT) scans of those patients who required sternotomy in hopes of predicting which patients are likely to require sternotomy at the time of thyroidectomy. Preoperative prediction would allow for better counseling of the patient and better planning for the operating room team. The authors noted that extension below the carina (relative ratio [RR] 7.5), posterior mediastinal extension (RR 16), presence of nodular disease in the mediastinum (RR 2), presence of an ectopic nodule (RR 6), and conical shape of the goiter (RR 14) were predictive of the need for sternotomy.

In contemporary practice, the preoperative CT scan is ubiquitous. However, very little literature guides us as to how to use the CT scan findings to better develop the operative plan. Often coordinating a 2-team approach to a surgical procedure takes planning and foresight. Additional intraoperative concerns, such as patient positioning and available instrumentation, may change if a second team is to be involved in the procedure. This article helps us further form a framework as to when a 2-team surgical approach is likely to be required and both counsel the patient appropriately as well as prepare the operative teams and operating room personnel. This data-driven approach seems far superior to the current prevalent approach of merely asking for the second team to be on "standby" and evolving the plan as the operation proceeds.

C. T. Klodell, Jr, MD

Pre- and Postoperative Management

Role of Blebs and Bullae Detected by High-Resolution Computed Tomography and Recurrent Spontaneous Pneumothorax

Casali C, Stefani A, Ligabue G, et al (Univ of Modena and Reggio Emilia, Italy)
Ann Thorac Surg 95:249-256, 2013

Background.—The prevention of recurrence after a first episode of primary spontaneous pneumothorax (PSP) remains a debated issue. The likelihood of recurrence based on the presence of blebs and bullae detected on high-resolution computed tomography (HRCT) imaging is controversial.

Methods.—We evaluated patients conservatively treated for PSP who underwent chest HRCT scan in a single-institution retrospective longitudinal study. Absolute risk values and positive and negative predictive values of recurrence based on HRCT findings were the primary end points.

Results.—We analyzed 176 patients. Ipsilateral and contralateral recurrence developed in 44.8% and 12% of patients, respectively. The risk of recurrence was significantly related to the presence of blebs or bullae, or both, at HRCT. The risk of ipsilateral recurrence for patients with or without blebs and bullae was 68.1% and 6.1%, respectively (positive predictive value, 68.1%; negative predictive value, 93.9%). The risk of contralateral pneumothorax for patients with or without blebs and bullae was 19% and 0%, respectively (positive predictive value, 19%; negative predictive value, 100%). The risk of ipsilateral recurrence was directly related to the dystrophic severity score: recurrence risk increased by up to 75% in patients with bilateral multiple lesions. Multivariate analysis showed that a positive HRCT was significantly related to ipsilateral recurrence.

Conclusions.—The presence of blebs and bullae at HRCT after a first episode of PSP is significantly related to the development of an ipsilateral recurrence or a contralateral episode of pneumothorax. Further studies are needed to validate the dystrophic severity score in the selection of patients for early surgical referral.

▶ Primary spontaneous pneumothorax remains relatively common in clinical practice and usually requires hospitalization. Although conservative treatment is the traditional approach to the first episode, this may become prolonged and lead to a significant socioeconomic effect.

The risk of recurrence after an initial conservative treatment has been reported to be between 16% and 52%, increasing to 65% after a second ipsilateral episode. Although there is very little controversy as to the effectiveness of surgical pleurodesis in preventing recurrence, there is clearly not currently agreement on the indication for surgery after the first episode of pneumothorax. In general, intervention after the first episode of spontaneous pneumothorax is appropriate for patients with persistent air leak, with hemopneumothorax, or at high risk for occupational reasons, such as divers or pilots. I have often added to this group those patients who may be in remote locations and have difficulty finding medical care, such as deployed active duty military personnel and those traveling to remote locations for mission trips. Outside these aforementioned conditions, surgical pleurodesis after the first episode of spontaneous pneumothorax is not recommended.

The authors postulated that because the rupture of blebs or bullae is thought to represent the main cause of spontaneous pneumothorax, the presence of these lesions on high-resolution computed tomography (CT) scanning may be predictive of future recurrence. They, therefore, conducted a retrospective study to evaluate the predictive value of blebs or bullae on CT scanning on future ipsilateral or contralateral recurrent pneumothorax.

During the study period, the management of the initial episode of spontaneous pneumothorax was standardized. Small pneumothoraces were treated with bed rest, whereas larger ones required chest drainage. Management followed the guidelines with a threshold for surgery for air leak with persistence for 4 to 5 days. All surgical procedures were thoracoscopic and consisted of stapled resection of apical blebs when indicated and mechanical pleural abrasion.

The retrospective review of the CT scans was conducted by thoracic surgeons and radiologists using the same novel scoring system for severity of bleb and bullae identified. The authors found that the presence of blebs or bullae had a high-risk value of recurrent ipsilateral recurrence (68%) and that risk increased (82%) when multiple air-containing lesions were detected.

Although this is a single study and does not change the guidelines currently available for management of spontaneous pneumothorax, it does raise some interesting clinical questions. First, should every patient with spontaneous pneumothorax have a high-resolution CT scan? Second, if that CT scan shows multiple air-containing lesions, should earlier intervention be considered? While this area remains fertile for further investigation, it may be reasonable to obtain CT scans on any patient in which there is some controversy on proceeding with surgical pleurodesis at the time of the first episode of spontaneous pneumothorax.

C. T. Klodell, Jr, MD

Amiodarone Significantly Decreases Atrial Fibrillation in Patients Undergoing Surgery for Lung Cancer
Riber LP, Christensen TD, Jensen HK, et al (Aarhus Univ Hosp, Denmark)
Ann Thorac Surg 94:339-346, 2012

Background.—Postoperative atrial fibrillation occurs in 5% to 65% of patients undergoing thoracic surgery. Although postoperative atrial fibrillation often is regarded as a temporary, benign, operation-related problem, it is associated with a twofold to threefold increase in risk of adverse events, including transient or permanent stroke, acute myocardial infarction, and death.

Methods.—A total of 254 consecutively eligible enrolled patients undergoing surgery for lung cancer were included in this randomized, controlled, double-blinded trial. Patients received 300 mg of amiodarone or placebo intravenously over 20 minutes immediately after surgery and an oral dose of 600 mg of amiodarone or placebo twice daily during the first 5 postoperative days.

Results.—The patients in the amiodarone prophylaxis group had a reduction in the risk of atrial fibrillation of 23% (12 to 31); number needed to treat was 4.4 (3.1 to 7.8). A total of 38 in the control group and 11 in the amiodarone group experienced atrial fibrillation ($p < 0.001$). Adverse effects were observed in 10 patients equally distributed in both trial arms.

Conclusions.—Postoperative prophylaxis with a high dose of oral amiodarone after an intravenous bolus infusion is a safe, practical, feasible, and effective regimen for patients with lung cancer undergoing surgery. It significantly reduced the incidence of postoperative atrial fibrillation.

▶ The incidence of atrial fibrillation after pulmonary surgery is significant and can reach as high as 46% after pneumonectomy and 30% in patients requiring lobectomy for lung cancer. One series reports a mortality rate of 25% in patients with atrial fibrillation following pneumonectomy.

The treatment of postoperative atrial fibrillation varies and can include beta-blockers, calcium channel blockers, or class III antiarrhythmics such as amiodarone. Short-time amiodarone prophylaxis is characterized by a very low risk of side effects and few contraindications. The most feared noncardiac side effect is pulmonary toxicity. Most often, amiodarone-associated pulmonary toxicity is seen with chronic administration but has been reported in short-duration therapy.

The authors hypothesized that prophylactic amiodarone significantly reduces the risk of atrial fibrillation following pulmonary resection. Their trial enrolled patients following elective lobectomy of pneumonectomy and administered a bolus of 300 mg of amiodarone followed by an oral dose of 600 mg in the treatment arm or placebo in the control arm. The primary endpoint was time to atrial fibrillation, with a secondary endpoint of time to symptomatic atrial fibrillation.

From this randomized, controlled, double-blinded trial, they found a significant reduction in the rates of atrial fibrillation in the treatment group. They stress the importance of the high-dose treatment over the first 5 postoperative days, during which the patients are at highest risk. Although the use of prophylactic amiodarone after cardiac surgery has been well-documented, this may be the first trial of this type to report this finding following lobectomy, bilobectomy, or pneumonectomy for lung cancer.

One caveat to the authors' reported experience is that the bulk of their operations were performed through an anterior thoracotomy. It is unknown how well this directly translates to the United States, where much more pulmonary surgery is conducted either via posterolateral thoracotomy or via thoracoscopy.

However, given the impressive reduction in the rate of atrial fibrillation as well as other reports confirming similar results in cardiac surgical patients, it may be prudent to consider amiodarone prophylaxis in patients requiring major anatomic pulmonary resection for lung cancer.

C. T. Klodell, Jr, MD

Article Index

Chapter 1: General Considerations

Chapter 2: Trauma

Chapter 3: Burns

Chapter 4: Critical Care

Chapter 5: Wound Healing

Chapter 6: Transplantation

Chapter 7: Surgical Infections

Chapter 8: Endocrine

Chapter 9: Nutrition

Chapter 10: Gastrointestinal

Chapter 11: Oncology

Chapter 12: Vascular Surgery

Chapter 13: General Thoracic Surgery

Author Index

A

Abecassis M, 120
Abu-Elmagd KM, 246
Adam R, 314
Adibe OO, 287
Adkinson JM, 41
Agarwal A, 73, 152
Agopian VG, 244
Ahlin S, 239
Ahmed Ali U, 9
Ahya SN, 129
Ajibola O, 206
Alberro JA, 296
Alexander EK, 185
Almashanu S, 219
Almoudaris AM, 20
Amar L, 168
Amersi F, 274
Anand T, 78
Ancona E, 11
Anderson S, 79
Andriulli A, 325
Ardoino I, 297
Arianayagam R, 328
Arora VM, 7
Arriaga AF, 21
Arroyo A, 150
Asoglu O, 309
Aspalter M, 377
Ausania F, 116
Azuh O, 90

B

Bachelet T, 134
Bader AM, 21
Badiel M, 31
Bagshaw PF, 276
Baicker K, 15
Bainbridge D, 14
Baker T, 129
Bakker OJ, 165
Balch CM, 318
Ballman KV, 293
Ballow SL, 79
Baloch ZW, 185
Barnato AE, 32
Barnes JL, 217
Baron RB, 23
Barshes NR, 375
Barton FB, 125
Bastarache JA, 209
Becher RD, 88

Begum SSS, 409
Belghiti J, 118
Bellin MD, 125, 126
Belyansky I, 265
Benedetti JK, 308
Benjamin S, 408
Bennett C, 279
Bennett JL, 146
Bensimon CM, 145
Berendt AR, 162
Bergman J, 279
Bertok M, 270
Beutner U, 255
Bhangu A, 77
Bhangui P, 314
Bharara M, 374
Bhullar I, 42
Biere SSAY, 229, 342
Birkhäuser FD, 197
Bittner RC, 407
Blackbourne LH, 27
Bloemen MCT, 58
Bokhari F, 386
Bond CD, 408
Boneti C, 300
Boracchi P, 297
Borozadi MK, 99
Bosma E, 260
Bösmüller C, 123
Botteri E, 325
Bourjault M, 142
Bousamra M II, 411
Brault-Noble G, 35
Braverman AC, 356
Breuillard C, 220
Bridges ND, 120
Brind J, 201
Brölmann FE, 101
Bruggink JLM, 383
Bryant AS, 405
Bui TD, 370
Buitrago D, 176
Bujko K, 334
Bukur M, 28
Bull AL, 160
Burlew CC, 208
Burns B, 42
Burton TP, 100
Butler FK Jr, 27

C

Cajaiba MM, 122
Calland JF, 45

Callum J, 54
Cameron PA, 56
Campanelli G, 266
Carey TS, 29
Carlson GW, 320
Carlsson LMS, 239
Carsten CG, 348
Carter C, 131
Carter YM, 408
Cartotto R, 54
Casali C, 416
Cassivi SD, 403
Castilla DM, 74
Castillo MA, 61
Cauley CE, 174
Cerfolio RJ, 405
Côtre J-C, 142
Chaim E, 234
Chale S, 95
Chan PC, 37
Chang DC, 364
Chang GJ, 334
Chang R, 170
Chang S-C, 272
Chang WK, 151
Charbit J, 35
Chardon P, 35
Charles AG, 29
Chen C-C, 52
Chen C-L, 71
Chen L-C, 52
Cheng T, 290
Cherukuri A, 131
Chhitwal N, 262
Chindris AM, 191
Chiu PWY, 285
Choi JJ, 153
Christensen TD, 417
Chu CK, 247, 326
Chu H-P, 201
Chua TC, 337
Chung R, 28
Cima R, 159
Cima RR, 143
Ciraulo D, 104
Citton M, 167
Clancy CJ, 120
Cody H, 294
Coffey JC, 9
Colavita PD, 265
Cook C, 164
Coralic J, 262
Cornia PB, 162
Costa G, 246
Costa MA, 156

433

Printed and bound by CPI Group (UK) Ltd, Croydon, CR0 4YY

08/05/2025

01864755-0013